I Lost 160 Pounds, Now It's Your Turn!

Slim down
LEVEL UP

**INCLUDES
SLIM DOWN
PROGRAM AND
MEAL PLAN**

Discover Weight Loss Tips From a
Healthy Thick Chick

MYLITTA BUTLER

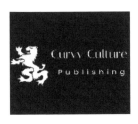

Copyright © 2021 Mylitta Butler

Slim Down Level Up

Discover Weight Loss Tips From a
Healthy Thick Chick

ISBN 978-1-7358238-5-0 *Paperback*

978-1-7358238-1-2 *Hardcover*

978-1-7358238-2-9 *Ebook*

978-1-7358238-4-3 *Audiobook*

Cover and Typesetting by (www.hmdpublishing.com)

Published by Curvy Culture Publishing

DISCLAIMER

This book is a general education health-related information product. It is intended for healthy adults age 18 or over.

This book is solely for educational and motivational purposes. The information and tools presented do not constitute medical advice and are not a substitute for consulting with a Physician, Nutritionist, or Dietitian, prior to changing your dietary or exercise regimen. Any diet, exercise or health advice in the book is not intended as a medical diagnosis or treatment. Prior to starting any dietary, or exercise advice from this text, you should consult with a professional before you begin or if you have any questions about your health.

ACKNOWLEGEMENTS

To my rock, my husband, and my best friend, thank you for sticking with me through thick and thin, literally. Thank you for believing in and trusting in my visions and supporting me while I continue pursuing my dreams. Win, lose, or draw, I know you always have my back. I am honored to be your wife.

To my heart, my son, for being so supportive and loving while Mom was busy working and following my passions. Thank you for all the times when I was writing this book and you came in and checked on me, to see if I was okay and needed anything. You make me proud to call you my son.

To my family and friends, who never stopped believing in my ability to overcome my struggles. Thank you for being support- ive and understanding not to ask me to make my five-meat baked beans, deep fried chicken, and baked mac & cheese, while my *weight loss food shift* was taking place. Thank you for the encouragement and support and for never seeing me as the fat family member or friend.

Lastly, to all the women, mothers, and grandmothers, the ones I know and do not know. The ones that have passed on and the ones who are still here. Over the years, I have drawn strength from seeing and hearing your stories. Your testimonies. Of how, despite being knocked down, counted out, and seen as invisible, you still found the strength to keep going. You found your voice to keep pushing and to keep making the world a better place. I am grateful to be on earth with women like you. Thank you for the strong arm of women empowerment and for letting your light shine.

CONTENTS

EAT THE CHEESEBURGER & CHOCOLATE CAKE

THE 4 STEP WEIGHT LOSS FOOD SHIFT

THE SECRET SAUCE

THE 6-WEEK SLIM DOWN LEVEL UP PROGRAMS

YOUR GET MOVING PLAN

SLIM DOWN LEVEL UP QUICK START GUIDE

SIS YOU'RE NEXT,

Sometimes, you do not even realize how bad you are hurting until you are not in pain anymore. My battles with weight and the number of times I abused my body with unhealthy diet behaviors was countless. I had struggled with my weight since I was nineteen years old, going as high as 304 pounds. Then too low, down to 143 pounds, and everything in between.

The vicious cycle of excessive eating and then depriving myself had put me on a destructive path. If I wanted to keep living, my life needed to change.

When I first set out to write *Slim Down Level Up,* I was not even sure how much of my story I was comfortable sharing with the world. That was until I sat down and kept writing. The words were flowing like a faucet, and so were my tears. That was because, in the early part of writing the book and laying out the formulas of how I lost the weight, I realized something. Losing the weight was not just about the physical shedding of the pounds that made me feel lighter. Rather, it was the emotional healing that lightened the heavy load I was carrying along with the weight.

Because when you push down years of trauma into the bottom of your core, when you block out bad memories for a long time and mask it with food, you do not know the burden that is lifted off, of you when you finally release the hurt. I realized dieting was so much more than just physically losing weight.

Before discovering the *Slim Down Level Up Formulas,* for a long time, I felt trapped in a place of feeling powerless to the excessive weight gain. I was sinking deeper into a depression looking for a way out. I know what it can feel like to deal with the emotional hurt that can come with being obese. The insurmountable body shame many of us feel when we walk around carrying an unhealthy amount of weight. The feeling of binge eating to numb the hurt. The dreadful thoughts of starting another diet only to fail *again*. Not even understanding why it did not work in the first place.

After years of trying and failing, using numerous diets, supplements, weight loss pills, potions, and excessive workouts, I figured out what works best for me. It did not involve abusing my body or the need to take extreme measures. What it took was getting creative and thinking outside the *traditional* diet box.

Using the *Slim Down Level Up Formulas* helped me find my way out of the mental and physical obesity prison, I was locked in for so long. I used it to conquer my weight loss Goliath. **I can tell you, if I would have continued fighting to lose weight with the same old one diet philosophies, I would have not defeated him. Because what I later realized was, using one diet only addresses one part of the obesity equation.**

You may have struggled and tried to lose weight several times in your life and were unsuccessful in getting and keeping it off. You may be facing a weight loss Goliath in your own life right now and not know where or how to get started *again*. You may need help in figuring out what really can work this time to get the weight off for good.

This is what drove me to want to write this book. The way many people have been dieting for years is not working, as far as achieving long-term weight loss results. The vicious cycle of picking *a diet*, losing some weight, and then gaining it back, needs to stop.

I wanted to share with you the tips and tools of how to effectively combine different *diets* together. Not just mixing one diet with another per say, but there are techniques and scientific reasons behind why it works. Specific steps you will be able to use to take losing weight to a whole different level, for long-term success. That was how I took back my health, lost the weight and won. You can, too. I know our weight loss journeys might be slightly different, but our goals are more than likely the same. The desire to feel good about ourselves. To get back to who we once were before the guilt and shame of the weight gain set in. Just know in these pages, you will find the truth of my struggles and what I used to triumph over obesity. Luckily for me, with time, self-love, acceptance, and these same weight loss tips and tools, my truth set me free. **Now, it's your turn.**

As you read through this book, my hope is that it encourages you, guides you and gives you strength. Some of the stories and exercises in the book may resurface feelings from your past. If, so, I implore you to sit with those feelings. Allow yourself time to process those emotions. Always remember, no matter where you are on your weight loss journey, it is okay to start again. The best way to do that is: **start by starting.**

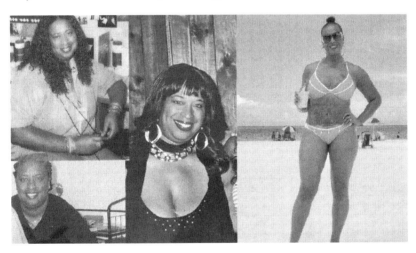

WHAT YOU CAN EXPECT

This book is written to speak to and guide the tired dieter. It is designed to work, specifically, for the tired, *experienced dieter*. The one who has had multiple attempts at losing weight and was unsuccessful in keeping it off. I am talking about water fasting dieters, yo-yo dieters. Cabbage soup dieters, and *I have tried every diet known to man.* **This book is for the one who is looking for *the missing piece* to the dieting puzzle.**

The one who feels unmotivated on how to get started again. The one who needs help in discovering, healing, and removing the *dieting hurt* that has been a heavy burden carried for far too long.

Ultimately, it is written for the one who wants to understand why they keep gaining the weight back. To the one who wants to learn the power of combining different diets together, so they can lose weight for good. YOU are who I aim to speak to in this book. I want to show you how I won against the battle of the bulge by learning how to combine a variety of diets together, in various ways. And how you can, too.

By the end of this book, you will have three *Slim Down Level Up Formulas* and a 6-Week Program that can set you on a path to feeling more in control of your health and your body. You will hear testimonies, research and stories from other people who have been successful, in losing and maintaining weight by using the power of combining different diets together.

My hope is you will not just rush through the book to say you "completed" it. Instead, spend time really learning the different weight loss techniques and how they can help you on your journey. Then, start applying them to your daily life.

It is one thing to say you read something or learned something new. It is a completely different situation when you apply what you learned and become what you read.

You may have started and tried many other diets before, but probably not like this. Because the key to the *Slim Down Level Up Formulas* is:

A. The power of identifying *your WHY'S* of gaining the weight (the keys to getting started again).

B. Getting to the *WHAT, WHEN, AND HOW* of dieting (how they are all connected).

C. The mixing and matching different *DIETS TOGETHER, SI-MULTANEOUSLY*, to lose the weight. And lose it for good (We will discuss how weight loss is more than one-dimensional and requires multiple tools to fight and win).

Your struggle is my struggle. It is why I am eager to share my journey with you in the coming chapters. What you will hear in some of the stories are years of pain, not wanting to face my "whys," binge eating and feeling shame and guilt. Falling down, getting back up. Feeling deflated, then restored again. Ultimately, finding my strength to start over with the right *formula*s to succeed.

Struggling, falling down and having tough days, are going to be a part of the journey. Accept that reality and process it, even before you get started again. Because that is what being human is all about. In the bigger picture, when starting a diet, perfection is not the goal*, progress* is.

From my pictures and stories, you will be able to see, I lost the weight. But I did not get it *right* every day. What I did do, more days than not, was find the strength to keep going. And so, will you. One meal, one day and one pound at a time.

In the book, we will go over the importance of acknowledging the triple **WHYS** of your relationship with food. The relationship it has with your weight. As well as how they can be essential in making this time different than any other time before, when you set out on a diet.

Long-term weight loss takes a detailed planned strategy to win. That is why we will cover the four essential parts that can help you in losing weight successfully:

1. The *why* of the weight

2. The *what* of the diets

3. The *when* of the foods

4. The *how* they can work together

Look at this book as your guide. It is designed to empower you, so that when you are ready, you can set yourself on a path to win. In certain parts of the book, there will be some questions that ask you to go within and answer from your heart. So that the mental part of losing weight can also be addressed. Doing this can help you with not just being physically ready to lose weight, but mentally prepared as well.

Are you ready? The competition you are in is with yourself, to fight for your health. And only you will be the hero in this story. Only you can take this information and apply it in your life until you reach your goal. And, ultimately, *learn* how to maintain it.

"Don't give up, the race is not won by the swift, but rather to those that keep running."
-Unknown

PROLOGUE

"It happens to a lot of people. It's ok, the doctor will give you something to clear it up." Her voice sounded anything but reassuring to me. She seemed unsurprised and a little annoyed. And it showed on her face. Her voice sounded even more aggravated when she asked me to sit back down so she could take the rest of my vitals.

She was the nurse at my doctor's office. I would normally only see her once a year at my routine checkups. My regular appointment was not scheduled for another month. But I called to see if I could be seen sooner. I told the receptionist, "I think it could be an allergic reaction to something I ate. I'm really not sure." I'd had a breakout on my chest, under my breasts and on my stomach for the past few days. And it was not going away. It needed immediate attention because it was itchy, red, bumpy, and it had started to hurt. I was relieved when she said they could squeeze me in the next day. However, I would need to come early to do bloodwork.

It was exactly two weeks after my 24th birthday. I was sitting on the awkward examination table, wearing nothing but the too small, too tight, hideous examination gown and my pink grandma panties. I thought, what results will I hear today?

"You are going to die an early death. Is that what you want?" I could still hear those words coming out of my doctor's mouth a year prior. We were always very candid with each other.

He told me I had high blood pressure and high cholesterol and that I needed to lose weight. Same song and dance I had heard at my three previous checkups with him. When I left his office the last time, **my vicious cycle of fad diets began again**. They would normally last about 3 weeks on average. I would start a diet, cut out a few of my favorite go-to foods, and I would lose a few pounds. Then something would come up at work or school that stressed me out. And the weight would start coming back on. **I would fall off the horse again, eat extra-large portions of food, and bake a chocolate cake**. I would try again, cut my calories more, drink lots water and even exercise a little. But after hitting several plateaus and feeling frustrated, I did not stick with it and would give up.

It was hard trying to lose weight because my family and friends would come visit me a lot. And that would always involve loads of food. Like, my famous five-meat baked beans, macaroni and cheese, fried chicken, ribs, potato salad and corn on the cob. When that happened, I would throw the diet out the window with the kitchen sink.

I would tell myself that I would start over again on Monday, or after the next holiday. But that would never happen. **I turned right back to what was comfortable and familiar, eating and more eating**. And I would bake another chocolate cake.

"The doctor will be in shortly. To discuss further about what can *help* you." She put an emphasis on help as though she knew something that I did not know, and I was in trouble.

I started fidgeting as she walked out and closed the door. The crinkling sound from the annoying paper, on the examination table was starting to get on my last nerve. I sweat all the time. But especially when I am nervous. So, it was no shock that my thighs were sweating from sitting there so long. And I could start to feel the knot in my stomach get tighter as I watched the minutes go by on the clock. And, of course, because they are not made for someone my size, that too small, too tight examination gown, (they force you to wear) kept coming untied. The longer I sat there, I could feel sweat dripping down from my face and under my breasts. I attempted to get off the table to grab a paper towel to dry off, but of course, that was when the door flung open and my doctor walked in.

He gave me his usual greeting, "Hi, how are you? Good to see you." I respond but kept my answers to a minimum because I wanted to hear what he was going to say. He pointed his finger at me and said, **"You can only be one of the big O's but not both!"** Those were the exact words that came out of my slightly overweight, middle-aged doctor's mouth.

I thought to myself, What?! Now I am really confused. It was bad enough I had to wait so long to see him. I had already felt enough shame and really wanted to hear whatever he was going to tell me so I could go home.

The nurse who took my blood pressure and weight, prior to guiding me to the exam room, had already done enough to make me feel guilty. She had rolled her eyes and shook her head in disgust when taking my weight. That day, **I tipped the scale at 304 lbs.** Even after begging her to retake it without my shoes and bracelets on, it did not take off but a few ounces at best. I shamefully saw the number and pretended I did not see it.

It was the heaviest I have ever been. In fact, I had gained 17 more pounds since my last visit. The nurse made sure to tell me, as she documented my chart. And now, my doctor was giving me a lecture with verbiage I do not understand.

I began to look more perplexed and annoyed, so he continued on, "Listen to me very clearly. **You can either be Obese or you can be Old**, but you can't be both!" I turned towards him and was about to speak when he said, "And the rash on your body is because of the excess moisture coming from all your skin folds. Remember, we talked about this before. Bacteria loves moisture and heat." I let out a loud sigh. And then he finished off by saying, "If you get rid of the rolls, you can eliminate getting the rashes." Now, I was the one rolling my eyes.

THE BIGGER PROBLEM

I was still sitting there, waiting for my doctor to finish reading my lab results. I crossed my arms and took a deep breath. The doctor moved a step closer to the examination table, and I could feel his disappointment. He pointed his finger at me and started shaking his head. As though I had just gotten in trouble for something I should have *known* better not to do. I mean, I did have to admit to myself that I did not hold up my end of the bargain from my last appointment. I told him I would work on getting my weight down. And, honestly, I did try. **But life, cheeseburgers and chocolate cakes kept getting in the way.** And clearly, the scale reported my failed attempts at changing my eating habits. As my doctor always says, "The numbers on the scale do not lie."

As he flipped through the pages of my medical chart and blood work results, my heart began to race. Instinctively, I knew the news was not going to be good. His body language and his demeanor suddenly changed as he looked at the last page of the report. "The rash isn't the worst of the problems you are facing today." And then, he hit me with it. **I could have fallen off the table hearing the results.**

Of course, I knew I still had high blood pressure and high cholesterol. I figured that went hand and hand with my additional weight gain. But what got my attention was when I heard the doctor say, "You are borderline type 2 diabetic, and if you don't do something soon, you are asking for a host of additional problems." I froze. Because I knew people who had diabetes, and they dealt with a host of daily struggles. I knew some who had to give themselves insulin shots daily and take all types of medications. Others who had to have their foot or leg amputated. That was not the future I had envisioned for myself. I did not one, want to think of, being without my feet or legs, or two, needing to take even more pills than I was already taking to survive.

SUPER-SIZE COMBO CRIES

As I got dressed to prepare to leave the doctor's office, I felt relieved and sorry for myself all at the same time. I did not want to keep going down the same unhealthy path. Honestly, I felt like I did not know who I was anymore. Especially whenever I looked in the mirror.

Over the years, somehow, the weight had buried my inner soul and dimmed my light that used to shine so bright. I felt empty inside.

I was not excited about hearing any of the lab results. The reason I felt any type of relief was because the doctor told me my numbers were not high enough, to have to take any medications for the pre-diabetes. I still had to take them for the high blood pressure and high cholesterol. If I were to avoid a fate of taking insulin shots and a host of additional medications for the rest of my life, I needed to seriously heed his words *this* time.

"If you just lose at least 30% of your body weight, you can avoid a lot of these problems." And that was where the feeling sorry for myself set in.

Because as he was writing up a prescription to get rid of my rash, I did the quick math in my head and realized 90 pounds was a lot of weight to lose.

But losing my legs, or worse, my life was not a reality I wanted to face either. So, I went home to put a plan together on how I would get the weight off.

"Sometimes the weight we need to lose is not on our body."
-Unknown

I would be telling a lie if I said I did not stop off at one of my favorite fast-food restaurants on the way home, because I did. I got two super-size cheeseburger combo meals to take home, to *help me get through* the evening. And help me process the results I had just heard. Of course, after arriving home, I baked a chocolate cake.

After eating, I went upstairs to get myself ready for bed. I figured I would sleep on the results and work on my plan the next day. I would either start *one* of the popular diet programs again, or at least cut my calories and start exercising.

I picked out my pajamas: a pair of leggings and an oversized T-shirt, and I headed to the bathroom. As I was taking my clothes off, something happened. I started to cry as I was stepping into the shower. I mean, the kind of cry where wailing sounds were coming out my mouth, while gasping for breath. I could feel my jaw trembling. I placed my hand over my mouth in an attempt to get me to stop crying. It did not work, I cried more. The mirrors and glass shower door were fogged up. I had to be in there for at least a good 20 minutes or more, just sitting on the shower bench. **I sat there feeling empty.** Letting the hot water hit my body so long that the water had started to turn cold.

At first, I did not know why I was crying. After getting out and starting to dry off, I replayed the doctor's words from earlier that day in my head. And I realized why. He told me,

"Take a good look at your life. And I want you to decide if this is the future you want for yourself."

I really did not know what I wanted other than not to keep feeling the same way. I did not want to carry the guilt and shame anymore from being excessively overweight.

As I finished drying myself off, I did something I had not done in a long time. Normally, when I get out of the shower, I quickly put my pajamas on. But this time, I did not. Instead, I looked at my body. I stared in the mirror looking at every inch of me. And I did not like what I saw.

It was not about all the stomach rolls, cellulite and stretch marks that were looking back at me, or the hideous itchy red rash on my chest. Nor was it seeing how my heavy, elongated breasts hung down so low, which made it look like I had three nipples instead of two. (Back then, before my breast reduction, my nipples were almost even with my belly button). But it was the fact that I had lost myself in all that weight. I did not recognize who was staring back at me in the mirror.

On the days I would overeat, it normally involved me making a chocolate cake and trying to drown out the feelings I was having by using food (somehow, eating chocolate cake always made me feel a little better).

The variety of emotions I was carrying with those 304 pounds often made me feel like I was standing in a crowded room, full of people, screaming at the top of my lungs for help. But no one could hear me.

THE WEIGHT SHIELD

After leaving the doctor's office and crying in the shower, I realized I still had a lot of unanswered questions. Mainly about how, exactly, I was going to get the weight off.

I had to stop hiding behind my weight. I knew I had to stop using the same dieting techniques I was using because they did not last long. And if I was going to escape the feelings of being trapped, it had to start with me. I needed to truly figure out a way to lose the weight for good.

The first step needed to be, for me to stop being mad at my body. Because being mad was not taking the weight off. And I had to stop telling people I had a medical thyroid problem and that was why I gained so much weight.

Seriously, the sad part was, I had my thyroid tested three times before. And knew I did not have that medical issue. But it did not stop me from telling the ones I was the most embarrassed around that I did.

Second, I knew the time had come for me to stop waiting for a miracle diet pill to be invented, before I got rid of the weight. I kept telling myself, I could pop some magic weight loss pills, go to sleep, and wake up slimmer. But of course, that never happened. If such a pill existed, I would have done whatever it took to get ahold of it.

It was time to stop using food as my therapist and for instant comfort when I needed it. I realized what I needed to do and what I wanted to do were two different things.

I needed to own up and acknowledge I was turning to *comfort foods* every time I felt depressed, angry, or inadequate. **Most of the time, my eating was not because I was hungry. But because I was hurting.**

Lastly, the toughest one of them all: I needed to address the *root cause* of my addiction to my drug of choice, food. I knew why I turned to it so quickly in my times of need. Food did not doubt me, it did not let me down or put me down. And it did not make me feel useless or insignificant. But the real reasons behind the *why*

I kept turning to it would need to be dealt with. Especially if I was going to work on losing the weight for real.

The depth of emotions that came over me as I stepped out of the shower that night, made me realize my food choices were putting me two steps closer to the grave, than I wanted to be. It was all due to the unhealthy relationship I had developed with food.

After I stopped crying again for the third time and gathered my thoughts, I made a conscious decision. Somehow, **I was going to change my relationship and break up with my long-standing first love, food.** I needed to figure out how to develop a new healthy relationship with *how* and *why* I ate.

I would commit to doing some type of exercising. Even though I knew that, at my size, it would hurt a little at first to move. I would figure out a way to do something daily. Because I had heard it enough from my doctor to know why I needed to. He told me the more weight I lost, the less pressure I would be putting on my bones and joints. It would mean a lot of the pain and discomfort I was feeling would be greatly reduced. I was ready to get started. But what this new lifestyle would look like and how I would get there, I did not know.

After putting on my pajamas, I laid across my bed and tried to let go of everything that took place that day. It was long and exhausting, and I needed to get some sleep. After laying there awake for about an hour, I accepted the fact that sleeping was not going to happen. My mind was full of too many things, and sleep was the last thing I would be able to do.

I got up and did what I often did when I needed to get something out. I grabbed my journal. Right there, sitting on my bed, close to midnight, I made a decision that would change the rest of my life. I decided to truly fight to find *her*. The her that I had lost over the years while struggling with the weight. Her who had been there for me through thick and thin.

I wanted to fight to find her, because she always believed in me, even when others counted me out. Her who was constantly giving others pep talks and motivational words, even while she was hurting herself. I decided to fight for her because she used to be so positive and could find the silver lining in everything. She saw the glass half-full instead of half-empty. I needed to find her again if I was going to truly take control of my life and get my fire back. She had been buried long enough in the weight. She had carried past pains and hurts for too long. It was time to find her and fight for *her* return.

The magic to fight for and find her happened, right there, inside my favorite pink, sparkly notebook. All the lights were turned on in my room, and I silenced the TV. I took out a pen, and my fight for *her* would come in the form of a letter. A pep talk letter about getting back to who she once was. About loving herself more and accepting her body, every inch and every pound. I wrote non-stop, and after finishing the letter, I signed it. To show I was making a commitment to myself. Then, I stood in the mirror and read it out loud. It was the letter I needed to write and needed to hear.

I finally realized, even at 304 pounds, I was worth fighting for, and I wanted to win. That night, the letter gave me the push I needed to battle my weight like I never had before. I had lost weight previously, but it was not with the power of her. It was not with the much-needed words in the pep talk, or with the refocusing of what I was fighting for. Which made a difference because it was on that weight loss journey that my dieting philosophy was changed. It all started with my determination to win. Coupled with the creative side of my brain, and feeling tired of failing with using one diet, I discovered the makings of the *Slim Down Level Up Formulas*. I learned different ways to combine diets together for successful weight loss.

I kept the letter all these years and often referred back to it on tough days. As a reminder of why I started losing weight and took control of my health. Why my journey would always be different than any other time before. Because I was different and had decided to stop letting the weight define me.

THE WEIGHT LOSS PEP TALK

Hey you. There you are. Born into a world that you did not realize was waiting on your arrival. It took months to create such strength, and fire. You are meant to be here. You are somebody. You are beautiful, even at this size. Yes, I am talking to you. **I know a big part of your weight problem stems from your past.** You have experienced some unpleasant situations. There was dysfunction, feelings of brokenness and inadequacies. Verbal and physical abuse at times. Which led to feelings of shame and worthlessness that set in, like seeds planted long ago. But here you are, still standing.

Because your worth is not tied to your weight. You are priceless. The strength you have within you and the light that radiates all over you, is exactly why I need you to embrace the beauty of who you are again.

Over the years, some people tried to break you. Others counted you out. Because of the weight, you felt invisible in certain situations. As though your presence did not matter.

You were broken and then put back together, and then broken again. All in a span of a few years. And yet, here you stand.

Listen to me. Like you have never listened to anyone before. You are beautiful. You are wonderful. You are the answer to somebody's prayers. Stop hiding behind the weight. Because the universe needs what you have. Hear me clearly, you are going to figure out what to do and make time to get the weight off, for good. You will not do it for anyone else other than yourself this time.

This is about you. It has always been about you. Your weight is not allowed to define you anymore. You must know how fabulous and wonderful you are, without the need of a scale. Or being able to squeeze into a certain size. You. Yes, I am talking to you. I need you to do the world a favor and stop hiding your magic, your light. Stop cancelling events and outings because of the shame of the weight. I believe in you. And I know you will get control of your health.

You can no longer hide behind the weight. You can no longer self-medicate with food. It is time for you to come out and embrace your beauty again.

Starting now, I want you to make this the beginning of a new day. A completely new way of looking at and having an appreciation of yourself and your body. You are somebody! And you will remove those shattered glasses you have been looking through for years. You know, the ones that make you look at parts of your body and only see them as flaws. Take them off!

You will start looking in the mirror and see her. Her who has been through so much. Her who has tortured her body long enough. With countless diets and eating habits that set you on a vicious cycle of unhealthiness. Yet, through all the ups and downs, through all the tears you cried, when no one was looking, you are still standing. You can do this. **You are strong.**

You were made for this. I need you to see her. Her who has a heart of gold and the kindness of a gentle soul. I need you to see her. Like you have never seen her before. Because she holds the key to unlocking the obesity prison you allowed yourself to be trapped in for far too long. I know when you see her, I mean really see her, you will love her in a way you have not before. **You will start loving her every curve. Every inch and every scar or imperfection you once saw as a flaw, you will now embrace as your story.** Your journey. They are your survivor scars. Showing everything you made it through. They are beauty marks, of a life that has touched others in ways that are immeasurable.

Also, I need you to stop dressing how you feel. I know how you feel most days. Depressed, insignificant, and disappointed in yourself, for allowing the weight gain. You are going to start dressing how you want to feel. You will dress how you want to be addressed. You deserve to feel beautiful, confident and to have self-love. So, I need you to get up tomorrow, fix your hair and put your lipstick on. Put on your favorite pair of leggings. You know, the ones that make you feel your best. And rock those cute high heels that you have not worn in a while. And go tackle the world.

Starting today, I need you to love her, celebrate her. Because by loving her curves where they currently are, on the journey to where you want them to be, you will truly embrace your beauty again.

You are also going to stop waiting to buy that cute dress and those sexy shoes. The ones you wanted but thought you were too heavy to wear. Schedule that hair appointment you have been putting off for a while. Do not wait until when you get to your goal weight to start feeling beautiful. You are beautiful.

Lastly, you will no longer play victim to the weight. **You will be victorious.** Remember your self-worth and strengthen your self-love daily. Your future self is already so proud of you. She knows you are going to do it. This time, you're putting yourself and your health first.

Love,

Me

Writing the letter was one thing, and it seemed to just flow out of me when I began. But reading it out loud was a whole different story. It was so hard for me to get through the letter. Because every other sentence, tears were streaming down my face. My eyes were red from me wiping them so much, and my voice kept cracking, but I made it through. Such a burden seemed to leave my body even before I read the last word. I had not lost a pound yet, clearly. But for some reason, I felt lighter and I could breathe better. I felt different. That was when the journey to fight for my health began, *again*.

PART ONE
THE MISSING PIECE

1

YOU DON'T KNOW WHAT YOU DON'T KNOW

Most people will never know what it feels like to be trapped in your own body. To struggle with a mountain that seems too hard and impossible to climb. To carry an astronomical amount of weight. Not knowing where to start to get back to a feeling of being in control.

When I sat down and started writing to share my weight loss formulas, several things flashed back in my mind. Particularly, about some of the situations that brought me to the point of needing to find a *different* way to lose weight. Which made me think about certain real-life physical and emotional struggles of being obese.

Before, I could even get to the point of searching for a different weight loss solution, I had to get real with myself. It was a hard pill to swallow. I admitted I was out of control. I had allowed my feelings to be dealt with by using food, excessively eating all the time, and it was sending me down an unhealthy, dangerous path. For some reason, back then, I could not find the strength or motivation to do something about getting the weight off and taking control of my health.

Confession Time: **It was so bad, I remember standing up in my kitchen cooking dinner, and at the same time, I was eating a footlong sub and a whole bag of potato chips. Yes. I was eating while preparing to eat!** (Please tell me I am not alone in doing this because it turned into a daily ritual for me).

When I got on the scale, the 304-pound number that stared back at me was, unfortunately, not shocking. Because I could painfully feel every one of those pounds. Specifically, in my back, knees and especially coming from my oversized 44 DDD chest. In the evenings, when I took off my bra, my shoulders were red. It often looked like they were beaten with a hammer. I knew it was from the straps digging into my skin from the weight of my breasts.

I hurt all the time. I suffered from chafing problems when my inner thighs would rub together raw. But I was in a constant state of denial. My eating kept spiraling out of control. Painfully, I had to calculate and admit I was easily taking in over 8,000 calories a day.

My health kept declining, and I was slowly dying because I was more focused on who was cooking the ribs, oyster dressing and chicken for the next family get-together. I was also more focused on when the next girl's trip would be. Not a vacation, per se, but rather to my favorite all-you-can-eat buffet, with my *food* friends (the kind of friends that every time we got together, it involved eating). I was dying because, instead of making time to exercise, I made excuses. I also somehow never made time to figure out how to cook and eat healthier meals for myself. I was more focused on spending hours getting my hair and nails done because it made me feel better to focus on anything other than my body. **My habits were sending me down a path that would only ensure two things: 1. I would need a larger coffin when I died, and 2. My hair and nails would look good at the funeral. Yet, I was still in denial and kept excessively eating.**

I had trouble sleeping at night and could only lay down with my head elevated. Because I had a hard time breathing when lying flat.

I suffered from terrible migraines from the amount of pressure I felt, from carrying all the weight.

Towards reaching my highest weight, I stopped taking pictures. I stopped wanting to go out with friends. I became a closet eater (again) and found myself binging on large amounts of food when no one was around.

I felt extremely embarrassed around my family. Who, unlike me, were mostly super tall and thin! I mean, well over 6 feet tall. They would not be considered obese, let alone overweight. Which is why often I did not share with them when I was dieting. I knew they would not understand and could not relate to my struggles.

The time came and I hit the wall and needed to figure out another weight loss solution. Because I was emotionally and physically drained, and tired at failing using endless diets. I had been for a while. But I did not tell anyone.

Why would I? It would only make me feel more guilty about my weight. They would judge me and wonder why I did not just get control. "Stop eating so much and start exercising."

A little over a year and a half prior to me losing 161 pounds, I had overheard those words in the grocery store. And it stuck with me. Two elderly ladies were talking and pointing at an overweight woman shopping. Thinking back, the overweight woman was probably close to my weight. At least 290-300 pounds.

The frail looking elderly lady, with a full head of grey hair and too much red lipstick on, seemed to find humor in how heavy this lady was, and how the overweight woman needed to get around the store on the motorized shopping cart.

For whatever reason, they felt the need to solve her weight problem, right there in the middle of the bread aisle. Because, *of course,* they knew exactly what she needed.

With the signature two step recommendation, **"She is too fat; she needs to stop eating so much and start exercising."**

For those of us who have battled our weight several times in our lives, we know those statements are only part of the answers to losing weight. Especially losing weight long-term. Because most people have tried to use several diets before but kept failing.

Figuring out the physical part of dieting and losing weight is one thing, and it can be challenging. **But sometimes, losing weight is so much more than just shedding pounds.** It is about acknowledging the need to get to the heart of *why* there is a weight problem in the first place. This can be more difficult because, more often than not, there is a need to address the emotional and mental part of weight loss, *before* starting another diet (I spent years in therapy before I figured that part out. I will share more about that later in the book).

The reality of how to successfully lose weight is a little more complex than most people realize. For example, you could pick another diet and start battling your weight again. You could get mentally and physically prepared to succeed. By deciding to eat less and move more. However, due to the way the dieting culture is set up, more than likely, you would not win. You would regain the weight back. That is because there is something bigger that has been happening in the on-going weight loss battle. Guess what? It is exactly what has been keeping you from being successful in losing and maintaining weight.

I am talking about a weight loss formula, techniques that I want to share with you. I can tell you one thing, the signature two-step recommendation is not the answer you are looking for. At least, not for successful weight loss.

THE WEIGHT LOSS PICK-A-DIET-TEAM BATTLE

What happened to me all those years when I kept failing at losing weight goes back to an old saying my grandmother used to say, "You don't know what you don't know, that is, until you know."

What if I told you, one of the key missing pieces from the weight loss equation, to be successful long-term, was there all along? Would you want to know if it was true? Would you believe many of us did not know to use this technique or thought about doing such a thing, even during all the failed diet attempts we had?

Breaking news! It is true. The weight loss techniques have been and are being used by many people for years. The kind of people who have experienced long-term weight loss success, using the same techniques. Because they are not *dieting,* they have figured out what the best formula is, and they stick with it.

Successful Weight Loss? Yes, and there are some entities that may not want me to tell you this, but I am going to give it to you straight. A big reason why you did not know is due to how the multi-billion-dollar health and fitness industry is designed. It is because of the way they created the *diet code philosophy.* Which, unfortunately, are the same philosophies many of us have followed and believed in for several years. Let me explain.

Over the years, because of how the weight loss industry has positioned itself, the pick-a-diet-team process, is one of the main reasons why many of us have failed, multiple times, at losing and maintaining weight. By choosing one diet team to play on, we are often doomed to lose.

For example, we sign up and commit to dieting and eating one way. Because dieting traditionally is set up to be compartmentalized, we pick a team to be on. We join the team and become completely engrossed in that diet's eating style. I did it repeatedly over the years and even would recruit some of my family and friends to join in on my team. To name a few: Team Intermittent Fasting, Team Keto, Team Paleo, Team Vegan, Team Weight Watchers, Team Low-Calories, Team Jenny Craig, and Team Low-Carbs.

We buy and eat all the food necessary for our success with that team. We follow what the diets' *eating style* and culture tells us to do, faithfully. Initially, we lose weight. However, when it stops working, we often quit. We blame ourselves, thinking we must have done something wrong. We take ourselves off the team, and in a short period of time, the weight comes back on. The frustration sets in, and this is where the need to solve the problem begins.

You did not fail at losing weight because the diet you chose cannot work. The problem was the diet you chose was not designed to work, long-term! You were set up to fail.

Let that sink in a minute. Because truth be told, you only had part of the equation to be successful. Let me explain a little bit more. The way the *diet code philosophies* are set up, you (probably like me) were diligent and remained faithful on your diet for a while. Waiting for it to keep working. The first few pounds came off, and you were excited and proud of your hard work. But it was probably short lived. That is because they are specifically designed to only work short-term for you. No more and no less.

You were previously unsuccessful because you did not know it would be more than okay and **necessary** to "add to your team" and to their diet code philosophy. By doing so, you would have changed the outcome of your journey and continued losing weight, by choosing another diet to have used in conjunction with it. At the same time. Utilizing the power of combining different diets together. All while unlocking the secrets, to being successful and the various ways to stop regaining the weight back.

Combining Different Diets? Yes! Let me say that again, Yes! Because one diet cannot address the *two key factors* that are required for you to be able to successfully lose weight, long-term. **It is the reason why you would have started a diet and failed every time.** When I realized the key to stop failing was to tap into the power of using this technique, it blew my mind at first. Because when I started using it, it was so effective in helping me to continue losing weight. I was ecstatic at how it worked and I could use it not just to attain but also maintain my weight loss!

After discovering and seeing the technique in action, I kept thinking, where had this key dieting information, this missing piece, been all my life? Especially where had it been all those times when I was miserable, struggling, and eating diet food I mostly did not like. Failing by losing then gaining weight constantly. All while blaming myself the whole time. Not realizing using the one diet technique was the problem.

Why Did We Go So Long Not Knowing This Technique?
The reason is because we did not realize how strongly we were programmed by the *diet code philosophy*. In essence, we followed the leaders, and they led us astray. We believed, in order to lose weight, we needed to pick *a Diet*. Be faithful to that diet philosophy. End of story, no questions asked, and that is exactly what we would often do.

We trusted in the professionalism of the diets, and for some of us, we were even encouraged or recommended by our doctors, nutritionists, or dietitians. They suggested we use a certain diet. Or they agreed with one of the ones we selected. Telling us to stick with the set parameters and use it to get the weight off.

Here is how it would typically play out for many of us on a traditional one-diet journey. We would start the diet, follow the steps, wait for the pounds to come off, and most of us already know how the next part of the story would normally end. Weight loss followed by a repeated weight gain.

Does Combining Different Diets Together Work? Yes! A Resounding Yes! I can tell you firsthand, and I will share with you, additional stories, and examples of how effectively it works. And how it can work for you. Combining different diets together can be the most beneficial weight loss tool you learn to use. And it can help you finally lose the weight for good. Let me share with you how I first found out about the power of using this technique.

During a part of my weight loss journey, I was using one diet *eating style*. I called it my *Base Diet*, since it was the foundation for what I was using. My Base Diet was to follow a Low-Calorie Diet. I reduced my food intake as low as 1200 calories and 40 fat grams a day. After initially losing some weight, I kept hitting plateaus. No matter how much I reduced my calories, my metabolism slowed down, and the weight stopped coming off.

I thought, if different diets work individually, what would, happen if I used more than one at the same time? Could it help me with losing more weight and stop slowing my metabolism down? So, I set out on a mission because those were the answers I needed. I was determined to find out.

THE POWER OF THE DIET REMIXX

Back then, I had been dieting so long, at one point I labeled myself during the journey a *professional dieter*. Somehow, I had mastered the art of losing and then regaining weight. Neither one of my degrees are in nutrition or fitness. However, over the years, I have read, studied, researched, and used so many different diets. Mainly, because I wanted to learn their effectiveness to help me lose weight, and then I kept wondering where I was going wrong.

With all the information I found, it prompted me to want to figure out solutions. The kind that would last.

What I did was take some of that knowledge and started experimenting. After consulting with my doctor about advice and safety with what I wanted to keep doing, the magic continued to happen.

It was the power of combining different diets together that showed up and showed its true strength to me. Strength? Yes, because using multiple diets can address the two key factors that are in play, when it comes to losing and maintaining weight.

What Are the Two Key Factors in Losing Weight? They are the body's ability to lower, insulin levels, *and* insulin resistance. Which are directly tied to what, when and how much we eat (We will talk about the key roles they play and their importance with losing weight in Chapter 2).

I discovered lowering *both* needed to be a priority for successful weight loss, so I used the strength of different combinations to keep fighting my battle. I realized when I was only using one diet, no matter which one it was, it was not doing the job.

By using the Base Diet with the Remixx Diet, my weight continued to come off. When that started to happen, I formed my own team, *Team Diet Remixx*. Ever since that happened, losing weight has never been the same for me.

How Did I Use the Diets Together to be More Effective?
What I did, was combine in a second diet, which I later called the Remixx Diet. I chose to add Intermittent Fasting (time-restricted eating). I used a 16:8 schedule, only eating in an 8-hour window, and combined it with the *Base Diet* (Low-Calorie) that I was already on. By doing so, not only did the fasting schedule tell me *when* to eat, but it also filled in one of the key missing pieces to the diet equation. It addressed lowering my insulin resistance.

The Low-Calorie Diet created the calorie deficit I needed to lose weight. But eventually, it caused my metabolism to slow down. By adding Intermittent Fasting to the mix, it helped increase my slowed metabolism and decrease my hunger at the same time, which was associated with the reduction in caloric intake.

The power of the *Base Diet* and the *Remixx Diet*, lowered, both, my insulin levels and my insulin resistance. As well as reduced the large amount of belly fat, which I call the dangerous weight, I was carrying. (We will discuss more about fasting and its benefits of helping to reduce stored body fat later in the book).

Since I was on a roll with losing weight, I consulted with my doctor one more time. After getting the green light, I took it a step farther, and moved to adding what I later called the *Bonus Diet* to my mix.

For example, I kept doing the 16:8 Intermittent Fasting with the Low-Calorie Diet. But I took a technique out of the Vegan Diet philosophy. I went meatless three times a week, added more fruits and vegetables and ate more whole grains. I also started having smoothie dinners two times a week. **In a month, my 15 pounds weight loss turned into 33 pounds.** Those small changes made a huge difference and increased my weight loss success.

You may be thinking, besides my example, is there more proof that combining diets together can work? Yes. Several. For instance, years after successfully following the technique, I came across a few studies that were conducted on the effects of using more than one diet together. It made me realize the validity of the power of the different combinations and why they had worked.

Here is one of the results from the research I found:

"Further studies confirm that the combination of intermittent fasting with a caloric restriction (diet) is effective for weight loss." (1)

The main reason this technique is effective is because using both diets can address the need to lower insulin levels and insulin resistance. Which if both are not addressed weight loss stalls.

WEIGHT LOSS SUCCESS STORY TIME

Here are three individual testimonies showing examples of the effectiveness of using a combination of diets. They are success stories from women who shared their journeys of finally discovering, the power of combining different diets together. After years of struggling with their weight, they were able to figure out what finally worked best for them.

Charmaine: "I chose a low-carb and intermittent fasting eating plan because after trying several methods to lose weight, this combo was the only one that I felt I could sustain over my lifetime. I have lost 70 pounds in about seven to eight months." (2)

Perris: "I combined Keto and Intermittent Fasting with HIIT Workouts to Lose 55 Pounds."

Linda: "When I put a low-calorie and low-carb diet together, I lost 62 pounds in seven months. And felt so in control of my eating and my weight for the first time in my life. Because I know how to keep it off." (3)

Yes! Three snaps in the air, happy dance for them. Their success came from lowering both their insulin levels and insulin resistance, by combining different diets. I do not know about you, but I love hearing stories like those because it shows weight loss is not just attainable but maintainable. The same power of combining different diets that worked for them, can also work for you in helping you lose weight long-term.

Isn't that the goal when we diet in the first place? Long-term weight loss, to say goodbye to yo-yo dieting for good? To use a diet that really works. For most people, the answer would be yes.

The way I used the previously mentioned Base, Remixx, and Bonus Diets, coupled with the results from the research study and the success stories, are all examples of *Slim Down Level Up Formulas* doing what they can do best. Which is maximizing weight loss for optimum results. More importantly, helping people win against the battle of the bulge.

In the world of weight loss, fitness, and health, learning to combine a variety of different diets together and understanding why the techniques can work is, by far, the missing piece many people have been searching for far too long.

Even when I decided to share my weight loss story in this book, I got to thinking. Why don't more people know about combining different diets together? Why are there so many uninformed dieters? Process those questions for a moment.

If you are like me, you have tried several diets in the past. We could probably sit down and compare notes on what to eat or what not eat for hours. However, why can we not sit down and compare notes of using the power of combining different diets together?

Prior to you reading this book, have you ever heard of using the techniques before? Or has it ever been recommended by a professional for you to use in helping you to lose weight?

For example, have you ever thought about combining Intermittent Fasting with Weight Watchers? Keto and Low-Calorie? Or Low-Calorie and a Vegan Diet? Intermittent Fasting and Low-Carb with alternating One Meal a Day and a 36-hour fast? But did not know how to do it. How about using Intermittent Fasting and Keto? Or, eating Vegan three times a week with Intermittent Fasting to maximize your weight loss?

Probably not is my guess. If you had received that information already and knew about the techniques, you would not have necessarily needed to read this book. Unless, that is, you just wanted to hear about other success stories from those, who also discovered the power of combining different diets together.

With a growing population of people either overweight or obese, and who are dieting or getting ready to start a diet, why haven't many of them already discovered or been told how to use this powerful technique? Even with all the technology and the research we have in the world to date, the combining of different diets together is not widely known or shared. It was not until I was looking for additional data to use in this book, did I recognize it.

Even though I was in my own little bubble and knew it worked for me and continues to work for several others, my assumption that more people knew was wrong. The more I researched, I discovered there are a lot of individuals still in the dark about the effectiveness of using this technique.

How do I know that? Because the obesity epidemic rates are still rampant. Which is why I consider myself even more lucky, that my doctor co-signed on my *Slim Down Level Up* combinations years ago. It is why I was so appreciative that he also gave me some insight on why it could work so well. Because unfortunately, what he did was rare. But why is that?

Why are there not more doctors, nutritionists, and dietitians looking into the *missing piece,* and talking about it? Why are they not sending out reports, publishing more papers or books and telling all their overweight and obese patients or clients, new ways to lose weight successfully? Why have there been no recent advances in the world of dieting yet?

What has been happening, unfortunately, with the *advances* in the world of dieting, is most of us have been left up to our own devices. Trying various ways to get the weight off. Year after year, many of us wishfully brought items from the weight loss trilogy. Praying they contained some form of magic pixie dust that would melt our excess weight away.

What is the Weight Loss Trilogy?

1. Pills, 2. Potions, and 3. Programs. Many of which, when used, did not bring us much success, or if it did, it was short-term.

Think about that for a minute. Do the professionals want us to remain obese or, is it they do not have the answers or viable solutions, on how to help fight the disease? I often wonder why are doctors waiting to treat the obesity disease by prescribing us medicine after the fact, instead of figuring out how to stop the cause of the increased and repeated weight gain?

Thanks to a lot of research studies already conducted, most doctors know what causes obesity. Most know, obesity rates are continuing to go up. If you ever struggled or are still struggling with being overweight or obese, you know the weight is not going to go away on its own. Nor is it going to go away with the current weight loss trilogy or the *popular diet solutions* given on how to lose weight. Most are the same techniques, just dressed up with different names.

Thought Provoking Questions:

Have you ever thought about why the professionals are not searching for more answers to share with us? Think about it right now in this very moment. You just read, the diet code philosophy is not designed to work long-term. Why are they not giving better solutions to what they know is an out, of control disease?

In an article I recently read, it gave me some of the answers to those questions. It was not what I thought I would hear. The article was titled, "Why I Stopped Telling My Patients to Lose Weight." While reading it, I came across some interesting comments about some of the advice doctors were giving their obese patients and whether, or not it was working.

One doctor shared his insight as to what is the current state of how obesity is being treated in the profession. "We need to get serious and stop pretending that telling patients to lose weight, without giving them the tools to do so, is an acceptable intervention."

He later goes on to say, "Many doctors agree we need to change how we approach obesity but are divided about how." (4)

What? Lord help us! (My brain, "Doctor please tell me that is not your final answer?") Seriously, I wanted to scream after reading the article, for all those people who, in the past, turned to their doctors, nutritionists, or dietitians for help in losing weight. But did not get the tools they needed to be successful, past the *expected* short-term weight loss timeline.

The professionals and experts seriously need to come together and figure this out. Because the reality is, the traditional, "eat less, increase your exercise, take these pills, learn more discipline, pick another diet, and go home" techniques are still not working.

Final Questions: Now that you have seen a few examples of how combining different diets together can work, do you think if more people had already known, about using the techniques, it could have helped them fight their weight loss battle? Could it have increased their success? Lastly, do you think it would have been helpful to have known the techniques on the last diet *you* were on?

If your answer is yes, great. Stick with me because I have a plan. By the end of this book, you are going to gain a better understanding of the missing piece. And see several other examples of why combining diets together can work. You will also learn a variety of different weight loss combinations you can use. Ultimately, you will not be an uninformed dieter anymore. Because you will know reasons why you should not start another diet again without using the techniques in this book. In the next chapter, we will talk about the *Diet Trap* and how to avoid it.

Side Note: Have you dieted in the past using any Low-Calorie Diet and wondered why you were told to cut your eating off at 6 pm? Did you think it was to help with reducing late night snacking and then realized it was contributing to you losing weight? If you followed the cut off times, and stuck with it, you were partially using the power of a (mini), *Slim Down Level Up* technique and may not have realized it. For example, if you stopped eating at 6 pm and did not eat breakfast the next day until 7 am, that would be a 13-hour fast combined with your Low-Calorie Diet. A 16-hour fast or more is ideal for maximum weight loss. However, even with the shorter fasting timeframe, by not eating, you would have allowed your body to reap some of the benefits, of creating a calorie deficit *and* fasting at the same time. Now, imagine if you were dieting and added the additional recommended time-restricted eating and only consumed non-caloric, approved liquids during the extended fasting window. That coupled with a Low-Calorie Diet could increase your weight loss success, like it did for me. We will talk more about fasting, approved liquids and how using this technique can be done in the coming chapters.

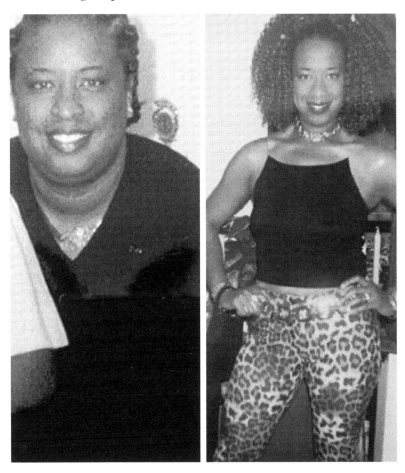

You ever see a picture of yourself and not even recognize who it is? That somehow, the weight made you look so much older and different. The picture on the left is me tipping the scale over 300 pounds. The day the picture was taken, I had lunch with my oldest brother. We went to one of my favorite restaurants, because they had some of the best chocolate lava cakes around. I remember that day specifically because I went home deflated and angry. That was because the waitress who took our order thought my brother was my son. To highlight the significance of why I was not happy that day: my brother is just two years younger than I am. When I got home later that evening, **I couldn't start Fasting fast enough!** I knew Intermittent Fasting had health benefits, but I had also heard it had anti-aging properties. I wanted to do something to get the weight off and to help me look younger. Thanks to the *Slim Down Level Up Formulas,* the picture on the right is the result of fifteen months later and going down to 143 pounds.

2

THE DIET TRAP

Question: If "Fewer Foods + Healthier Foods + Fewer Calories = Calorie Deficit" will choosing just one Low-Calorie Diet get you to your weight loss goal?

| Intermittent Fasting Keto Vegan Paleo Jenny Craig Nutrisystem |
| Low Calorie Weight Watchers Mediterranean South Beach Any Diet* |
| **Fewer Foods + Healthier Foods + Fewer Calories =A CALORIE DEFICIT!** |

Calorie deficit, calorie deficit, calorie deficit. When it comes to weight loss, you probably have heard those words more times than you can count. For most of the top diets, those words are usually their number one theme used to tell us how to achieve weight loss.

Low-Calorie Diets can work for us by creating the calorie deficit needed for losing weight. We can choose Vegan, Paleo, Weight Watchers, South Beach, etc. When we do reduce our overall caloric intake, we start experiencing weight loss. Then, in a short amount of time, we hit a plateau and are not exactly sure why the diet stopped working. Especially since we were taking in fewer calories like we were told. We continue reducing our daily food intake lower and lower, but nothing seems to work. This is when the ineffectiveness of using one diet sets in.

The reason they stop working and do not work long-term is because, with a large decrease in calories, there is an increased appetite that can take over. Followed by a decrease in the metabolism, which takes place usually within a few weeks of first losing weight.

The process of reducing your calories is one of the main reasons why you initially lose the weight. But, once the decreased metabolism kicks in and your hunger takes over, the fight to see who is stronger begins. Then the constant growling stomach and hunger pangs can awaken, and the decrease in your energy levels can overpower you. Making you want to give in, binge eat, or quit.

It can be frustrating and can make you feel your efforts of reducing your calories and *starving* do nothing to help you *really* lose the weight. The reality is the need to understand what is happening in your body when you reduce your calories is what holds the key to you being successful going forward.

The calorie deficit, in fact, is a key powerhouse player in your ability to lose weight. But it is only one piece of the weight loss puzzle needed to continue losing and to keep it off. When your diet choice and calorie deficit go into full gear, it causes your body to respond to the reduction of food intake. When this happens, the metabolism will resist to receiving less food and adjust to the changes in your eating.

For example, my dietitian once told me an average size woman in a coma burns 700-800 calories at rest. That is just for her to have basic body function, heart, brain, kidneys, lungs etc. Since she is in a coma and receiving fewer calories, her metabolism would not be running at the same rate than if she were up and moving around. As well as if she were eating a higher caloric intake. Therefore, to continue normal body function accurately, her metabolism, adjusted to a slower rate to be in alignment with her energy expenditure and her body's needs. The human body is so amazing and designed to protect itself, and it will adapt and respond based on what we are experiencing.

When you are on a Low-Calorie Diet, it is inevitable, your metabolism will slow down. Because the body thinks you are depriving it by only taking in a limited number of calories. Therefore, your hunger senses are activated, so the body can ask for the additional calories it needs. Since calories equal energy, the body needs energy to operate all your major body functions. What happens is your brain sends the signal to activate your hunger senses and tells your metabolism to slow down. Not to punish your efforts but as a way to preserve energy.

This process can be the most frustrating part in losing weight because no matter how low you keep taking your calories, your body will keep making the adjustments. It will continue to slow your metabolism down even more to protect itself. This reoccurring process in the body is created by you following the ever so recommended and required, calorie deficit to lose weight. Trying to overcome this obstacle by using one diet is not a viable long-term solution. It becomes a vicious cycle of repeated decreased calories, slowed metabolism and increased hunger. The *all you need to do is create a calorie deficit,* theory needs to stop being told to people without the other key missing piece to the equation.

This has been one of the main reasons why the battle rages on in the weight loss ring, with obesity being the undisputed winner. Due to the fact that, no matter how much discipline you have, or which *one diet* you use, you can and usually do stop losing weight. What often happens next is you regain the weight back that you lost. Mainly, because eventually your body's metabolism wins the fight.

Before we go any further, I want to tell you something, in case no one else has ever told you. **If you have failed at losing weight, by following a one diet philosophy technique in the past, it is not your fault. You are not a weight loss failure. The way dieting has been traditionally designed sets you up to fail.** It will work for a while, but as I said before, it will eventually, stop.

If you have heard any of the terrible statistics about the high weight loss failure rates and short-term weight loss being inevitable and became discouraged, it is not your fault. These are two of the main reasons many people do not want to start a diet again to only fail.

Truth be told, your previous weight loss failures cannot be put on your lap any longer. A key piece has been missing, and the need to find it has been ignored long enough. Continuing to use the same dieting techniques that have constantly failed you, will not help your struggles with losing weight get any better.

"The definition of insanity is doing the same thing over and over again, and expecting different results."
-Albert Einstein

With the obesity rates projected to be one billion worldwide in the next few years, and with so many people struggling with being overweight, something has to change in the way people are being taught to fight against obesity. If nothing changes, the numbers will only continue to go up and, unfortunately, so will the death rates.

Follow me here for a minute as we look at some statistics. Sadly, if something does not happen in how dieting is approached, more people will continue to struggle, with losing weight and to fight for their lives.

According to a published report by the United Nations conducted in 2017, worldwide there were almost eighteen million people who died from cardiovascular related diseases in one year. (5) It is a shocking number to hear. The main associated causes were heart disease, obesity, unhealthy diets, strokes, and heart attacks. The next leading cause of death worldwide annually, which is almost 50% less than cardiovascular diseases, was cancer. Equating to a little over nine and a half million deaths.

Over the last several years with the advances in medicine and technology, cancer has been highly researched by the professionals. They have developed a *variety* of ways to fight against a disease that, unfortunately, has and will continue taking so many lives annually.

What do they do to fight cancer, to reduce the death rates? They attack it using multiple layers and different techniques to increase the patients' chances of beating it. They do not rely on *one* technique to win against such a massive multi-layer disease. They look at fighting the diagnosis in its totality. How do I know this? My husband is a cancer survivor. A big reason why is because, thankfully, when he was first diagnosed, they did not give him one treatment to fight the disease. It was a combination of different techniques and treatments that was able to help him win and be cancer free.

Question: If cancer is the number two killer of people worldwide, and a multi-layer approach is used to attack it, why isn't the *number one* killer of people, (cardiovascular disease) being fought the same way?

Why Does this Matter? The way the diet code philosophy is set up, make no mistake about it, cardiovascular diseases associated with being overweight or obese have been and will continue to be the leading killer of people worldwide.

Unfortunately, unlike cancer, it is not being attacked using a multi-layered approach. Why? Most people have not been told or understand how to win against the disease using more than one weapon. They have gotten stuck in the diet trap and need help getting out. Are you stuck? If so, it is time to get unstuck.

The unrelenting rise in obesity rates, the diet trap, the failed diet code philosophies, have gone on long enough. There needs to be a reduction in the awful yearly statistics of the number one cause of death. How do we do that? **It is time to *Level Up* on obesity and fight it head on with a variety of techniques. Just like millions of people do every year with fighting cancer, it is time to square up, punch obesity in the face and stop letting it win.** It is time for you to dominate losing weight.

When I discovered how to fight using more than one weapon, by using the power of combining different diets together, I was able to positively affect some of the associated *dis-eases* I had with being obese. Like how I was able to reduce one of the risk factors associated with yo-yo dieting, (heart disease), lowered my blood pressure and cholesterol, as well as reduced my inflammation. I also was no longer pre-diabetic, and my sleeping patterns improved.

The major victory came from taking it one day and one pound at a time. By doing that, I reduced my chances of becoming one of the yearly death statistics.

Why Make Changes in How You Diet? **For you to continue fighting your weight loss battle using one of the current diets, is like a boxer in the ring with one hand tied behind her back.**

She is going to reduce her daily food intake and create the required calorie deficit. She will get a few punches in, move around the ring, and even feel good about herself, for standing up to the opponent. She might make it a few rounds. Before the disadvantage knocks her out.

Frustrated and bruised, she stays down and does not get back up, so she loses. Not because she did not have the strength or the motivation to succeed. But she entered the ring to a fight she could not win. Fighting using one diet alone is not the way to victory.

When I started my battle to lose weight years ago, using more than one diet and breaking down the diet code philosophies weakness, it gave me both my hands to fight with in the ring. I am married to someone who used to box, which made me pause and think about the strength it takes to stand up in the ring and go toe to toe with an opponent.

All the more reason I understand why, having both hands gave me a better advantage in the fight and increased my chances of winning. It was the key factor for me losing and keeping the weight off. Once I learned how to create and use the *Slim Down Level Up Formulas,* the boxing scorecard turned in my favor. Making me the undisputed winner.

The reason most people have failed with dieting in the past or found themselves being frustrated with experiencing repeated plateaus and weight gain is because, they were unknowingly fighting a losing battle.

That is why having the right information can be so powerful in making sense of how to successfully win at losing weight. There are two facts to keep in mind when it comes to dieting:

1). All diets *can* work for a period of time

2). The degree to which they can work is tied to our body's ability to lower increased insulin levels as well as reduce insulin resistance

I mentioned in Chapter 1, how combining different diets together, to address the needs of lowering insulin levels and insulin resistance, was key for me in losing weight. You may be wondering what causes increased insulin levels and insulin resistance in the first place? More importantly, how does that relate to your weight loss journey? To name a few, increased insulin levels and increased insulin resistance can be due to stress, sleep deprivation, *what, when,* and *how* much we are eating and drinking or a combination of all of them.

Diets can work in different aspects by helping us fight the associated risk factors linked to the obesity disease. For example, heart disease, high blood pressure, inflammation, high cholesterol, and diabetes. For many of us, it is why we start a diet in the first place. Not just to move the scale. But because we are facing multiple medical issues linked to the excessive weight gain. We use dieting as a way to help us on the journey to getting healthier by getting the weight off.

There is a problem in the dieting puzzle as it relates to what we often believe diets are supposed to do and how they are supposed to work. The problem is the habitual diet trap that no one seems eager to fix.

For a long time, I was on the diet trap rollercoaster, signing up for or following multiple weight loss programs. Dreaming and waiting on the industry professionals, to come up with the next great weight loss tool and diet products. That somehow, they would miraculously create different types of special techniques and food, that I could use and wake up thinner. I would be able to use their special code and get the products to my home quickly. That way, I could lose weight for good.

You probably already guessed, that dream never came true. Here is the kicker of why there is no sense of urgency to help us *really* lose weight long-term. Especially with using the current popular diets and weight loss products.

If the weight loss concepts and products keep selling, even with the participants' long-term success rates low, the desire to fix what is broken is not a priority, if what is broken continues to be a money maker.

THE DIET TRAP! Pump the brakes. Pause and take that in a moment. You may even want to read it again, out loud. The reason I say that is because once I realized what was going on, it was eye opening to me. It was a lot to take in and process. **Because it is in their best interest to keep us obese and constantly struggling to lose weight.**

I understand companies are in business to make money. However, to recognize how the bulk of an entire industry *knows* their products and services do not work long-term, yet they are not fixing them. How do they know? Because the success rates of most dieters are low and the promised results they make, do not last.

Diets and weight loss products are promoted almost everywhere as a way to help us lose weight. We see them on TV, in magazines, on billboards and on social media. After seeing several advertisements, and often after checking with our doctors, nutritionists, or dietitians, we got our hopes up and decided to start losing weight. Using some of the products or services.

Think back to the times when you were dieting, do you ever remember reading, even in the fine print, when you signed up for either pills, potions, or programs, that it said, "You will lose weight, but it will only be short-lived."?

I sure did not read or hear anything like that, because it would have been a statement I would have remembered. Who knowingly wants to pay for things that do not work for long?

What I do remember reading and hearing are the two ever so faithful disclaimer statements, the weight loss and fitness industry is notorious for putting on their products. As well as attaching to their services.

You probably have heard or seen both.

1. **"Results not typical."**

2. **"These statements have not been approved by the Food and Drug Administration."**

Bam! That is their carte blanche disclaimers to be able to sell us anything, whether it works or not.

How can they get away with it? They have and they will continue as long as we keep buying from them and falling into the diet trap. Do not hold your breath waiting on the weight loss cavalry to come in and fix the situation. We do not know how long it will take before the FDA steps in and tells them to stop selling us *weight loss dreams*.

The trap is one of the reasons why diets and products can work at first but then stop. We often pay our hard-earned money to lose weight, then turn around and gain it all back, because they are not set up and designed to last.

You may be thinking, did she not just say earlier that diets can work? Yes, you heard me correctly, I did. A diet can work, short-term. Later in the coming chapters, I will show you the powerful techniques of combining different diets together and the reasons why they can work long-term, successfully.

Just to be clear, I am not saying there are no weight loss products on the market that can help with losing weight. There are some, but unfortunately as stated, most will only work for a while.

Questions: On the subject of using diets, have you heard the answers to why they truly do not work long-term from anyone in the weight loss and fitness industry? How about from the professionals? Or was the blame put back on you as to why the diet did not work?

A few years back, I read a very interesting book called, The Obesity Code, by Dr. Jason Fung. In the book, Dr. Fung highlights the reality of the diet situation, as it relates to the out of control obesity epidemic. And why people continue to fail at losing weight, using traditional diets. He says,

"But none of (diets) them work for very long because none of them address the *totality* of the disease." (6)

Pump the brakes and wait a minute again. In a nutshell, all this time, the way people have been traditionally dieting would be similar to halfway treating cancer, wondering why it keeps coming back. We cannot *partially* fight a monster like obesity and think we can win. It is too big and too powerful of a giant. It is why we lose weight, plateau, and regain it back, every time.

Do your previous failed attempts at losing weight using one diet make more sense now, as to why they could only work short-term? Sadly, when you started those diets, you were not expected to succeed for long, nor could you. Without having all the right tools, you were set up to fail.

I am not blaming the professionals or the health and fitness, diet industry, per se, but they are continuing to do as they have always done. Unfortunately, their weight loss solutions have only been able to focus on and treat one part to losing weight. With doing so, they are not addressing all known parts associated with the obesity equation. Which goes back to the saying, "You don't know what you know don't, that is until you know."

The time has come for them to know and to realize we can win by attacking this problem from multiple angles. Using the follow-one-diet technique is not helping. Continuing to use the same pills, potions, and programs can be an inevitable trap that far too many people can still fall into. And that needs to stop.

After learning about and using the *Slim Down Level Up Formulas,* it will be one trap you will not fall into anymore. This is why I am happy that by the end of this book, you will have the techniques that can be used to win the battle of the bulge in your life.

When did I know I could win my battle? After years of struggling with my weight, coupled with hearing the high weight loss failure statistics, the way the diet code philosophy was set up, and once my eyes were opened to the infamous diet trap, I had to find another solution to losing weight. Over time, by putting certain pieces together, I did.

I knew some of the previous diets I used had worked to a degree, and they had some good attributes, as far as food choices and a variety of dieting techniques. Some of which I could draw from to use in creating a recipe to win.

Besides sharing the previously mentioned steps I took, over the years, while losing and maintaining weight, I strategically used six different diets, in a variety of combinations. As well as in different time sequences. I learned, the concept of *there is power in numbers* also applies to mixing diets together.

The Slim Down Level Up techniques of combining different diets helped me lose even more weight than when I was using them individually. It was the missing piece that enabled me to get off the diet trap rollercoaster, for good.

In the process of losing the weight by combining the benefits of what worked best in various diets, I became what you see today: **A Boss, Vegan, Keto, Low Calorie, Weight Watchers, Intermittent Fasting, Mediterranean Diva!!** It was the process of learning how to combine and use different diets at certain times that was key.

Using the techniques addressed the need to lower my insulin levels and my insulin resistance. It also made my long-term success with "food options" limitless. I opened myself up to new recipes that I otherwise would have not known about. That special weight loss food I was waiting for was there all along. It was in a variety of other diets and their food choices, waiting for me to discover them, and use as resources, in helping with reaching my goal.

The unwritten rule that has kept people from trying different foods from other diets needs to go away. There is no reason why you cannot mix the foods from a variety of *diet eating styles* together. You can look at it as your Diet Buffet, with endless options to choose from, all of which are designed to help you lose weight.

For instance, by experimenting with the food from different diets, I discovered ways to cook plant-based, Vegan recipes. Like sesame tofu with broccoli, which was surprisingly delicious. It allowed me to learn how to pick tasty low-calorie, dense foods, like Teriyaki Vegetable Stir-Fry with cauliflower rice (I will share a few weight loss benefits to having meatless meals later in the book).

I also discovered other food options I could use from some of the other diets. For example, I ordered food from the South Beach,

Jenny Craig, and Nutrisystem Diets because it was convenient. I used recipes from Weight Watchers, because it helped with keeping my food portions in check and made meal planning easier. I used Keto recipes because using a Low-Carb Diet helped me lose more weight.

The food you eat while losing and maintaining weight will play a vital role in your success. When you have access to multiple eating styles and their options, it will allow you to not feel pigeonholed to only eat certain foods.

Besides learning how to master using different foods from a variety of diets, the key to my success was utilizing the power of mixing any diet I chose, with *varying* Intermittent Fasting schedules. As well as combining a variety of Low-Calorie and Low-Carb Diets together. They were the tickets to a world that forever changed eating and dieting for me.

There was a reason why I used varying Intermittent Fasting schedules. **Your body will require change as you are losing weight.** Using the same schedule is not a long-term diet plan as your body, over time, will adjust to what you are doing. For example, there was a time when the fasting schedule I used to lose 25 pounds could not be used to lose the next 15 pounds. I plateaued. My body had gotten used to the fasting schedule of using the 16:8 timeframe. By varying my fasting time, adding in 3 days of an 18:6 schedule and a 24-hour fast once a week, I was able to keep my body guessing and continued to lose more weight. We will go over later in the book various ways and options as to how you can keep your body guessing, by making small changes as you are losing weight.

Going forward, you can conquer the diet trap by gaining an understanding of the power of combining different diets, in various ways, to reach your goal weight. As well as, be able use those same techniques to stay in maintenance mode.

The weight loss combinations will be your introduction to the *Slim Down Level Up Formulas* you can use, to be successful. In the coming chapters, you will see a series of additional stories and research data on using the power of these techniques in different ways.

Side Note: Whenever referencing the eating styles in the book, it is either referring to the actual foods, which are key to that diet, the way in which the foods are eaten and *when* and *how* they are eaten.

WINNING AGAINST THE WEIGHT LOSS ODDS

It is such a good feeling when I hear or read about how other people are winning the weight loss battle, even though the diet code philosophy has traditionally been stacked against them. We will look at a variety of success stories throughout the book. By reading them, it may change your diet perception, helping you realize there is a path forward for you to also succeed.

For example, here is some encouraging news in the world of weight loss. There was a research study back in the early 2000's that was conducted over a five-year period of time.

When completed, it showed promising long-term weight loss results. The reason for the random study was because the researchers wanted to show the world, successful weight loss was possible. And it did not necessarily need to come from a controlled study.

The study was done by the National Weight Control Registry on collecting success stories from over 2,500 participants. Most of the volunteers were solicited through newspapers and magazines. And even the researchers were surprised. Dr. Wing, one of the leading researchers says, "On average, the participants were able to maintain a 67-pound weight loss for five years. And between 12 and 14 percent had maintained a loss of more than 100 pounds." (7) All of the participants found various ways to lose weight and keep it off.

She later goes on to say, "They are compelling detailed histories of successful long-term dieters."

After reading the data, it put a big smile on my face. I do not know about you, but when you have been beaten down for so long, as I was, with trying to lose weight, and you finally win, it is very exciting to hear about other people winning the battle of the bulge as well.

While writing this book, besides sharing my own story and the people I previously knew of, I wanted to be able to share with you the excitement and testimonies of additional weight loss success stories. From people who also discovered combining different diets together, to lose weight successfully. Real, everyday people who knew firsthand what it was like to struggle. How through it all, even with the diet code philosophy not in their favor and the odds stacked against them, they still managed to find a way to win.

I browsed the internet, reached out to people on social media, through Facebook groups, and Instagram followings and looked through several fitness and health magazines. When I did, I was ecstatic to hear the numerous personal weight loss success stories. Of course, the stories I connected with the most were from the people who showed the power of combining different diets together, to reach their fitness goals. How using the technique was life changing for some of them.

WEIGHT LOSS SUCCESS STORY TIME

Here is an example of one woman's success story that was shared:

Chineye E.

"With Keto and Intermittent Fasting, I lost 90 pounds in 9 months and erased my joint pain and discomfort." (8)

Yay! Hearing, her testimony, of course, made me smile as I read it. As someone who spent years in discomfort and pain before I lost the weight, it can be life changing when you finally are not hurting anymore. I especially enjoyed reading, not only did combining the diets positively affect the number on her scale, but it helped with relieving some of the physical ailments from carrying the excessive weight. She found the *technique* needed to fight her obesity battle and won.

Guess what? Weight loss success stories like hers are not rare. For instance, there was a study in 2019 that highlighted the positive health and weight loss outcomes of combining different diets together, at the same time. Over the 8-week randomized trial, "Overweight or obese women who fasted three days a week and ate a lower-calorie diet, lost more weight, and had better cardiometabolic makers than those who only fasted, or only restricted their calorie intake." (9)

Excitement! I loved reading that study as well, because using fasting alone or a low-calorie diet by itself was not as effective than when using them *together*. It showed how the participants used the power of combining more than one diet, to maximize weight loss. It is not a coincidence that combining different diets together helped the people in the stories I read or the participants in the studies. Like me, they found their missing piece combinations. It increased their overall success by addressing the disease in its *totality*.

Side Note: I am not saying no one has ever, or cannot, be successful using one diet in losing or maintaining weight. Everybody is different, and what may work for one may not for another. What I am saying is using one diet for me did not work, for long. Both my insulin levels and insulin resistance were not addressed, and I kept regaining the weight back. It was not until I started combining different diets together, in various ways, did it work for me.

Throughout the book, as I continue to share stories, and tips on the power of using these same types of techniques, as well as additional steps I took, my goal is to speak to you. Especially if you have been frustrated over the years with trying to successfully lose weight. But have not been able, to use one diet, to achieve your long-term weight loss goals. Dieting frustration is not your friend, and it is time to eliminate it from your weight loss equation.

MEATLESS, NO CARBS, AND WEIGHT LOSS PROGRAMS?

Before we dive further into the book, I want to make something very clear so there is no confusion. In order to be successful using the *Slim Down Level Up Formulas*, you **do not** have to join a weight loss program, or become a Vegan and completely give up eating meat. Nor is this about telling you to only commit to a Keto Diet and to never eat carbs again. Or to use Intermittent Fasting every day and eat break- fast at 11 am.

You do not have to only eat Weight Watchers or Mediterranean Diet food either. The formulas are all about choices. When we discuss them later in the book, there will be examples and a guide on how you can use the food from a variety of diets to help you lose weight. How combining them together is a powerful tool.

For instance, there is a reason why you will see a variety of Vegan, food and snack options in the book. Even on a Low-Calorie Diet, combined with Intermittent Fasting, by choosing to add *Meatless Mondays* or *Try Tofu Thursdays*, it will not only mix up your meals but expose you to more healthy eating options. They can help you lose more weight. How? You would be choosing low-calorie, dense plant-based foods, that can make you feel fuller longer, causing you to eat less, allowing the weight to come off.

The Keto eating style is shown not because you have to be full-fledged Keto necessarily. But if, while using Intermittent Fasting, with a Low-Calorie Diet, you take a page out of the Keto philosophy and hold the bread or the bun sometimes, when eating a sandwich or burger, or lower your processed carbs intake, like rice, pasta, refined grains, you can create a larger calorie deficit. Another bonus is, when a Low-Carb Diet is combined with Intermittent Fasting it puts your body into Ketosis, helping you to burn stored fat as fuel (we will talk more about Ketosis later in the book and the powerful weight loss benefits of being in that stage).

Another example is the Weight Watchers eating style, in which food options are shown, not because you have to join the program or only eat their food. But if you are using a Low-Calorie Diet combined with a Low-Carb Diet, by adding food options from any one of their Color-Coded Plans, it can be helpful with meal planning. They offer a variety of low-calorie meals, snacks, and recipes that can take the guesswork out of how much you are eating. If and when you want to try any of them, the options will be there for you to use in that chapter. (The Weight Watchers Program is based on a points system assigned to food; however, each meal, food option or snack also comes with nutritional information, so you can see how many calories, fat grams etc. are in each item).

The three *Slim Down Level Up Formulas* we will go over, are about empowering you. So, you can decide which combinations will work best for you, at each stage of losing weight. Your selections will be based on your lifestyle, the amount of weight you want to lose and your food preferences.

Recap: The two key factors in losing weight will be controlling your insulin levels and insulin resistance. Learning how to combine multiple diets together can address both. The three different formulas will show you how to do just that in various ways. They will all answer the, what you are eating, when you are eating and how much you are eating. Which is essential to your weight loss success. In the next chapter we will talk more about how this works.

3

THE POWER OF COMBINING DIFFERENT DIETS

L et us take a look at the three key reasons why the people in the previously mentioned studies and success stories were able to lose weight combining different diets together.

When you gain weight, it is associated with persistent, increased insulin levels. Which can come from eating at all times of the day and at night. Also, from excessively indulging in empty calories, like junk food, and *lots* of processed foods. Unfortunately, those types of choices can lead to a decrease in your insulin sensitivity. When this happens, it can cause weight gain, heart disease and diabetes.

But on the flip side, by design, when you start a diet, it reduces or removes certain types of food from your options. Especially the ones that can cause increased insulin secretion. When dieting, by not typically eating those types of foods, and by reducing your caloric intake, it can lower your insulin levels. The key here is getting the body to lower insulin levels and increase insulin sensitivity, so weight loss can occur. This step is also a way to ensure that the weight keeps coming off. A part of this process can take place in the body when you start using one diet. But it is important to point out, again, to achieve *both,* you need a multi-dimensional diet strategy. As discussed earlier, one diet is only addressing one part. By now, you probably realize, that is why your previous weight loss success was short lived.

If this is not your first time, dieting, you are probably beyond ready to specifically figure out how to make both parts of the diet equation work, so your frustration and diet disappointment can end. This is why I want to unpack this a little bit more. For most people when they hear the word, insulin they think it only applies to someone with diabetes.

This is not the case. Every time you eat, whether you are on a diet or not, it increases your insulin levels. If your insulin levels and insulin resistance are both linked to your ability to lose and maintain weight, what will be the key to you dieting and efficiently lowering both?

Yes, if you guessed using more than one diet, we are on a roll and you got it right. **If you were to use a low-calorie diet, for example, like Jenny Craig, it can help with lowering your insulin levels by reducing or eliminating the types of food that causes high insulin secretion. Combining it with an Intermittent Fasting Diet can help with reducing your body's insulin resistance. And the two can work together in helping you lose weight, long-term.**

Side Note: Insulin resistance occurs, when excess glucose in the blood reduces the ability of the cells to absorb and use blood sugar for energy. It is when your insulin levels tell your cells fuel is on the way, but they do not open up, to receive the glucose. Which means, sugar stays in the bloodstream and after a while your body stores it as fat. This is the main reason why it is essential to control both insulin levels and insulin resistance, for successful weight loss. You can lower your insulin levels by using one diet, however, if your insulin resistance is still high, it will cause your body to continue to store the extra glucose as fat, instead of using it for energy.

Before we go on, I want you to keep in mind besides using Intermittent Fasting, to lower insulin resistance, there are also other ways this can be done. By using different sets of diet combinations, which I will explain later in the book. There will be other options to choose from, if for whatever reason you do not want to utilize fasting in one of your main diet combinations.

Recap: Successful long-term weight loss is about understanding the importance of the key roles insulin levels and insulin resistance will play in your weight loss story. Because when both are managed properly, success can be inevitable.

WEIGHT LOSS SUCCESS STORY TIME

Here is another success story that used the power of combining different diets to help one woman reach her weight loss goals. And she did it by combining two of her favorite diets together.

Alexis H.

"I lost 42 pounds combining Weight Watchers and Intermittent Fasting." (10)

Super excited for her! Weight Watchers has been used for years in helping people count points (calories) to keep their intake low. Hence, the faithful calorie deficit is created. However, as we learned in Chapter 2, after a certain point, due to the reduction in calories, the slowed metabolism will kick in and weight loss can be stalled. By adding Intermittent Fasting to her mix, Alexis, used the power of combining different diets together to control her insulin levels and insulin resistance.

When I first started combining diets together, I did not have a deep understanding of the significance, of the roles insulin levels and insulin resistance played in weight loss. But because I was pre-diabetic at the time, I made a point to know the importance of how they both needed to be addressed.

In doing so, I developed a better understanding of the human body and how complex yet amazing it is. But I will be the first to admit to you, I do not know everything about losing and gaining weight, even though I labeled myself a professional dieter.

Over time as I did more research, had additional personal weight loss victories, and spoke to others and heard their testimonies, I realized why combining diets together worked so well. I also realized why continuing to use one diet would have not gotten me to my goal weight. No matter how hard I kept trying, my efforts were not the problem. The technique was.

For example, the way in which Dr. Fung explains insulin levels and insulin resistance in the previously referenced book, The Obesity Code, sheds more light to the realities of this issue.

The book explains more in depth, how most people have been missing the need to understand, these key factors in fighting against the obesity epidemic. How using one diet has not typically worked, or at least did not work long-term.

This is how Dr. Fung explains what has been happening with traditional dieting:

"Most diets restrict the intake of foods that cause increased insulin secretion, but don't address insulin resistance. You lose weight initially, but insulin resistance keeps your insulin levels and body set weight high. By fasting, you can efficiently reduce your body's insulin resistance, since it requires both persistent and high levels." (11)

Wow! That was a mouthful and a lot to take in initially. I read it out loud twice when I first saw it and highlighted it in the book. It made perfect sense. When you address the need to reduce your insulin resistance, (the very thing, keeping your body's set weight high and prevents you from losing more weight), you can win.

For years, I had combined different diets together, because using one did not work for me long-term. I knew the benefits from using Intermittent Fasting because it was one of the common denominators I often used. I also knew firsthand combining different diets worked for several other people. Mainly, because their combinations did what one diet was not able to do.

But to hear it from an informed, medical professional's point of view, who did not hold back on making direct connections to a significant root cause of a failed weight loss philosophy, was powerful. One diet does not work long-term. In his book, he provided detailed research pointing to why there is a need to address the *totality* of losing weight. As a path to defeat the obesity epidemic.

"Regular fasting, by routinely lowering your insulin levels, has been shown to significantly improve insulin sensitivity. *This finding is the missing piece in the weight-loss puzzle."*

This reiterates the fact that, your weight loss is tied back to a two-part equation, with the two key factors needing to be addressed for long-term success.

Does That Mean We Only Need to Use Intermittent Fasting to Lose Weight? No! While losing weight, the missing piece is all about controlling your insulin levels and insulin resistance. You now know this as your true weight loss gospel. However, there is a second piece to the puzzle that is important for you to learn about. Intermittent Fasting by itself does not answer the three key questions to losing weight. What, we are eating? When, we are eating? and How much, we are eating?

The answers to those three questions, need each other to work successfully long-term. No matter which diet, you choose, if you cannot answer those three questions, it can eventually pose a problem for you. For example, even if you were to just use Intermittent Fasting to lose weight, it is technically only dictating when, you will eat. The, what you will eat and how much you will eat also needs to be addressed. Combining Intermittent Fasting with a different diet, will be able to answer all three key questions to losing weight.

What Does All This Mean For You? You may be thinking, does that mean initially one diet (Low-Calorie, Vegan, Jenny Craig, Keto, Weight Watchers, etc.), can help you lose only some weight? But you would need additional tools, like Intermittent Fasting, or in conjunction with a different eating style (going meatless 3 days a week, lowering your carb intake, having liquid dinners), to help you lose more weight or maintain it? Is that because your body's own insulin resistance will try and fight against the weight loss, by wanting to return to its comfortable *higher set weight?*

Yes. Yes, and yes. Because unlike previously, when you probably used one-dimensional dieting, learning multiple ways to use different diets can help you fight the disease in its totality. Ultimately, your body's ability to lower your insulin levels and reduce your insulin resistance, by combining different diets together, is key. So that weight loss and weight maintenance is a reality you can attain. When we dive deeper into the three *Slim Down Level Up Formulas* later in the book, the what, when and how much you are eating will be laid out in a variety of ways. You will be able to see, learning multiple ways of battling the totality of losing weight, is the answer you have been waiting for all this time.

SOME DIETING PITFALLS TO AVOID

A few months before writing this book, I joined some Facebook weight loss support groups. One of which was an Intermittent Fasting group for women. I enjoyed seeing other women cheer for and support one another while on their journeys to losing weight. Besides seeing the motivating, before and after pictures and stories, I kept seeing several posts from women who were still struggling.

After reading some of the comments and questions coming from other members in the group, I realized what the issues were. They kept hitting plateaus or were not losing any weight at all when first starting and often wondered why. They were only eating inside of their approved timeframe and were frustrated and confused as to why the weight was not coming off faster.

There is a commonly floated unwritten rule about how Intermittent Fasting can be used to lose weight, but it is not really a diet. But rather a way of eating. If you Google Intermittent Fasting, you will find a variety of articles spouting similar words. Technically, the thought process can be seen as truthful. Unlike most fad diets, fasting is something you can do for life. It can shape and change your eating patterns by limiting the time in which you eat.

However, as we have talked about as it relates to being successful with losing weight, Intermittent Fasting alone does not answer the three key questions.

Remember: The **What**, you are eating, the **When** you are eating and the **How** much you are eating.

Here is an example of one of the common problems that was shared in the Facebook group. By a woman using Intermittent Fasting by itself and how by doing so, it was hindering her weight loss success.

NO COUNTING CARMEN

Carmen started out dieting using Intermittent Fasting with a 16:8 eating schedule. She read that fasting can be a great way to get rid of stored fat and lose weight. Her starting weight was 205 pounds, and her goal was to lose 50 pounds.

She ate two meals and a snack during her 8-hour eating window. In the first two weeks, even though it was a little tough getting used to not eating breakfast and cutting off her late-night snacking, she lost 2 pounds. But was frustrated because she felt she should have lost more weight.

However, Carmen fell into a common dieting pitfall and believed, Intermittent Fasting was not a diet. She *really* did not *need* to watch what she ate. No foods were necessarily off limit. That is where the problem in her ability to lose more weight derived from.

Since Carmen did not have any idea, how much she was eating each day, she thought just cutting back on her eating and fasting would be enough to lose weight. But the problem was, her usage of one diet could not answer the three key questions.

Prior to starting Intermittent Fasting, Carmen's daily intake was about 5,500 calories and 450 fat grams. With multiple meals and snacking, all throughout the day and at night, it was easy for her to get to those numbers.

Even though she pushed back eating breakfast until 11 am and stopped eating past 7 pm, she still was able to take in, on most of those days, 3,700 calories and 330 fat grams. A large part of which was processed and high carb food (she later was able to figure out her food intake using a fitness tracker app).

If Carmen would have known about the *Slim Down Level Up* techniques and added one more dieting eating style to her mix, (like any of the Low-Calorie Diets, with recommended daily food intake), it could have changed her outcome. By her using both diets together it would have addressed the two key factors with losing weight: lowering her insulin levels and her insulin resistance.

For example, based on Carmen's weight, if she would have adjusted her food intake to about 1800-1900 calories, and 60-63 fat grams, she could have seen more weight loss results. By doing so, maybe she would have felt her decision to change her lifestyle by using Intermittent Fasting was a good choice.

What Carmen did was change one piece of the dieting puzzle by reducing *when* she was eating, down to an 8-hour window. However, even though she reduced her overall food intake, it still was not low enough to create the calorie deficit needed to lose more weight. Also, her food choices to break-fast were not ideal for optimum results, and she was eating primarily a high carb diet throughout the day.

Carmen fell victim to the same one-dimensional dieting pitfall that has failed so many people. After speaking with her, she learned the key to successful weight loss is, to make sure her choice of diets can answer, the three key questions needed to lose and maintain weight. (Carmen went on and lost 17 pounds in her first month after figuring out her right combination of using Intermittent Fasting, Low-Calorie and Low-Carb Diets together).

Here is an example of, like Carmen, how one of my diet attempts did not answer the three key questions and where I went completely wrong. Unfortunately, like, her, I started dieting using some misleading weight loss advice. Mine was "don't count calories, just eat less."

First let us take a look at what I was eating before starting *the diet* and following *the advice*.

MY FOOD INTAKE EXAMPLE

BREAKFAST	LUNCH	DINNER	SNACKS
Pancakes, sausage, eggs: 1340 calories, 64 fat grams Frappe coffee: 420 calories, 18 fat grams OJ: 150 calories, 0 fat grams	Double burger with cheese, mayo, ketchup: 660 calories, 82 fat grams, Large French Fries: 430 calories, 18 fat grams Coke: 510 calories, 0 fat grams Dessert: 410 calories, 19 fat grams	Large Alfredo sauce: 870 calories, 87 fat grams 5 breadsticks: 700 calories, 125 fat grams, Soup: 220 calories, 15 fat grams, Chicken shrimp pasta: 1390 calories, 94 fat grams, Cheesecake: 730 calories, 42 fat grams	A bag of chips: 140 calories, 10 fat grams, Snickers candy bar: 280 calories, 14 fat grams, Bag of peanut M&M's: 250 calories, 13 fat grams
Total=1900 Calories, 82 Fat Grams	**Total=2010 Calories, 119 Fat Grams**	**Total=3910 Calories, 363 Fat Grams**	**Total=670 Calories, 37 Fat Grams**

MATH TIME: My grand total for one day = **8,490** Calories, **601** Fat Grams.

*The average person takes in about 2,000-2,500 calories and 80-150 fat grams a day.

You probably have your mouth wide open in amazement on how much I was able to consume in one day. I know I did when I first saw it written down. But those were most definitely my numbers.

The sad part is that example was only a snapshot of what a typical day for me used to look like. Per my confession in Chapter 1, my daily intake was: 7,000-8,000 calories and 500-600 fat grams. How do I know that?

After failing using Intermittent Fasting with the "eat less" advice, I owned up to my daily calculations and accepted the reasons why I was not losing weight. For example, in the beginning I followed a similar pattern to what Carmen did and reduced what I was eating by half. Or at least I felt like I was eating a lot less in my eight-hour window.

The reality was, when I started tracking, my daily intake was still around 4,000 calories and 350 fat grams. Not low enough to create the calorie deficit needed for me to lose weight. Also, not low enough for me to take complete advantage of the fasting benefits of burning my stored fat as fuel. Unfortunately, I was adding more fat to be stored by still taking in excessive calories and fat grams.

This is, why I cringe when I hear someone say, "You don't need to count calories, just eat less, and you will lose weight".

To say, "just eat less," to someone, like me, whose eating had been out of control for so long, without cognitive accountable of caloric and fat grams intake, is like telling an alcoholic to just drink less. What does *less* mean?

Being told to eat less is a subjective phrase. Because depending on who is on the receiving end of those words, it can have different meanings and produce different outcomes. For you, it could be you think **you do not need to count calories**. For me, I may think **I only need to cut my portions in half**. As my eating example showed, half of 8,000 calories, was not good advice for my weight loss strategy.

It is one thing to not understand the need to combine different diets together for successful weight loss. A lot of people do not know that yet. It is a whole other situation when statements like "eat less and you don't need to count calories" are some of the biggest dieting pitfalls advice that keeps circulating. It can hinder you from being able to lose weight. By preventing you from acknowledging the importance of two key things: 1. Knowing correct portion sizes and 2. The significance of counting calories. (In Chapter 10 are Daily Body Budget Charts for calories and fat grams intake recommendations based on your weight, age, and activity level).

Most of us, when setting out on a diet, need parameters to help us help ourselves. This is another key reason why combining different diets can be beneficial for you. They can set the parameters of what, when and how much you should be eating. **I have yet to come across one diet that can answer those three key questions**.

If you are on a diet right now or if someone recommends you try one, if it cannot answer those three questions, it is time to go back to the drawing board and look for a different solution. One that can save you from frustration and being disappointed.

This is why I am excited that you are learning about the importance of using the techniques. And about why you should not set out on another dieting journey, no matter which one, only using one diet. Because unfortunately, if you do, it can be the reason why the desired weight loss results you want, will not be seen.

Side Note: Using Intermittent Fasting for weight loss has benefits beyond moving the scale. It has healing properties that can help improve your overall health. Besides aiding in reducing insulin levels and insulin resistance, it can lower, blood sugar levels, inflammation and help reduce blood pressure. As stated, fasting has no dietary restrictions; however, it does not mean calories do not count, or that the types of calories selected do not matter. For best results, combining another diet choice with fasting can help you make better food choices inside of your eating window.

By combining Intermittent Fasting with a variety of different diet eating styles, it can be your first-class ticket to better health and to reaching your weight loss goals.

In the next chapter we will talk about the importance of preparing you for the weight loss journey, mentally and physically and how by doing so, you can set yourself on a path to transform your life.

4
WEIGHT LOSS DESTINATION AND JOURNEY

My excitement for you will continue to grow, as we prepare you to start on your new journey of taking control of your health and slimming your body.

The weight loss journey is an interesting subject and one that also requires attention in order to be successful. There are so many different goals we set in our lives that have a starting and ending point. When it comes to the goal of deciding to lose weight and take control of our health, did you know it does not necessarily have an ending point? It is so important to process all the necessary steps in losing weight long-term. Because what do we do, when we get to our goal weight?

This was a big step for me to learn and accept. Weight loss is a destination and a journey. There will be no point in my life when I will be able to *not* continue the lifestyle change because I will see the weight come back. Losing weight is one part of a two-piece puzzle. Maintaining it is the other.

This is why, in the book, I provide a variety of different diet combinations you will be able to choose from, because this step is critical. Like some of the previous success stories we read about, figuring out which combinations will work best for you is going to be the key to your long-term success.

Even though you will be dieting, the combinations you choose, can be ones you can do for life. I will show you various ways they can be used and mixed and matched together. They are not going to be short-term fixes. This is not a fad diet. But rather **a recipe created for your success.**

Learning the techniques is how you will create a long-term weight loss, weight maintenance strategy. That will be specific to the things you like and prefer and will also be able to answer the three key dieting questions. I wanted to cover this key point with you because maintenance is just as important as losing weight.

Over the years when I have shared my weight loss story with people, it amazes me that I am often asked one question in particular. Matter of fact, since sharing my story through social media, I am asked this same question at least once a week. "Do you still have to work out and watch what you eat since losing the weight?"

Don't I wish that somehow my body magically does not remember my previous set weight at 304 pounds, my size 28 pants and my 44 DDD chest! You know, the obese girl who still lives inside, who would love for me to go back to my old unhealthy habits. Like devouring whole chocolate cakes, with two double cheeseburgers and a basket of French Fries so, she can take over again! (**Full Disclosure:** The *Slim Down Level Up Formulas*, work when we work. When we stop using them, the power they give us to lose and maintain weight, will also stop working. After discovering and following the formulas, I kept my weight off for over 8 years. That was until I got pregnant with my son and totally lost my mind with eating, again. In those nine months, I went up to 285 pounds! Luckily, after forgiving myself for gaining that much weight back, I knew what to do once I gave birth to him. And used the formulas to go back down to 170 pounds in 11 months).

My response is always the same: I absolutely, still have to work out and be cognitive of why, what, when and how I am eating. What I also tell them is, since my body has gotten used to my new comfortable "set weight," it is a modified version, with fewer workout days. That I continue using the *Slim Down Level Up Formulas* of combining different eating styles together, so I can maintain my weight. Also, how being exposed to a variety of different food options makes maintenance mode a lot easier and convenient.

Here is the key step to why I had to acknowledge weight loss as a *Destination and a Journey*. Because:

"IF YOU CAN GAIN WEIGHT, YOU CAN ALWAYS GAIN WEIGHT."

Let that sink in a minute. Because I do not know if you heard, from one of the other diet programs, once you reached your weight loss goal, you were done. That there would be celebrations all around. You would cross that finish line, collect your medal, and go home.

Sorry, but I will not be telling you that anywhere in this book, because being weight loss real with you is important to me. Just because you reach your goal weight does not mean your work is done. Yes, I look forward to hearing your success story of how you used the *Slim Down Level Up Formulas* and conquered the weight loss dragon in your life. Matter of fact, for additional support along the way, you can even join my Facebook weight loss support group called-Slim Down Level Up and share your testimony there. I look forward to seeing your transformation pictures. I want you to celebrate, do the happy dance and shout and sing when you reach your weight loss destination. But, when you do, try not to get so comfortable in your new weight that you forget what it took to get there. The maintenance stage requires work.

For example, there is a reason why most of the people who do extreme dieting, like on the show *The Biggest Loser,* cannot maintain their weight loss. Because the excessive and extreme measures they took to get there (extremely low-calorie diets, excessive workouts and cutting out all fun foods), is not something they can do long-term. Unfortunately, once they go back home and revert to their old eating and lifestyle habits, without a realistic maintenance strategy, the weight comes back on.

It is probably why they have not done a follow up show, like "Where Are They Now," or a Reunion Show, because most have not been able to maintain the weight they lost.

Unfortunately, the actions the contestants took to lose the weight are not rare in the world of weight loss. I think more often, than not, when people start a diet, they put extreme pressure on themselves and only focus on the number on the scale. To the point, they become obsessed and take whatever healthy or unhealthy measures to get there.

Starvation, deprivation, binging and purging, extreme exercises, laxatives, unknown potions, and excessive use of diet pills, to name a few. All while not realizing, once they do arrive at the destination, that is when the fun and games really begins. The *lifetime* journey starts.

If you have ever gone down any of those extreme paths, do not do it this time. Please do not feel the need to speed up or beat yourself up, if your journey is not going as fast as someone else's. If you put in the time and allow the power of combining different diets together to work for you, your body will make the adjustments in due time and the weight will come off.

You will not have to use any extreme measures. You can eat real food because the dieting combinations you choose will be catered to you. And it will be a technique you can do long-term. This, is why, before you start using any of the three *Slim Down Level Up Formulas* and select your diet combinations, stand in the mirror, look yourself in the eyes, and say these words out loud:

"HOW I ATTAIN IT WILL BE HOW I MAINTAIN IT."

Key Points to Acknowledge to Yourself Before Losing Weight This Time:

1. If I Can Gain Weight, I Can Always Gain Weight

2. How I Attain It Will Be How I Maintain It

Processing those two keys points is a way to look at your new way of eating and living as a *destination and a journey*. The destination is the weight loss and all the benefits that come with the changes you make. The journey will be the maintenance stage for life. By keeping this in mind, you will realize, it will be a series of marathons, not sprints.

ARE YOU READY TO WIN?

Are you ready? Figuring out if you are weight loss ready to win, before starting a diet, reminds me of the time when I used to play basketball. My old high school coach used to ask us a similar type of question prior to the team warming up.

Before each game, he would have my teammates and I huddle around him in a circle, real close, and as he spoke these words, he would look at us to see if the determination was there on our faces:

"You can have your head in the game but are you ready to win?"

Successful weight loss is about you being ready this time when you start. Not just ready, but ready to win. By the end of this book, with the additional testimonies, research, and stories of how to fight your weight loss battle, you can start with a different dieting mindset and the tools that can set you up to be victorious in this game we call life.

This may be your 1st or 121st attempt at losing weight. It does not matter. All those other times were just practice and brought you to this very moment in your life. The number of times you attempted to lose weight, but were not successful, in either reaching or maintaining your goal, does not mean you cannot start again.

Because this time, when you are ready, you can succeed.

Notice I said *when you are ready*. Because, as you are reading this book, I do not know if you are ready to start. You may not be ready for the shift. In the coming chapters, we will continue to talk about the mental and physical steps to being successful with losing and maintaining your weight.

There is a mental switch that will need to be turned on in order to prepare yourself to make daily, weekly, and monthly changes in your eating and lifestyle habits. The changes will not all happen at one time. It is not realistic to think all your previous eating and lifestyle behaviors will vanish overnight. Mine did not, it was a process. However, when the switch in your mind is turned on and you are ready, you can start heading in the direction of positively making changes. One day, one meal and one pound at a time.

You may have read a weight loss transformation story or book that tells you things like, "You can do it. Let's go. Start today!" I used to catch myself saying those same types of things to people whenever they asked me about my journey. But I have stopped doing that over the years. Because of one key reason.

I thought back to a time when I started to lose weight and was unsuccessful. Mainly, it was because my mental state was not in line with my body's plan to make a change. And I was not ready to win.

The body cannot live without the mind. If you are not mentally ready to do something, but you start it anyway, that could be the main reason why you are not successful. Especially as it relates to losing weight. I have started out on several different diets in the past and failed because my mind was not in the right place. Usually, I only started one at my doctor's urging or because one of my friends wanted a *diet buddy*.

I completely understand if, while you are reading these words right now and anticipating or entertaining starting a new diet, you are not ready. Not ready for the *shift* towards the new ways of eating and being more active. You may not be in the right mental place currently in your life. That is okay, do not get in the ring if you are not ready to fight, because losing weight is a physical and mental battle.

Wait until you are ready to make the change. When you can make the commitment to yourself. Especially, wait until after you have transitioned your mind to let go of any guilt and the shame you may be carrying. It doesn't matter how or why you got to your current size. All that matters is when you are ready to fight for your health, you will! **Most importantly, allow time, to forgive yourself for the weight gain.**

When you are ready, the tools in this book, (the *6-Week Slim Down Level Up Program* which is laid out in an easy-to-follow guide), along with the grit and determination, I know is inside of you, can and will see you through. Not only can you reach your goal, you, will have the knowledge and feel empowered to maintain and stay there for years to come. Because you ARE going to dominate losing weight!

You can never go back and undo all the times you threw in the towel and were mad at yourself for the weight gain. Or all the times you did not realize you started a diet and were missing the key piece to your weight loss tool bag, of combining different diets together.

The wonderful thing about life is, there is nothing wrong with starting over. You can look at each day as a reset and a refocus. Because it is the restart that gives us an opportunity to make each day better than the day before. You deserve to look and feel your best. To cease the opportunity of picturing a healthier and happier you, right now.

Recap: When you are ready to get started again, if you happen to stumble, learn to make it part of the dance. Remember, do not aim for perfection, aim for progress. Life is a stage. Count each one of those steps as practice for when you *will* nail the performance. Because the show will continue to go on, as long as you keep showing up each day in your own life.

Side Note: 6 key words-*Create Your Weight Loss Vision Board.* My, weight loss vision board was a big inspirational tool for me and was one of the keys to my success. Prior to getting started this time, create your vision board, and see yourself already at the weight loss finish line. Cut out, staple, tape or glue, motivational quotes, your weight loss goal and things that will make you happy. Let your board include pictures and words that will inspire you. A big part of creating the board is to love your curves exactly where they are. Write down positive words about yourself. Refer to the board throughout your journey as a positive reminder as to why you started in the first place. Set realistic goals for yourself and let *size healthy* be your motivation. The power of visualization is so important. For example, my weight loss vision board had pictures of me at my heaviest, and pictures of me not so much at my lowest weight, but included pictures of when I was smiling and happy. I also added pictures of my husband and son. Because I wanted a better quality of life to be able to spend more time with them and not be so tired all the time. And it had inspirational quotes and pictures that told me I can achieve anything and that I deserved to be happy. As do you.

By creating your weight loss vision board, you are setting the stage and creating the vision for what is to come, success. We can't be what we can't see. I have a saying, **"See It, Want It, Believe It, and You Will Achieve It."** You can and you will reach your goal this time.

In the next chapter, we will talk about how to go about setting your weight loss goal, the reasons behind the goal and how it is tied to you maintaining it, once you arrive at your destination.

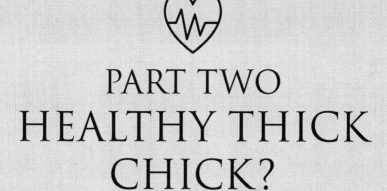

PART TWO
HEALTHY THICK CHICK?

5

WHEN THE BMI TELLS LIES

Underweight: BMI is less than 18.5	
Healthy Weight: BMI is 18.5 to 24.9	
Overweight: BMI is 25 to 29.9	
Obese: BMI is 30 or higher	

Being optimistic and having a positive attitude coupled with creating a weight loss vison board, are all wonderful things to have on your journey. What will be key is being realistic about the weight loss expectations and requirements you place on yourself. Even more important is *where* the desire to set the expectations will come from.

Your goal weight can be set, using several different factors. For instance, like looking at the numbers on the Body Mass Index Chart. However, that may not always be a good thing.

Specifically, because, the old faithful BMI Chart has been fooling us and telling lies for years. It sets the standard of what is supposed to be a healthy weight. It has also been a tool used to tell us if we fall in the overweight or obese categories. Will your goal weight be based on this chart? If so, it can cause you to set unrealistic weight loss goals for yourself. To the point, you could relentlessly try to fit in on the chart in the *right* section. Doing whatever it takes.

Questions: Have you ever strived for a weight loss goal, based on the BMI Chart, and when you reached it, you were miserable doing the things it took to stay there? You ever set an unrealistic goal to reach a certain size or number on the scale that you were years ago, and did not factor in either your current, age, stage, and lifestyle? I have, and it did not turn out well either. I'll elaborate more on that in a moment.

Just for the record, I am almost 5'10," tall and back when I was over 300 pounds, my BMI was 42. That was the number my doctor told me, and I remember it specifically, because it was my age at the time, in reverse.

Twenty-four years old with a BMI that classified me as obese. In case you didn't glance at the chart, anything over 30 is obese; I clearly had surpassed that number. That was why my doctor told me to lose 30% of my weight to improve my health and decrease my chances of being diabetic. He wanted me to aim to get down to about 205 pounds, so that my BMI would be below 30. Hearing those numbers at first made me feel like it was a mountain I would not be able to climb. It was intimidating, and on most days, I had to dig deep to find the strength to keep going. But I was determined because I wanted to start feeling better.

Luckily, at that time, I was able to reach the goal. My doctor was right, with the ninety-five pounds weight loss, my blood pressure and cholesterol dropped, and to my relief, I was not pre-diabetic anymore. I felt unstoppable and healthy. To the point I was even running in 5k and 10k races, with a goal to run in marathons one day.

With the ninety-five-pounds weight loss, I could have just focused on continuing to live a healthy lifestyle and maintained my weight. Do you think that is what happened? Of course not. I remembered what the numbers on the BMI Chart were and where I needed to be, in order to be *healthy*. So, what did I do? I completely went extreme weight loss crazy and aimed for an unrealistic weight loss goal. I went from the 205 pounds down to 143 pounds, all before I even came up for a breath. I did not even wait and check to see if my body liked my new set weight along the way. Or if I would be happy once I got down there on the scale. Wrong move on my part.

What are you going to base your weight loss goal on this time around? A chart, a certain size, or a number on the scale? **How about setting your goal based on listening to how your body feels, not what a number says?** Ever thought about that?

What happened to me when I didn't listen to my body was, I remember stressing, eating less, detoxing, and working out excessively to get the last 20 pounds off to reach that 143-pound mark (I was aiming to weigh 145-pounds). Why was I doing that to myself? At 143 pounds, my BMI would be 22, which said I was *healthy*. But I was not. I was eating very little food, and when I finally came up for air, I realized I was not happy continuing to do the things, it took to get to that low of a weight.

To get to that weight was attainable, but it was not a maintainable weight I could healthily sustain, long-term. Instead, I needed to allow my body to dictate where it was going to be the most comfortable at, which was key for me in being happy and healthy. I learned to love my curves at the set weight, where I did not have to take extreme measures to be within a certain range on the scale. Which for me is 170-180 pounds. Size 12-14, or 16 depending on the designer.

My BMI stays between 25-27, and it still classifies me as being overweight. Regardless of what the chart says, I feel the most comfortable and healthy at this weight, not the 143-pound, high school weight I unrealistically had set for myself. In reality, as an adult, I was too thin at the 143-pound mark and had the bobblehead look going on. (Seriously, my head looked so big on my thin body).

During that time one thing I learned, was instead of fighting against where my body felt the healthiest at the higher weight, I had to stop holding on to the *squeeze back in* wishful thinking that was not going to happen in my closet. I accepted the fact that I needed to go ahead and donate my smaller clothes. I was not going to be a size six or eight anymore. I did not want to be either. I had gained such a new appreciation for keeping some thickness to my curves and not having to take extreme measures to be a smaller size.

On paper, what my BMI number said about me was lying, because in real life, I was healthy. One of the weight loss health benefits I was the most, proud of was, even with being *overweight*, I was still able to reach my goal of being able to run in half and full marathons (in case you did not know, I was proud because that is 13.1 miles for half marathons and 26.2 miles for full marathons).

Later in the book, besides talking about the various ways you can utilize the power of combining different diets together, we will also discuss things like, how much should you eat to lose weight, how to dine out, meal plan and cook at home with ease. As, well as tips on preparing for special events and the holidays. All to prepare you, to dominate losing weight. However, before we can move on to those sections, there are a few important questions I want to ask you first.

When you set out on your journey, what size will make you *happy* and why will being that size make you feel good? Is it because you want to fit back into your old clothes, return to your high school weight, pre-childbirth weight, pre-marriage weight, or just a number you have in your mind that you think will make you happy?

I want to say four things to you that may be helpful, **so, you do not set out on your journey, planning a trip to get off at an exit, based on a dream destination you will not enjoy.**

1. Do not set a goal weight that is too low or unrealistic that you will have to take extreme measures to attain.

2. Recognize, once you do arrive at the weight loss destination, you may not be happy doing what it will take to stay there.

3. Understand, healthy is not a size as much as it will be about how you feel and how your vitals will have improved.

4. Make sure you will be happy with living the life you created, centered around being that size, because your, eating and activities will have to match what it took to get there.

What could happen if you do go on that trip is, you could get off at that dream exit and need to turn around and come back, because you realize it is not a healthy place for you to stay. That is basically what happened to me when I lost those 161 pounds. I drove 30 miles past my exit (30 pounds) before I realized I needed to stop and turn around. To head back to exit *healthy*.

This time around on your weight loss journey, let your body dictate what is going to be your new set weight. Your new happy weight. Not a number based on a size.

When asked next time how much weight you plan to lose, or what size are you trying to go down to, say, "Size healthy and happy." Your goal weight should be more about how you feel, not the number on a chart.

The chart can be misleading anyway, and there is more proof that there is nothing wrong with being a **"Healthy Thick Chick."** Matter of fact, more studies are showing, people with a little extra meat on their bones, who are classified as overweight, are living longer than those who are supposedly in the healthy category on the BMI Chart.

For example, in 2013, there was a meta-analysis on mortality rates, using the BMI of overweight and obese people, in comparison with those considered to be of normal weight. The results point to the fact, that we cannot let a single number on a BMI chart, or a number on a scale, dictate what size classifies what health is or what it is supposed to look like.

"We also continue to equate normal weight with good health in spite of mounting evidence that this is not true. In fact, in some studies, patients who are classified as overweight live longer than those who are a normal weight." (12)

Bam! There it is, another reason to love our curves. Being a Healthy Thick Chick is not bad at all. Even with carrying a little extra thickness, we can still live long.

Let me say this, before you think I am promoting obesity. I am not saying obesity is healthy, because it is not. I knew the health risks associated with it when I initially lost the 95 pounds.

Which was one of the main reasons why I was glad I stopped having the physical complications and I improved my health.

What I am saying is, the health reasons behind needing to lose the weight and the pressures we can put on ourselves to reach a "normal" point, on the BMI Chart can be counterproductive. Sometimes, setting unrealistic goals to lose a certain amount of weight can cause more harm than good.

Research shows when we lose large amounts of weight and gain it back, (yo-yo dieting) we are putting ourselves at a greater risk of heart disease and depression. (13) By increasing our chances of experiencing a heart attack or a stroke. In essence, we are working against ourselves when we do this. And during the process, it can make us feel like failures when we don't lose the weight or because we can't maintain the loss.

The reality is, setting an unrealistic goal weight that can cause you to yo-yo diet, could put you at risk. It could be more dangerous than if you were to just maintain a lower amount of weight loss. Even if that meant you would be classified in the same category that I am in, as a *healthy* overweight person. That would be so much better than constantly putting yourself at risk of a heart attack or stroke. Yo-yo dieting will never be your friend, and it is not good for your health, mentally or physically.

Instead of trying to reach a number on the scale, or a certain size, that will only cause you to regain some, if not all, of the weight you lost back, you can try a new technique this time. Losing weight should not be a stressful situation for you. **Stress can mess with your progress, and that is the last thing you want to do.** Stress-free, convenient weight loss is going to be your new friend.

Focus on heading in the direction of living healthier, picture it in the distance and start walking towards it. The weight will come off each day as you make better choices with your eating, as well as by lowering your stress levels and being more active.

Allow your body to speak to you regarding what number it feels its best. For example, that could mean instead of you setting a goal to lose 85 pounds, it may only need to be 60 pounds to get to a point where your body feels healthy and happy. Those 60 pounds down may help improve your overall health, help you sleep better and improve your quality of life.

With easing or removing joint pain or any other discomforts you may be experiencing from carrying the extra weight. Did you know, for every, one pound of weight we lose, we take five pounds, of pressure off the body? It's true and it can help ease so much.

In the 60 pounds weight loss example, the important thing would be to celebrate your curves and do not stress over the additional 25 pounds that you did not lose. You can work on maintaining the loss and continue making healthier choices daily. In time, your body will allow you to lose any additional weight at a pace it is comfortable with, and one you can maintain.

There is one more key point I want to make, as it relates to setting a weight loss goal and aiming to reach it. What is important is not so much about the amount of weight you lose but rather about *where* will you still be carrying the weight. Being curvy is not a bad thing. As long as you are not carrying visceral fat, which is the excessive weight coming from the belly area, you do not need to be so concerned with the scale necessarily.

The number on the scale may just be a little extra thickness in your chest, buttocks, hips, and thighs. Which are all the normal places a lot of women can have fat deposits. It is not an automatic diagnosis that says you are unhealthy due to the extra curves. Your blood work, how you feel and how your clothes are fitting, can be the other important factors you can look at. As, well as, if you are incorporating weight training into your routine, keep in mind, muscle weighs more than fat. As you continue to work out, you can increase your lean muscle mass and lose inches. This will help with slimming and sculpting your body.

The time when you should be concerned about losing additional pounds is if your waistline is thirty-five inches or more. That would mean you are at risks for additional health problems. Like heart attacks, strokes, type 2 diabetes, breast cancer, Alzheimer's disease, and colorectal cancer.

The good news is, you can take action to reduce excess belly fat and reduce your risks if you are still carrying some of the weight there. Later in the book we will talk about one of the key benefits to using Intermittent Fasting, for its effectiveness to burn up belly fat, (visceral fat) that otherwise may be difficult to lose.

Recap: When you set out to lose weight, this time, it can be more beneficial long-term, if the focus is not so much on the weight loss goal itself and which size you will be. But, rather, on your decision to start **living healthier**. If you are carrying a little, extra curves but are feeling good and are healthy, remind yourself, "My extra curves and thickness is not a sickness."

DRAW A LINE IN THE WEIGHT LOSS SAND

Now that we have talked about the importance of setting realistic goals, expectations and having stress-free weight loss, let us talk about weight loss parameters. As, well as how not to gain the weight back. This is key because I know you are going to lose the weight, and I want to prepare you for the victory dance before you start the race. Here's why:

Picture this, you use the *Slim Down Level Up Formulas*, change your eating habits, exercise, and are determined in doing what it takes to get the weight off. Family, friends, and even strangers cheer you on along the way and share in your success. After reaching your goal weight, and with the excitement of crossing the finish line, you celebrate your hard work. Now what and how do you continue to be victorious? By having a plan in place, **prior.**

I can tell you what happened to me, when I crossed the finish line without a plan of action, because that was where my regaining the weight troubles would begin. Slowly, I would slack off. My *sometimes* treat foods became more regular, my active workout schedule became less active, and in time, ten pounds crept back in on my scale.

Which would not have been a problem had I reeled it back in then. But of, course, you probably already guessed, that did not happen. The problem was those ten pounds would turn into twenty and then thirty. Before I knew it, my hard work was fading away and I was back in the 200-pound club heading towards the 300's again. Sound familiar and can you relate?

So, far, we have established that your set weight will be the number, your body feels its best and happy. Now it is important to talk about and establish a maintenance mode range ahead of time, that you will stay within, because this is directly tied to your goal weight.

Why Do You Need a Maintenance Mode Range? For the times when stress, hormones, age, vacations, or life happens, and the scale fluctuates. For example, if your body's new happy set weight is 165 pounds, you can give a range to stay between 165-175 pounds.

I gave myself a ten-pound range for my weight loss cushion. It helps me not to stress out when I weigh myself and there is a fluctuation. **I accepted the fact, there will always be a little fluctuation on the scale, and it is okay.** I realized several factors can be involved to cause the change. Stress, my time of the month, eating too many processed foods, hormones, etc.

Previously, when I did not give myself a maintenance mode range and establish it ahead of time with my goal weight, it was a main contributor to why I gained the weight back so easily. Like how I could lose 15 pounds but then turn around and gain back 25. I did not draw a line in the sand and establish my weight cap, or what to do when and if I crossed it (this same technique can also apply as you are losing weight).

I made an agreement with myself that when I did cross the range to take it as my *weight loss gut check* (no pun intended). To not make a big deal about it and, under no circumstances, to be stressed about it either. Learning to control our stress levels can be beneficial, especially while losing weight (stress releases the hormone cortisol, which in excess can cause weight gain and be counterproductive to your weight loss goals).

For me, crossing over the range just meant it was time to take care of business. I would just go back and reset my eating habits. Using the same things and techniques I used to get the weight off. By making the adjustments and corrections to my eating habits and increasing my activity levels, my body would reset back within my range. All would be well again in my weight loss maintenance world. The same technique and philosophy can be used for you as well and can be beneficial to your long-term success.

This is also why setting a realistic weight loss goal is important because it sets the stage for you to be able to allow yourself a *cushion,* that you can maintain without extreme measures.

By establishing your set range, you can make it easier on yourself with getting off ten pounds than if you let your scale continue, on to thirty pounds or more.

My best advice is, along with setting and then eventually reaching your weight loss goal, establish your set weight range. So, you can draw your line in the sand of what number you will not cross on the scale. Create a plan of action of what you will do when and if it happens. (FYI-the way the *6-Week Slim Down Level Up Program* is set up, you can always, if need be, restart at Phase 1 to reset your body back in your range).

Making this new *shift* in your life and deciding on what size healthy will look like for you, is all about preparing you for the before, during and after you reach your weight loss goal, so you can be successful long-term. These were the steps I took that allowed me to feel more in control of my eating, my weight, and my life.

If your weight loss goal involves getting out of being in the over-weight or obesity range, on the BMI Chart and to improve your health, you are on the right track. Just know, you will have the power to move the numbers on your scale and on the chart using the *Slim Down Level Up Formulas.*

In the next section, you will see a BMI Chart that is provided as a point of reference to know which category you fall in currently, based on your height and weight. (You can also use the BMI calculator on nhlbi.nih.gov for exact numbers). (14)

After the BMI Chart is a quick reference sheet on tips with weighing yourself. As well as which days are best to weigh in when losing weight. When getting started on your new weight loss journey, it is a good idea to get an accurate weigh of yourself. This will provide you a reference point, to track your progress along the way as, well as to see how far you will have come when you cross the finish line and reach your goal.

Remember, healthy is not a size, and if you decide to keep some of your curves while losing weight, I can tell you firsthand, being a Healthy Thick Chick is not a bad thing. Feeling healthy and happy is the best range you can strive to be at, on any chart or on any scale.

BMI: BODY MASS INDEX

Underweight: Your BMI is less than 18.5
Healthy Weight: Your BMI is 18.5 to 24.9
Overweight: Your BMI is 25 to 29.9
Obese: Your BMI is 30 or higher

BMI CHART

Weight (pounds)	Height (feet, inches)					
	5'0"	5'3"	5'6"	5'9"	6'0"	6'3"
140	27	25	23	21	19	18
150	29	27	24	22	20	19
160	31	28	26	24	22	20
170	33	30	28	25	23	21
180	35	32	29	27	25	23
190	37	34	31	28	26	24
200	39	36	32	30	27	25
210	41	37	34	31	29	26
220	43	39	36	33	30	28
230	45	41	37	34	31	29
240	47	43	39	36	33	30
250	49	44	40	37	34	31
	BMI	**BMI**	**BMI**	**BMI**	**BMI**	**BMI**

TIPS ON WEIGHING YOURSELF

To weigh or not to weigh, that is the question. Besides using the scale, there are other non-scale victories (NSV) you can celebrate while on your weight loss journey. Like mentioned earlier, how you feel and how your clothes are fitting. Having more energy, sleeping better, stress levels down and many more.

If you do decide to weigh yourself, here are a few tips I used that were helpful to me. The first one on the list came from a girl-friend of mine who recommended I only weigh in on Wednesdays. A great tip, because in case I had a treat day or travel day over the weekend, I could have a few days to get back on track with my eating before weighing myself. I have been doing it ever since and feel less stress stepping on the scale, since it is not the first day of the week.

1. Weigh in once- a-week: On *Wednesdays* only

2. It is recommended at the same time and always on the same day

3. The best time is first thing in the morning, before you eat or drink anything, and right after you use the bathroom

4. A naked weigh in is best or use similar clothing each time

5. Remember that the scale does not show all your body com-position, the inches you lost, neither does it show your mus-cle mass

6. Make sure your scale is on a hard-flat surface and try to weigh yourself in the same spot weekly

7. Test your scale monthly by either placing a dumb bell on it or a 5-pound bag of sugar to see if it is accurate

8. Remember that your weight can be different from morning to night or from day to day, but it is probably water reten-tion

9. As, long as, you are exercising and eating right, the benefits that you will gain will come from more than a scale

10. Remember to celebrate all NSV's as well (Non-Scale Vic-tories)

11. Be encouraged and focus on the long-term benefits of your lifestyle change and you will win and be successful

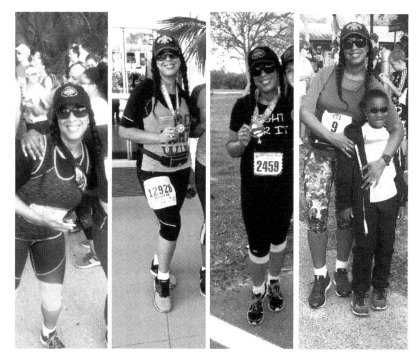

These pictures always make me proud and remind me that anything is possible. From a 300-pounder who hurt to walk, had high-
blood pressure, bad knees, and whose ankles were always sore, to
a marathon runner. Having my son at the finish line and seeing me
continue to fight for my health, by keeping my weight off and being active, is one of the best feelings in the world. In these pictures,
my weight is between 170-180 pounds. As I mentioned earlier, it is
my comfortable set weight and where I feel the healthiest (in case
you were wondering, I wear my hair in pigtails on race days for
good luck).

6

WHY WEIGHT LOSS IS NOT FOR THE WEAK

*"If losing weight was so simple, most people
would not have a weight problem."*
-Unknown

Anyone who has battled, and lost weight knows it is not an easy feat. Often you can feel like you are trapped inside your own body. Losing large amounts of weight takes lots of planning, grit, dedication, and a whole lot of mental strength.

By now, you have the basic concept of what the physical technique of combining different diets together is going to look like in the coming chapters. What about the other key pieces?

One of the other key missing pieces in successful long-term weight loss is, acknowledging and figuring out *Why* do we have a weight problem in the first place? *Why* do we eat so much? *Why* do we allow ourselves to get so out of control?

When we do not know the answers to those *Whys*, we sometimes minimize the mental strength needed for successful weight loss. Those why questions were the kind I avoided for a long time. I did not even want to entertain the thought that I had a problem and was trying to fix it with food. Asking why would have meant I needed to go within, to the core of my pain and depression.

Why Is Weight Loss Not For The Weak? Besides dealing with the frustrations of trying to figure out how to stop dieting wrong, more than not, there is an underlying reason behind the why of the weight gain. Behind the depression, the guilt and shame of being out of control. Unfortunately, I was one of those people who was walking around carrying the weight of those feelings. That, alone, took a lot of strength.

Understanding and facing the reasons *why* can be one of the key factors to taking the weight off. Getting to the heart of the why can be more difficult for some. I can tell you from past experiences, it requires looking within to see what is, the true reason behind the food. If you are anything like me, it has nothing to do with what we are putting in our bodies.

HOW IS IT NOT ABOUT THE FOOD?

A Flash Back Moment: I thought to myself, what am I doing? As I sat there on the couch, writing on the notepad that she gave me, I was not sure if I was ready to speak yet. "I want you to close your eyes, take a deep breath and release the words." She was standing in the far corner, near the window. She was my therapist, and she was speaking just loud enough that I could barely hear her.

I arrived at her office about 15 minutes early. As I sat in the waiting room, I thought of all the things I wanted to talk to her about. But for some reason, once I sat down and she began asking questions, no words came out of my mouth.

We were in the middle of the third session of a five-part series she created. It was designed to identify and get to the root of my excessive eating habits. As soon as the words left my mouth, it immediately felt uneasy to hear. **"I, am in love with food, and it has been my drug of choice for several years."**

My voice cracked a little and my hands were sweating, as I was pretending to still be writing on the notepad. I did it. I looked her right in the eye, and I said it. I was opening up to her and facing my hardcore reality, of the relationship I had developed over the years with food.

For a long time, I was in love with food. I thought food loved me back. Why wouldn't it? We had such a good thing going on for so long. At least, that was what I was telling myself when it kept giving me the love I needed.

At times, it felt like I was in a twisted abusive relationship with food. A relationship I could not walk away from. It had a hold on me. The kind I heard people talk about when they were addicted to someone or something.

I wanted out of the food relationship I was in. It was why I was in therapy. But what was out? And how would I get there? Unlike other drug addictions, food is not one I could just detox, delete, or completely remove myself from to escape. I could not just go cold turkey and wake up one morning and say I am not going to eat anymore. I did not know how I was going to get out of such an addiction. That was until, in therapy, I realized something. **Weight loss is a beast, and the battle to win starts within.**

I was still sitting on my therapist's couch. She had gotten up by now and walked closer to the window. "I need you to take a deep breath. And try to calm yourself down as much as you can." Her voice was low and calming, and she never spoke fast. Every word was with great intention and purpose. She had already started in with her next round of questions, and I started to cry. To the point I could not initially speak.

"Why do you think you keep gaining all the weight? And why do you want to lose the weight this time?"

I was not crying because the questions were not fair game. They were. We had spent weeks talking about the importance of getting to the core of my emotional eating state. But I was not ready to talk about it yet. I knew when I was ready, it would make sense to the pain and the emptiness I often felt.

You ever just start crying and not know why? Or have you ever just started feeling such a tightness in your chest, a lump in your throat and an empty feeling in your core? But did not know where it was coming from? Ever start binge eating to the point you vomit? And then feel so guilty for the next several days. And instead of making better choices moving forward, you eat even more, thinking it will make you feel better.

What if you figured out, the why behind those types of feelings and actions could be one of the key ingredients to losing weight for good? And even if you knew it might hurt a little and feel uncomfortable at first, would you want to find out your why?

My therapist had been trying for weeks to get me to do just that, identity my why. Because my primary physician, besides telling me to lose weight, recommended I talk with someone. To try and help me deal with the emotional part of being obese. So I could unlock what had been holding me back for years and causing me to struggle with my weight.

For some of us, we have gone several years to where we have pushed our why feelings to the side. Blocked them out, started another diet and pretended they were not there. Knowing good and well that what we were dealing with and avoiding on a regular had nothing to do with the food we were eating.

The food was just the effect of the cause. And because we often refused to deal with our emotions, the effect was we excessively ate.

"It is a psychological defense mechanism we use to protect ourselves from past traumas." That is how my therapist explained to me why I was not ready to discuss the heart of my why with her.

She said most people who suffered trauma normally embrace the "Soldier On" mentality. Which a lot of us could have adopted in our childhood. As a way not to deal with pain. Instead of dealing with our emotions, we would muscle up the strength to keep going and mask it with food.

After a couple more questions from her, I completed my session that day and went home and baked a chocolate cake.

SLIM DOWN LEVEL UP

Later that night, I thought back to her questions, and I was proud of myself for answering most of them. Even though I struggled, and it felt uncomfortable, it needed to happen. At that time, I couldn't answer all her questions, because I was still in search of and trying to understand my *why*.

CHOOSE YOUR HARD

Encountering struggles and figuring out how to overcome obstacles is a basic part of life for us. We have all faced different challenges at specific times throughout our weight loss journey. But if you have wrestled with your weight long-term, I discovered something I want to share with you. Sister to sister, woman to woman, girlfriend to girlfriend. A significant part of our weight loss problems is directly tied to us not wanting to address the triple **WHY** in the room. (Trust me, it can be ten times bigger than addressing the elephant in the room).

Before we get into understanding specifically how the *Slim Down Level Up Formulas* can work for you, let's talk about and unpack this **WHY**. Because I really want to see you win. No matter how many times you have failed at losing weight, I want you to be able to make the rest of your life, the best of your life. In order to do that, we need to first look at the triple **WHY**. Especially before you start another diet, so your overall success can be increased. Granted, you probably started your last diet without knowing the power of combining different eating styles together. But if you think you failed last time at losing or gaining weight because your only problem was with the diet food, or that you lacked discipline, you are sorely mistaken.

It could have been you fell down because you were dealing with personal issues with family or friends. Or you were dealing with pressures from work. Got frustrated and started hurting again. When that happened, your stress levels rose, and your insulin levels followed. You returned to what was comforting and familiar, *food*. Which made it easier for the weight to come back on and stay on.

How Do I Know This? Because that is what happened to me, more times than I can count. When it did, it was depressing and demoralizing, and it kept moving the number on my scale higher.

For many years, the pain I felt, the bottomless hole I was trying to fill and the healing I needed, was *not* coming from the food. Even though I thought it was.

The only thing that was happening was, I kept eating, kept increasing my insulin levels, and my set weight kept going higher. No matter how much I ate, I still never felt that good feeling I was in search of. I was sinking deeper into the obesity prison I had built.

Sound familiar? If so, just know we are not alone. Because most people eat and gain weight because of one or more of the **3 H's:**

1. We turn to food when we are: **Hungry**

2. We turn to food out of: **Habit**

3. We turn to food when we are: **Hurting**

Unfortunately for me over the years, and for several of us, number 2 and 3 are usually why we eat so much. We often struggle while losing weight because we are unaware of the direct connection, of the **3 H's** to the understanding of our *why* we keep regaining the weight back. Most of us do not know why we eat when we are hurting or why we keep eating out of habit. But it is linked, to our triple ***WHY,*** *in more ways than one.*

The FIRST WHY: **WHY do you think you eat so much?**

The SECOND WHY: **WHY do you think you have a weight problem?**

The THIRD WHY: **WHY do you want to lose weight?**

Answering, understanding, and processing the first two WHYs plays a huge role in the success, of how the third WHY will do long-term. Because the reasons behind wanting to lose the weight (to feel better, look better, etc.) will not matter, if the first two Whys are not identified and addressed. You may want to pause and read that again. Because it is a very powerful piece in the weight loss equation. This is why I want to talk about this before we go any further. If you have not yet identified *why* you turn to food and *why* your weight is probably connected to years of pain, guilt, and shame, your weight loss struggles can be a constant issue in your life. And no matter which diet you start, if it is not addressed, it can rear its ugliness when you least expect it. Showing up to sabotage your weight loss goals. Let's dive in a little more.

OUT OF ORDER

"How did you do it? What did you do? What is your secret?" We probably have asked similar questions when seeing someone who has lost a lot of weight. Hoping the answers could make our weight loss journey easier. Sometimes weight loss can be harder for us because the sequence of the questions we ask are out of order.

For example, while writing this book, and searching for additional success stories to use, I received several fitness related questions and messages. Most of them were from people on social media in response to my weight loss posts.

The number one question I was usually asked was, "How did you lose the weight?" The problem with me responding right away to the question was, they were starting out asking the wrong thing. When I would respond by asking a specific question, I sometimes received some push back. Or hesitation from them at first. Because most wanted me to immediately give them the *How* of my weight loss. How often did I eat? How did I exercise? How hard was it to lose the weight? How long did it take?

But instead of how did I lose the weight, I wished the first question would have been, "Why did you want to lose the weight?" Because that was the question, I asked them and wanted to know. I knew it would be the foundation to their weight loss success.

If we remain more focused on the how steps to losing weight, we will completely miss:

We cannot get to the "HOW" to lose weight until we know the "WHY."

I have discovered weight loss can be made easier or harder based on the reasons behind the *why* of the weight. Are you setting out to lose weight this time because you want to look better, feel better or for medical reasons? Most of us want to improve our health and look and feel our best. Those are all valid responses to want to get started on a diet.

However, if you do not get to and answer the questions of the "whys", the hard road you keep going down, no matter the diet, will only continue getting harder. Because you can start losing weight using the right techniques, but if something painful resurfaces from your past that has gone unresolved, it can derail the whole journey. In the process, you could potentially start packing back on the pounds, increasing your stress levels, and feeling disappointed in yourself, again.

For example, before my *awakening*, every diet I ever started was without me knowing **my why.** More importantly, *why* it was contributing to me being out of control with my eating. Instead of me starting with my why I was eating so much, and why did I have a weight problem, I ended with seeing several of the reasons *why* I failed. It came out in one of my therapy sessions.

Here are the questions my therapist asked me and the answers to why I kept throwing in the towel.

Why did you quit? It was too hard, and I got bored with the food choices.

Why didn't it work? I was stressed out and tempted by family and friends.

Why didn't you try something else? I was busy.

Why don't you want to start again? Because I feel like a failure.

Why didn't you prepare better? I thought I did.

Why didn't you have a support system? I do not know, but I did not ask anyone for help.

Why didn't you learn about better food choices? I only learned a few.

Why didn't you look for new recipes to try? Takeout was easier and tasted better.

Why didn't you want to exercise? It was hard and not fun.

Why did you stop believing in yourself? Because the weight started coming back.

Why did you use food when you were hurting? Because it numbs the pain and makes me feel better.

Answering and diving into the last question really pushed me to find solutions to stop yo-yo dieting. And to stop from easily quitting when I started hurting while losing weight.

I realized I could not move forward successfully until I paused and went back to see why I kept emotionally regaining weight.

When I said that last sentence to myself out loud, it was an aha moment. I spent several years looking for *physical solutions* to losing weight. Desperately searching for answers to why the diets were failing me. All the while, I completely missed the emotional part of why I kept regaining the weight. I would start one diet after another, not even realizing I needed to find the answers to my emotional *Why's*, of my weight.

Can you relate? If so, take another look at the why questions my therapist asked me. Spend some time asking yourself the same ones. Be honest and open to your answers. As I said, I want to see you win. Going within and facing your **Whys**, can be a major step in you making that happen. After answering the eleven questions, allow yourself time to process them *prior* to starting on this program. So that you do not fix one problem, (with bettering your health with dieting), but swap your why behaviors for another.

SWAPPING ADDICTIONS?

> *"The problem with removing one bad behavior, is*
> *you can unearth another."*
> *-Unknown*

A Flash Back Moment: "You seriously need help. I mean, who does this? Three?" She did not look at me when she said it, but her voice made me realize she was concerned. She kept rolling her eyes and kept looking back at me over her shoulder.

She was my beautiful, tall, thin, older sister. She had only been there for about twenty minutes but had already started in on judging me again. That was because she never had a weight problem. She would never understand my newly found obsession was just me enjoying my new life.

She had come over to my house to help me with reorganizing my closet. And of course, pick out a few items for herself. It was the first time since we were kids that we could wear the same size clothes. A big part of it was due to me losing so much weight. But she also was pregnant at the time and could use some of my size 8's as maternity wear. She needed something cute to put on because we were going to lunch later that day.

One by one, she kept pulling out several items and laid them on the leopard print, high-heel chair placed in the far-right corner. "You know these are the same dresses, right? And you definitely need help, because they all still have the tags on them!"

I remember how it all started. While I was losing the 161 pounds, multiple holidays, birthdays, and special events happened during the 15 months, it took me to lose the weight. During that time, my family and friends wanted to give me gifts. But instead of wasting money on things I would not need after reaching my goal weight, I asked for gift cards instead. Knowing I would be able to use the cards at, a later date, I stashed them away. Because I would eventually need a complete wardrobe for my new body. Going from a size 28 to an 8 would require all new undergarments, dresses, tops, pants, belts and even socks.

While losing the weight, I was so proud of myself. Because my issues with being addicted to food were gone. But by the time I had reached my goal weight, it was too late to stop my new issues. I could have not predicted what was about to happen in a span of just eight months. A jammed packed master bedroom closet, a guest bedroom turned into a walk-in closet and two spare closets later, I had let go of my food addiction and found my new love, shopping.

Back then, I did not even know it was possible to swap a food addiction for another. I wish I had known. Especially before I first set out to truly lose the weight. Because knowing could have kept me from being thousands of dollars in debt and from having multiple closets stacked with tons of clothes, shoes, and purses. Most of which I would never even use.

When I first started losing weight, I thought I was cured of my addiction. Because food *used* to be my problem. I convinced myself I was in complete control of my issues with excessive behaviors. Or at least, I thought I was. After a couple more conversations with my sister and seeing all the maxed-out credit card statements, I got control of my excessive shopping. But then I started excessively drinking, then the eating started again.

You see, the weight is not about the weight. The shopping is not about the shopping. Excessive drinking is not about the drinking. Do you see a pattern here? Addictions are tied back to the why. And contrary to what I thought, I did not completely address the triple **Why** before I started losing the weight. I would need to continue getting to the root of the problem to stop myself from the excessive behaviors. I do not know if swapping addictions has happened to you or someone you know. I hope it has not, because it can cause so many unforeseen problems. Sis, when it comes to losing weight, it is important not to start fixing one problem, without acknowledging that by doing so, another one could take its place.

If you need professional help to get complete control of it, like I eventually did, just know it does not make you weak. I believe in therapy and will always be a mental health advocate. As women, we carry so much on our shoulders. The importance of our mental well-being is the foundation for us to be successful at anything in life. In fact, talking with someone can make you stronger in the end. **It can be the start of a new beginning, without carrying the pains from the past.**

Recap: I can tell you firsthand, swapping addictions is real. If we do not address the core reasons of *why* we have a weight problem in the first place, addictions can remain. The pain can linger, and the emotional hurt can turn into something far greater than we can imagine.

Why Ask and Answer the *Why* Questions? Because we cannot fix what we do not know is broken. Sometimes we failed at dieting because we did not circle back and evaluate, WHY. If we did, we could have made changes and adjustments. Not just to the diet philosophy itself, but to the reasons why we were trying to make it work for us in the first place.

JOURNAL SESSION: Here are four *Why* questions that can be helpful going forward. Write your answers down and then say them out loud to yourself. I ask you to do this technique because this is why therapy is so powerful and is such a great tool to use.

When we speak to a therapist, it is not about them having all the answers. Rather, it is about us seeing our words and hearing our own thoughts out loud. Often for the first time.

QUESTIONS TO ANSWER BEFORE STARTING ANOTHER DIET

1. Why do you want to lose weight?

_____

_____

_____

_____

_____

_____

2. Why do you think you struggle with your weight?

_____

_____

_____

_____

_____

_____

3. Why were you unsuccessful on the previous diets? (Name at least three reasons)

_____

_____

_____

_____

_____

_____

4. Why do you think you turn to food when hurting and/or out of habit?

_____

_____

_____

_____

_____

_____

7

YOU DON'T HAVE A WEIGHT PROBLEM

*"That's right, it's time to change the narrative because
I do not like how I'm being seen!"*
-Unknown

Flash **Back Moment:** "Sign here and here and initial next to the four bullet points." As he handed me the clipboard through the little sliding window, I quickly filled out the paperwork. His words sounded robotic, as though he had said them, thousands of times before.

He was the jet ski attendant on duty that day on the beach. His demeanor and attitude seemed as if he wanted to be anywhere but working. Without even looking at me, he handed me the key and two life vests and asked, "How long will you be out today?" I was not sure. I was waiting on my husband to lock up our personal items in the lockers provided, while I checked us in.

Earlier that morning, he called the hotel's concierge desk to find out what time the rental shack would be open. So we could rent a jet ski for a couple of hours.

We had snuck away for a couple's weekend at the beach. Our son and the dogs were at home with the babysitter, and we wanted to spend some quality time together. I would have been fine just lying on the beach sipping on a cocktail, but my husband wanted to go jet skiing before having lunch and lounging by the hotel pool. I begrudgingly agreed to go. It had been so long since I was on a jet ski, and I feared I would not even be able to climb up on it because I was still carrying most of my pregnancy weight.

I stepped to the side to finish filling out my liability paperwork. Just as I was turning around to look for my husband, a young couple walked up and said hello. They were wearing life vests, dark sunglasses and what looked like two layers of sun block on their faces. They were giggling and talking about who was going to be the fastest driver. They handed the attendant their paperwork and headed down to his co-worker, who was standing in the water. He helped the two of them hop on the jet ski, and I watched them quickly drive off.

Finally, after a few more minutes, my husband walks up. "We good to go?" he asked me as I handed him his life vest and the key. After securing my vest, I started walking towards the other attendant who was standing next to the jet ski in the water. Before I could tell my husband, he could drive first, I was stopped in my tracks. "Oh! Wait, we have a problem. You both cannot ride on *one*. You need to rent one each. Unless you want to swim the whole time?"

What? I was confused. I had just watched the other couple take off on the same type of jet ski together, so I did not understand why we could not do the same.

He said, **"There is a weight problem, because the capacity is 450 pounds max.** So, unless you both want to keep swimming the whole time by constantly flipping the jet ski over, I'd recommend you rent two."

I looked at husband, who by now had already started walking back towards the rental shack. He knew he better quickly pay for the additional jet ski before I said I did not want to go anymore. I felt mortified. Especially because of the way the attendant looked at me.

Clearly, we were over the weight maximum. I knew it. And I did not need a calculator to quickly figure out the math. At the time, my husband was about 280 pounds, and I weighed 265 pounds. And to hear those words and know we were too big to ride together put a damper on the afternoon for me.

All I wanted to do was go lay on the beach, eat chicken wings and fries and drink countless cocktails. Which I did, soon after getting back from our hour-long ride.

We checked out of the hotel the next day, and on the drive home, I could not help but keep replaying the scene in my head at the beach. How the attendant and his co-worker kept staring at us as we drove off on the two jet skis. They were smirking.

I felt that once again, my struggles with my weight was the problem. Stopping me from enjoying activities in the same manner as someone of a smaller size would have.

I never said anything about it to my husband, but in the back of my mind, I was going to prove those jet ski attendants wrong. I did not have a weight problem because I was going to do something about my weight.

"Don't fat people know they are fat? And why won't they do something about it?" Of course, I knew I was fat. But I did not see it like a non-fat person may have seen it. I, surely, did not need the jet ski attendant whispering to his co-worker those questions to remind me of the fact. I especially didn't want to hear it that day.

Comments like that always made me mad. Mainly, because I was still in denial about my weight. I knew when my clothes were getting a little tighter and started to not fit me. But in my mind, the dryer had shrunk them. Or the dry cleaners used a special shrinking liquid (Please tell me, I am not alone, because seriously, I used to tell myself those things).

For a long time, I was mad that I had to buy bigger clothes. That I was only able to shop for them in a limited amount of stores. Matter of fact, I had a hard time finding something to wear for our trip. Which made me even more mad, that when I did go shopping,

I was subject to pay the **fat tax** that comes from retailers unjustifiably charging more money for plus-size clothing, *claiming* because it takes more material (I will tell you more about that in a moment).

I was mad at the way people stared at me in disgust when I ate at an all-you-can eat buffet. As I would head back to my table carrying multiple plates piled high with excessive food. I was also mad at all those times I had to *casually* check the strength of a chair before sitting down. To make sure it could hold me. Please tell me I am not alone on this one, either. I had broken one before and never wanted it to happen again. I spent a lot of time mad that I was the root cause of all my anger and frustration with my weight.

FAT TAX SIDE NOTE: If you have ever purchased plus-size clothing that was more than the standard sizes on the racks, I have something you may want to hear. You were subject to and paid the *Fat Tax*. It is another form of how industries profit off of us being overweight. As if it is a penalty fee for not fitting into the standard sizes. Let me explain.

For instance, in 2014, the retailer Old Navy came under fire for charging anywhere from $10-$15 more for a woman's plus-size pair of jeans, compared to the same jeans in standard sizes.

The argument was that the jeans required more material and it had *curve-enhancing* elements. A spokesperson from the company at the time, to justify the added cost, said, "This higher price point reflects this selection of unique fabrics and design elements." (15)

Questions: If a size 4 is bigger than a size 2, and a size 12 is bigger than a size 8, why do they cost the same? The size 12 uses more material and is designed for a curvier woman than the size 4. Yet they cost the same price. Why? Unless Old Navy was doing something different back then, compared to manufacturing clothing industry standards, their reasoning was not a viable excuse. Definitely not one that was worth charging that much more for the same type of jeans.

How do I know? I have the inside scoop in the world of manufacturing. Let me tell you how it came about, because it was out of necessity and years of being frustrated.

You ever dread when swimwear season would come around, hoping some new design would be available with better coverage that did not involve wearing a moo-moo? I did, specifically for the times when I felt insecure and wanted to feel less exposed. I stopped torturing myself waiting on the swimwear industry to finally design something new. Because I wanted swimwear that shaped and slimmed my stomach, hips, waist, legs, and thighs. I took matters into my own hands and decided to stop paying my hard-earned money on a swimsuit to only pay more money to buy a cover up. Especially since most of the swimsuits were working against my curves, rather than with them.

So, that is exactly what I did. I put pen to paper and started designing swimwear. In the process of working with manufactures to bring my creations to life, I learned the inside scoop. **The fat tax is not justifiable.**

When it comes to sizing and materials, there is an expected norm designers follow. Once you have decided on your designs and how many different sizes you want to make them in, it is a matter of grading the sizes up or down to fit into the desired measurements (Size 4 measurements are graded up to a size 6, size 6 measurements are graded up to a size 8, etc.).

That means the size 8 and the size 14 would be made with the same fabrics, using the same design. The only difference, if any may be, to add a higher waistband or thicker elastic to the larger sizes. The curve-enhancing elements they were referring to, is the added measurements (grading) from size to size that would be adjusted. Not an added cost to make the larger sizes, per se, because remember a size 8 uses more fabric than a size 4, yet they are charging the same price.

Imagine my surprise, when I was already mad from years prior, with being forced to pay extra for plus-size clothing for *more* material. Then to find out, it was not so much about more fabric being needed, or additional design enhancing elements. The additional plus-sizes could have been easily requested by the retailers and could have been done using the same techniques the other sizes were already being graded up from. The way it is typically done is by adding the additional measurements above the standard four to five sizes they usually make (XS, S, M, L, XL).

Knowing what I know, with Old Navy's situation, there could have possibly been an added cost if they were ordering smaller quantities of the plus-sizes. Which technically can make their cost per garment be slightly higher (However, it was very interesting how their men's plus-size clothing did not suffer the same fat tax as their women's collection).

I can tell you, once I realized how, garments are made and how the manufacturing process works, I thought back to all the times when I paid the *fat tax* for clothes. I have completely started looking at shopping differently. Causing me to compare items to see if I am being charged more, for being in the higher sizes. As you probably will now, after reading this.

The reality is, more industries, especially in the fashion world, need to understand being a plus-size woman should not come with a penalty fee. **The time has come for them to stop trying to body shame us into being a size we are not the healthiest at. Which can force us to diet excessively.** All to try and shove ourselves into fitting into the standard sizes of clothing (between a size 2 to size 12). Instead, they can get together as an industry and collectively start making the clothes to fit our curves. Include the plus-sizes in the standard grading system and stop charging more for being curvier.

Our curves are not going anywhere (just for the record sis, I am not hating on standard size women, as it is not their fault that manufacturers do not include the other sizes in what is considered standard sizes).

In the United States, almost 70% of women are in the category of being considered plus-size, which would be sizes 14-34. (16) We are not standard sizes, but that does not mean we are not worthy and should pay a *fat tax,* or struggle to find clothing because we are not smaller.

Whatever your weight loss goal is, I hope you do not aim to fit in one of the standard sizes just to say you fit into a standard size.

As discussed earlier, in chapter 5, allow your body to dictate where it will be the healthiest and the happiest. Even if that still puts you in the category of being plus-size (luckily in the past few years, more designers and retailers have started to provide a better variety of plus-size clothing to choose from, without the added fat tax).

CHANGE THE NARRATIVE OF THE WEIGHT

When I was mad the jet ski attendants spelled out, my weight was preventing me from experiencing life, as a non-fat person would, it hit me. I did not like how it felt. I thought when they looked at me, all they saw was the weight and me as a fat woman who *clearly* was in love with food more than herself. Someone who ate excessively and was out of control.

Subconsciously, what I blamed to be their degrading thoughts were some of my own. Unfortunately for me, those thoughts would play in my head on constant repeat. Especially whenever I felt ashamed of my weight.

Have you ever felt like this? That you identified with what you thought someone else's negative opinions of your weight were? That their thoughts became your thoughts? If so, it is not a good feeling to walk around carrying on the inside. That type of pain can fester. And often does not go away.

For instance, when the jet ski incident occurred, my desire to *prove* the attendant and his co-worker wrong was not about them. It was more about my own body shame and insecurities. The main problem was I needed to stop self-identifying with the negative words attached to the weight. They were toxic.

Things like, "You're humongous, disgusting, not normal size, too big to fit in anything in this store, you eat too much, do not sit there, I don't think the chair can hold you." Over the years, some of those words I heard, the others I felt.

When you look in the mirror, do you see the weight? Is that all you see, and do you identify with it, too? Is it to the point, that it's hard for you to picture yourself outside of the

weight? Because you think the weight is the problem. Like it was a jail sentence handed down to you after you were convicted of a crime. As though you were forced to serve your time and pay the penalties and consequences for your actions.

The problem is not the weight. The problem is how we keep letting the weight define who we are.

Questions: Did you, as you got heavier, look up and realize you allowed the weight to be front and center in your story? That all, of a sudden, it had the starring role to how you were experiencing life? Did it dictate what you would do and wouldn't do based on your size? And did it also have your voice, as though it was speaking to and for you? But you did not like what it kept saying.

It happened to me, and I did not like it at all because of how the weight had so much control over the scenes that would play out in my head and in real life. It felt like with each pound, the self-sabotaging thoughts and actions were mounting.

What bothered me the most was, over a period, of time, I realized how easily my weight and food addiction could make me irritated or mad about the smallest of things.

For instance, there was a time when the grocery store, I always shopped at stopped selling my favorite ice cream. What did I do? I had a full-blown complete meltdown in the freezer section. I even went up to the customer service desk and demanded they send someone to help me search.

I frantically walked back to the freezer aisle. Opened and looked inside each of the ice cream doors, as though it was not really happening. All while, the store manager watched in disbelief (seriously, I am not proud of that moment, but it really did happen). It was an example of how I allowed my food addiction and weight to continue running the show, and it wasn't a pretty scene.

That's why after some much needed soul searching, **I decided to change my thinking and it changed my life. I was no longer going to let my weight define who I was anymore. I was going to change the narrative.**

If your weight has been the star of the show in your life for too long, it is time for you to change the narrative. The negative, self-sabotaging character in your story needs to go. A new, more positive way of thinking and feeling can take its place. With you in the starring role.

In the process, you can take back your power of who you are. You can speak truth to power, *"Who you are has nothing to do with your weight."*

The weight you gained is real. It is a part of you. But going forward, you can *decide* you will no longer allow it to define you. You get to decide how you want to feel and how you want to show up in the world. The size of your hips, waist, legs, and thighs, should not be allowed to dictate your role.

I do not know how you may feel at this point in your life, but I want to tell you something.

When you look in the mirror next time, regardless of what anybody else thinks, your weight is not your identity. It does not show the beauty of your character, the strength of your heart and how amazing you are!

It is time to transition out and change the narrative of the weight. Your weight is not who you are. Your weight is the result of a combination of food and lifestyle decisions you made over several years. It does not get to introduce you or tell people who you are anymore.

How Do You Make the Transition?

1. *Decide* you will no longer be mad at your current weight. Because you know you can change that when you are *ready*.

2. *Decide* to no longer believe the negative thoughts or words used to describe your body. Because you know you are more than what meets the eye.

3. *Decide* to take the leading role in your story and fire the old character. Because they will no longer be allowed to speak for you.

FALLING DOWN IS NOT FAILING

Transitioning away from identifying with the negative cognitions is a key step on your weight loss journey. Developing a positive mindset to looking at being successful at dieting is another. It is about believing you can achieve your goals.

Our unconscious ability to feel overwhelmed with the failures of our past can derail our futures. Being obese, unhealthy, and with feelings of unworthiness can affect our mental state in ways we may not have realized.

For instance, when dealing with excessive weight, we, as women, can wrestle with mixed emotions. On one hand, we are constantly told through women empowerment, groups, magazines, and blogs to love ourselves. To feel beautiful at any size.

We see beautiful plus-size women "living their best life" online and in the news. They encourage us to celebrate and embrace our *curves*. But, on the other hand, on several days and in certain situations, we feel anything but worthy of a celebration. In fact, some of us feel as if we quit on ourselves, long ago, for not being able to get the weight off. The daily mental battle that goes on in our heads can be relentless.

Have you ever felt like this? If so, it is time for a change and to stop the mental self-sabotage from occurring. Because the weight will continue to try and make you feel empty, overwhelmed, defeated, and as a failure, if you allow it. As though you let everyone, including yourself, down. As though you will always fail at losing weight. The time has come to stop allowing that to happen. It is time to start believing in yourself again.

If you don't, your mind will try to continue playing tricks on you, to keep driving down obesity highway. Claiming you are not worthy to be healthy and happy. Making you feel your weight loss failures happened because you were not strong enough or good enough. It will work to convince you that there is no need to try another diet again, because you will not win. Whispering that when you do start dieting again, you will lose some weight, but your fate is inevitable. You will fail as you always have.

Those voices in your head that keep telling you, you cannot do it and you are a failure, they are lying! It does not matter that you were not successful in losing weight before. You can take control and fight for your health, now, with another battle, and fight another round.

How? **You can learn to master the S.T.A.R.** What does that mean? You ever wonder why, during an interview for a job, they ask you thought provoking questions? Like, "Tell me about a time when you encountered a situation at work with an employee, what happened and how did you handle it?" I can tell exactly why. One of my degrees is in Human Resources, and I spent several years as a recruiter while working on my masters. I spent hours going cross-eyed reviewing thousands of resumes and interviewing countless applicants. They are not asking you those questions just to get a better feel for your personality, per se. They are looking for a very specific thing. And if you cannot provide it, they usually do not hire you.

They're asking those questions because their main thought is, "Your past performance can dictate your future success." They are looking for you to complete the S.T.A.R to become the star and show them you can do the job.

Let me explain. They are looking for the: **S**ituation, **T**ask, **A**ctions, **R**esults of your past performances. If, while asking you those questions, you do not explain the four steps of the star, or if the results you took were not successful, their assumption is you do not have what it takes to succeed in the position.

Here is the thing, that past performance statement, does not, and will not dictate your future weight loss success because you are going to master the S.T.A.R. Watch how you can apply this same technique to almost any situation you face in life.

What is the **S**ituation? You have a weight problem. What is the **T**ask needed to take care of the situation? You need to figure out a way to lose weight. What are the **A**ctions you will take to get there? You will start a diet, make changes in your eating, and start being more active. What will be the **R**esults of those actions when you do? Weight loss! Done; the *star* is completed, and your results this time, will be different than any other time before.

Starting today, it is time to push aside any negative thoughts of you not being able to succeed because of the of times you failed in the past. Those thoughts need to go away. They are not allowed to live in your head space anymore. Kick them out! And on the days when you are struggling on your weight loss journey, and they think they can come back, you tell them, "Not today, negativity and doubt! Matter of fact, not tomorrow either or the rest of my life, because I am going to *dominate* losing weight and win this time."

You are going to get out of your own way and start be-lieving in yourself again. You are not going to fail anymore. Because, contrary to what you may think, falling down is not failing.

If you are not dieting right now, do not look at it as a bad thing, that you haven't started yet. Just call this, "The between time and in the meantime" phase of your weight loss plan. The journey will continue. Your past will not dictate your future success. As long as you get up and decide to go another round, you can win the battle. Winning is about not giving up. Even if you stayed down longer than any other time before, you can still get up and work on com-pleting the S.T.A.R. by getting started again.

Side Note: When you do start, try not to focus on your success being about how disciplined you will be. I often hear how people think they either failed or succeeded at something, because of dis-cipline or lack thereof. Your power can be in realizing, discipline can get you in the ring to start the weight loss fight. However, it will be your *determination* to win, that will keep you standing up in the ring and punching like your life depends on it. (In some situa-tions, as it was in mine, people diet not just to lose weight, but to fight for better health and their lives).

Recap: Falling down is not failing. Keep telling yourself that. Block out the negative voices in your head and hit the diet reset button. Do not beat yourself up for letting the weight gain happen in the first place. Forgive yourself for getting to this point in the weight loss journey (when I forgave myself, it was so powerful. It allowed me to lose weight guilt-free).

Most importantly, instead of being mad or disappointed in yourself, stand in the mirror and say, "I love you just as you are. I believe in you. I love you enough to want to start getting healthy again."

This time, your success is not about discipline or lack thereof, nor is it about your past performance. You can perform successfully. You have discipline and have used it in the past to reach other goals. Your weight loss discipline will get you to start the diet this time and show up for the race. However, make no mistake about it, it will be your *determination* that will get you to the finish line. Your determination trumps discipline, and it will be the same determination to win, that will see you through.

Remind Yourself Daily of These 3 Key Declarations:

One: I have made the decision in my mind to fight for myself and will hit the wall and come out swinging.

Two: I deserve to feel better, to lose the weight and to embrace my beauty, right now, even at the size I currently am.

Three: I am enough! I know enough, and I can do more than enough to make the rest of my life be the best of my life.

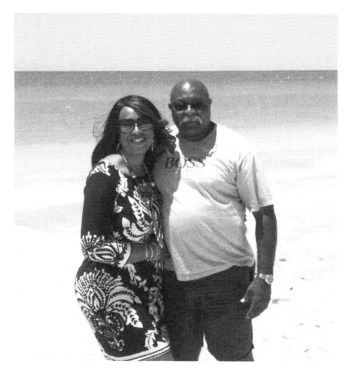

This is a picture of my husband and I the weekend the jet-ski innocent occurred. It was taken the day we arrived. As, you can see, I am all smiles. It was the first getaway after the birth of our son. And I remember being excited for the mini vacation. That was until the next day. You probably can see from the looks of it why we couldn't fit on the one machine and were over the weight capacity. Eventually, I got back in the ring, took control of my eating again, fought for my health and won. **It's Your Turn Next.**

In the upcoming chapter, we will talk about the role *the food* will play on your journey and how having access to a variety of options that are convenient and taste good, can be essential in helping you reach your goal weight.

PART THREE
THE WEIGHT
LOSS TOOL BAG

8

THE ULTIMATE DIET REMIXX

When you set out to lose large amounts of weight, it is going to take some time. For me, it took the fifteen months. For you, it could be months or even over a year before you reach your goal weight. *Food* is going to be important along the way.

Have you ever gone back to your old unhealthy eating habits while dieting because the food started all tasting the same? Bland and boring? I have been guilty of doing that in the past. Several times. I would lose interest in the food and find myself standing back up in my kitchen cooking everything in bacon grease, deep fried in vegetable oil and using heavy creams in my side dishes. Or I would constantly resort to getting fast food or takeout again.

A Boss, Vegan, Keto, Low Calorie, Weight Watchers, Intermittent Fasting, Mediterranean, Diva! You probably wondered when I mentioned earlier in the book about combining six different diets together to lose my weight, why did I use so many? Was it that I could not make up my mind?

No, that wasn't it. The main reason I experimented and tried so many was because I love to eat. Dieting did not change that, and no matter what size I am, I will always be a foodie. I did not, want to get bored with the food. Because I knew if I did, it would only be a matter of time before I would go back to my unhealthy cooking and eating habits permanently. The same habits that had gotten me to over 300 pounds.

So, instead, I made it my mission to find a good mixture of different food and recipe options to choose from. Especially, recipes and food I could enjoy cooking and eating.

After I cracked the diet code philosophy and created my own team, Team Diet Remixx, I used the different foods to my advantage. I discovered within some of the diets, there were food options that were delicious, low-calorie, low-carb, plant-based, and made losing weight more convenient.

At first, I was hesitant with using some of the diets because of what I had heard in the past and from my own experiences with their food being tasteless. But I was glad I gave it a second chance because the recipes and options were good. Not all of them, of course, but after experimenting with several, I found a host of my go-to foods I enjoyed. The best part was they not only tasted good but helped me lose weight. I had access to, a vast *Diet Buffet*.

Question: If you are only using one eating style of food from one diet, do you think you will get bored at some point on your journey?

Your success and failure rate of dieting can depend on your interest in the food. Eating tasteless food is probably not high on anyone's lists. Since the types of food will play a huge role in your weight loss story, you should still be able to enjoy them, even while dieting, and not feel limited in your choices. This is one of the benefits to using the *Slim Down Level Up Formulas*. Besides helping you to lose weight, it will give you a variety of food options.

Do any of the items listed sound delicious to you?

Italian-Style Sausage & Peppers	Chicken Fettuccine Alfredo
Chicken with Apricot Glaze	Lasagna with Meat Sauce
Tilapia Cacciatore	Homemade Meatloaf and Vegetables
7-Spice Shrimp & Chicken Stir-Fry	Chicken Carbonara
Dill Poached Salmon	Ham & Swiss Baguette

Beef Fajita Wraps	General Tso's Chicken
Blueberry Pancakes & Sausage	Cheesy Egg & Bacon Skillet
Chocolate Muffins	Cinnamon Rolls
Vanilla Buttercream Cupcakes	Triple Chocolate Cheesecake
Peanut Butter Banana Ice Cream	Apple Crisp
Lemon Cake	Chocolate Lava Cake

From the list provided, would you want to be able to eat similar types of food while losing weight? Would it be helpful if they came already prepared for you? If so, the chart is an example of the types of the prepackaged foods I ate, that helped me to lose weight. They were especially beneficial to have access to on the days and nights when I did not feel like cooking. The different options also kept me on track with eating less calories.

Food, delicious food, and more food is another key piece to your successful weight loss and we are going to go over several options. All of which, if you choose, can be combined in various ways on your journey. Prior to learning about, the three *Slim Down Level Up Formulas* and how the *6-Week Program* can help you reach your goals, we will briefly go over the food options. They are some of the keys to how the formulas are created and can be used.

To give you a variety of choices, and before deciding on which you prefer, we will look at the food options, in using the: Keto, Vegan, Weight Watchers, Low-Calorie, Mediterranean, Low-Carb and Intermittent Fasting Diets. Then later, in the Bonus Material section in the back of the book, you will be able to see key benefits of incorporating the foods from either the Paleo, Nutrisystem, South Beach, or Jenny Craig, Diets. **You do not have to use all of them to lose weight.** Some of the diets and foods you will like, others will not make your list of choices.

The three *Slim Down Level Up Formulas* you will learn about in the next chapter can be used in various ways and with various eating styles. You will be able to select from different combinations (in the coming pages, you will see a chart showing how the formulas are made).

Having a variety of food choices and different diets to choose from will allow you to cater the *6-Week Program* specifically to what you would like to eat while losing weight.

For example, the food in the chart on the previous page are all Low-Calorie and Low-Fat. They are the types of food that can help you create the calorie deficit needed for the first part of the equation to losing weight. The items on the list come from either, the Jenny Craig, South Beach, Nutrisystem or Weight Watchers Program. Their menus have gotten better over the years and I discovered some offer Keto, Vegetarian and Vegan friendly options as well. Again, you do not have to use them to lose weight. They are provided to show a variety of food examples.

Since we all have different food preferences, lifestyles, and are at different health levels, I wanted to provide you a list of diet eating styles that is vast. You may be the kind of person with a very busy schedule and need convenience with your meals. You may have certain dietary restrictions that need to be followed. Maybe you are someone who does not like to cook and needs a little help with meal planning. Or someone who would do better being a part of a structured diet program, with the added support while losing weight.

Remember when I asked earlier if you have ever thought about combining Intermittent Fasting with Weight Watchers? Keto and Low-Calorie? Or Low-Calorie and a Vegan Diet? Intermittent Fasting and Low-Carb with alternating One Meal a Day and a 36-hour fast? Using Intermittent Fasting and Keto? Or, eating Vegan three times a week with Intermittent Fasting to maximize your weight loss? I wanted to paint a picture of how using the power of combining different diets together can look. It is a small snapshot of the various ways you will be able to use the formulas to lose weight.

An advantage in using the formulas is you will be able to take a diet, maybe you used before, that only worked for a short period of time and combine it in a variety of ways with other eating styles, to make it work long-term. For example, after seeing the three formulas, and going over the diets in the book, you may decide to combine Intermittent Fasting with Weight Watchers or Intermittent Fasting with a Low-Calorie Diet. Just as, the combinations used by some of the women in the success stories we heard earlier.

The process of deciding on which of the diets and their food you would like to try is set up in a user friendly and convenient way throughout the book. The different diet eating styles all have multiple examples and easy to follow step by step guides. They are all self-contained.

It is set up that way in the event, you would like to utilize some of the food from any of the diets. For example, Vegan, Low-Calorie or Weight Watchers. It would be as simple as going to that specific chapter to find what you need. Each one will give you a list of the top go-to foods, example meal plans, shopping guides, recipes, and techniques to utilize with that eating style.

As you become more familiar with the techniques to follow, and see all the possible diet combinations, it can open-up a whole new world of eating and weight loss for you. So that you will have the tools to lose, and keep, the weight off for good.

After learning how the formulas work, the days of you setting out to lose weight using one diet at a time will be no more. Because by now, depending on how many times you have started and stopped a diet, you have realized, it does not work for long. Remember, one diet alone is not set up for you to be successful long-term.

BASE, REMIXX, BONUS, EXTRA, LEVEL UP DIETS

Before moving on to the three *Slim Down Level Up Formulas*, it is important to point out and give examples of how the formulas work. Similar to how I explained earlier in the book, they will all start with a *Base Diet*. In other words, that would be the main diet of your choice (any of the diets listed in the book can be one of them). Then, to add, power to your weight loss strategy, a Remixx Diet would be selected. Which can also be chosen from the list provided.

Combining diets together can maximize your weight loss, as it did for me. An example would be Intermittent Fasting as the *Base Diet* combined with Low-Calorie as the *Remixx Diet*. Then, to take losing weight to the next level, another combination would include a *Base Diet*, a *Remixx Diet*, and it would be topped off with a *Bonus, Extra, or a Level Up Diet* added. An example would be: Low-Calorie is the *Base Diet*, Keto is the *Remixx Diet* and a *Bonus Diet* of 3 Liquid Dinners or 3 Meatless Dinners a week.

Here are a few more examples of various *Slim Down Level Up Combinations*. Each has a Base, Remixx and Bonus Diet included (these examples were created from using the 3-Step Chart on the next page).

1. Intermittent Fasting with Keto and No Added Sugar Challenge

2. Intermittent Fasting with Vegan and 3 Liquid Dinners a Week

3. Intermittent Fasting with Weight Watchers and 3 Meatless Dinners a week

4. Intermittent Fasting with Paleo and 2 OMAD (24-Hour Fast added)

5. Intermittent Fasting with Jenny Craig and Platinum Low-Carb

6. Intermittent Fasting with Low-Calorie and 5 Days of an 18:6 Fast Added

7. Intermittent Fasting with Nutrisystem and Platinum Low-Calorie

8. Intermittent Fasting with Low-Calorie and 3 Soup Dinners a Week

9. Intermittent Fasting with South Beach and 1-36 Hour Fast a Week

10. Intermittent Fasting with Low-Carb and 3 Days of an 18:6 Fast Added

Take a look at the three-step process below. This is the foundation for how the formulas are made:

SLIM DOWN LEVEL UP FORMULAS CHART

STEP 1: PICK A BASE DIET

1. Intermittent Fasting 2. Low-Calorie 3. Keto 4. Vegan

5. Mediterranean 6. Weight Watchers 7. Paleo 8. Jenny Craig

9. South Beach 10. Low-Carb 11. Nutrisystem

STEP 2: PICK A REMIXX DIET

1. Low-Calorie 2. Mediterranean 3. Weight Watchers 4. Paleo

5. Jenny Craig 6. Vegan 7. South Beach 8. Intermittent Fasting

9. Nutrisystem 10. Low-Carb 11. Keto

STEP 3: THE BONUS, EXTRA AND LEVEL UP OPTIONS

The **Bonus, Extra,** and ***Level Up Diets,*** can be selected as *Enhancers.* They can be combined and used in conjunction with the **Base** and the **Remixx Diets:**

1. **Meatless Dinner** (3 Days a Week)

2. **Low-Calorie** (Follow Body Budget Charts)

3. **Sugar Free** (2-Week Challenge with no Added Sugars)

4. **Liquid Dinner Meal Replacement** (3 Days a Week)

5. **Soup Dinner Meal Replacement** (3 Days a Week)

6. **Low-Carb** (Reduce daily intake to 40-50 Net Carbs max)

7. **Platinum Low-Carb** (20-30 Net Carbs max)

8. **Platinum Low-Calorie** (Reduce to 1200 calories and 40 fat grams)

9. **Fasting Extra** (Add 3 Days of an 18:6 Fast Schedule)

10. **Fasting Extra** (Add 5 Days of an 18:6 Fast Schedule)

11. **Fasting Extra** (Add 1- OMAD= 24-Hour Fast)

12. **Fasting Extra** (Add 1- 36 Hour Fast)

13. **Fasting Extra** (Add 2- OMAD= 24-Hour Fast)

14. **Fasting Extra** (Add 2- 36 Hour Fast)

15. **Fasting Extra** (Add a 5:2 Fast Schedule)

16. **Fasting Extra** (Add a 4:3 Fast Schedule)

Why Are There Meatless and Liquid Dinners in the Combinations?

One of the key benefits from using the formulas is the power of adding in the *Bonus Diets* to your mix. For example, I did not suggest Meatless Mondays, Try Tofu Thursdays, and Liquid Dinners just to deprive you of eating your regular foods. Or to torture you. I promise, I wouldn't do that to you, there is a reason behind it. One that you are going to like. **They have the ability, to increase your success while losing weight.**

It is not just about reducing the amount of meat from your diet and reducing your caloric intake. There are other key factors involved when you have a lighter dinner.

For example, as it relates to eating lighter in the evenings, (Meatless Dinners), there was a study conducted in 2013 that highlighted how this can help you lose more weight. When people consumed a set number of calories and used them towards a larger breakfast, (or the first part of the day) and ate less at dinner, they lost two-and-a-half times as much weight in 12 weeks than people who ate the *exact* same calories but in reverse. (17) So, those who had a smaller breakfast, and a larger dinner lost less weight than those who ate lighter towards the end of the day. Which points to the fact that our bodies require and burn fewer calories as the day goes on. Eating lighter in the evenings can produce better weight loss results. When you start the program and have meatless meals, you can tell yourself, **"My Meatless Dinner Makes Me Thinner."**

Another example of using the formulas and the benefits of adding in Liquid Dinners as your *Bonus Diet* is, for weight loss and improved health. In 2012, there was a study conducted by the Nutrition Journal that highlighted the power of combining different diets together and with liquid dinners as an added plus. The conclusion from the study shows, Intermittent Fasting, combined with a Calorie Restricted Diet and Liquid Meals is, an effective strategy to help obese and overweight women lose weight and lower CHD, Coronary Heart Disease. (18)

When you start having your liquid meals, you can tell yourself, "My Liquid Meal Seals the Weight Loss Deal."

Having soup for dinner is also another option on the *Bonus, Extra and Level Up Diets* list that can be used as a way, to reduce your caloric intake in the evenings. You may want to take caution when selecting your soup options, as some are packed with excess sodium. But there are a variety of healthy recipes you can make and buy that can satisfy both your tastebuds and the lower calorie needs. When you are having your soup dinner, you can tell yourself, **"When Soup Appears, Weight Loss is Near."** (I know, I have these silly sayings, but they helped while I was losing weight).

The science and strategy behind the *Slim Down Level Up Formulas* and the combinations are designed to specifically maximize your weight loss. The various fasting schedules, the mixing and matching of the *Bonus, Extra and Level Up Diets,* are all structured in ways for you to be successful in reaching your goal weight.

Side Note: When fasting, I do not recommend using a Meatless, Liquid or Soup Dinner the night before starting a 24 or 36-hour fast. When preparing for a long fast, it is better to have a full meal the night before with protein, fats, and carbs. For best results, plan your meatless, liquid and soup meals around your fasting schedule.

WEIGHT LOSS SUCCESS STORY TIME

These are two success stories from women who discovered how to use the power of mixing and matching, different eating styles together. Their combinations are similar to the *Slim Down Level Up Formulas* just discussed.

Sophia from Wisconsin wanted to lose 45 pounds to look better and also because the weight loss could help with her being pre-diabetic. Her doctor recommended she try a structured diet program with premeasured low-calorie meals. That was because she needed help with portion sizes and did not like to cook. Sophia signed up for the South Beach Diet and ordered some of the food from their program. She combined Intermittent Fasting with her diet and started using a variety of different fasting schedules along the way. She used a 16:8 schedule and then added 4 days a week of an 18:6 fasting schedule after the first few weeks. This gave her better results. Her doctor told her Intermittent Fasting would help with lowering her insulin levels and insulin resistance. She also incorporated protein shakes for dinner two nights a week. Sophia lost 43 pounds in a little over three and a half months using this technique. She also combined the benefits of exercising by walking 30 minutes 4 days a week. Her doctor was excited about seeing her updated lab results. He encouraged her to continue using the Low-Calorie Diet and Intermittent Fasting to help keep her insulin levels under control. (19)

Nancy from New Jersey had been trying to lose more weight for weeks with little to no results. She hit a plateau and became frustrated. She found out a co-worker of hers lost a lot of weight using Intermittent Fasting with a modified Vegan Diet (Flexitarian), so she decided to give it a try. Her weight was 238 pounds, and her goal was to lose 70 pounds. Having tried Intermittent Fasting in the past, Nancy decided to give it another try to see if it would work. However, starting out using the 16:8 fasting schedule was too hard for her to stick with last time. So, instead, she chose to use the 5:2 schedule. Where she fasted two non-consecutive days a week and only ate 500-600 calories on her fasting days. On fasting days, to help with staying hydrated and to curb her appetite, she drank coffee, green tea, and sparkling water. She often broke her fast, using premeasured meals from either, Jenny Craig or the Nutrisystem program. Which included lean meats, vegetables, and very few carbs. She liked doing that because it ensured she was spending her 500-600 calorie budget wisely. To make sure she was not overeating, Nancy took her co-worker's advice and set an 1800 calorie and 60 fat grams budget. She used it to eat responsibly portioned meals on the other five days. Since she was following the Flexitarian Diet, on her non-fasting days, she cut out eating meat 3 days a week and focused on eating more plant-based foods. She also eventually cut out drinking sodas and juices. It took five months and exercising 4-5 days a week for 45-50 minutes, but Nancy was able to lose all the weight. (20)

Yes! Happy to hear their results. In Sophia's and Nancy's stories, they used the power of combining a variety of diets together to achieve their goals. As you may have noticed part of the time while losing weight, they ate food from structured diet programs. When asked why, they said because it worked with their busy lifestyles and it was convenient. It took the guesswork out of preparing meals and offered them nutritional weight loss options to choose from. Those factors contributed to their success.

In the next chapter, we will look at the three *Slim Down Level Up Formulas* and how they can be used. Whichever one you decide to go with can help you reach your goals and set you on a path to living a healthier lifestyle with a variety of food options. As you look at the formulas, you do not have to make, a decision on which one you will start with yet. There will be plenty of time to choose after looking at the different food options and diet programs later in the book.

9

THE SLIM
DOWN LEVEL
UP FORMULA
OPTIONS

Are you ready to be victorious? There are a variety of ways to answer the call and counteract the on-going fight against losing weight, and to win. The key step is removing the one diet philosophy technique from your regimen from here on out. Say good-bye to it. By doing so, regardless of which diet combination you decide to start with, it can be your ticket to being successful long-term with losing weight.

In this chapter, we are going to specifically lay out the three *Slim Down Level Up Formulas* that can be utilized to create multiple diet combinations. Up until this point, you have seen a variety of ways diets can be combined. However, now it is time to look at the three main formulas that you will be able to choose from. This will be what your combinations will be built around.

All three formulas will show how insulin levels and insulin resistance can both be controlled, so that you can lose weight using either one. We will briefly discuss them now, but you will see the combinations again later in the book, when we go over in detail and layout the *6-Week Program*.

One of the formulas involves using the power of combining Intermittent Fasting with a variety of low-calorie diet regimens. The second is about combining Low-Calorie and Low-Carb Diets together. The third will use Keto, Low-Calorie and Intermittent Fasting Diets to help you achieve your weight loss goals.

Why Should You Use The Formulas? The various combinations of formulas are what the body requires. If not, it can quickly adjust to using one diet and eating one type of way, and your weight loss can stall.

"The problem with most diets is they ignore the biological principle of homeostasis-that is the ability of the body to adapt to changing environments. If you try and keep a constant diet, the body will adapt to it. This means that successful dieting requires an intermittent strategy, not a constant one." (21) This is an example of how the body requires change in order to continue to lose weight. If you are using one diet, it can only take you so far before your body makes the adjustment to your new routine. All the more reason why combining different diets, at different times, with a variety of foods, can be beneficial to your long-term success. In the next section, *The What*, *The When* and *The How* much you will eat will start to fall into place.

SLIM DOWN LEVEL UP FORMULA #1

INTERMITTENT FASTING +LOW-CALORIE DIETS

Low Calorie Diets	Intermittent Fasting Diet
1. Decreases Metabolism	1. Increases Metabolism
2. Increases Hunger	2. Decreases Hunger

The first *Slim Down Level Up Formula* combination is **Intermittent Fasting with Low-Calorie Diets**. We have seen examples in the book using this powerful combination in a few different ways. The same magic can happen here when using this formula for you. Lowering your insulin levels happens when you follow a healthy Low-Calorie Diet, consistently. Your insulin resistance can be controlled and reduced when you combine Intermittent Fasting together.

As briefly mentioned earlier, another benefit to using Intermittent Fasting with a Low-Calorie Diet is, it puts the body into a state where it is burning stored fat as its primary fuel source. The best part is, it goes after the belly fat. The visceral fat. That area on the body that is considered to carry the *dangerous* weight and can lead to heart disease and diabetes. The super-stubborn fat, I call it. Fasting can get rid of it.

"A new study says, Intermittent Fasting combined with a lower-calorie diet may be the best plan for weight loss and a flat belly." (22)

Yes! Being in a fasted state can help you say goodbye to excess belly fat and help you lose weight. Most importantly, if you decide to use this formula, it can answer the three key questions for your successful weight loss. The what and how much you will eat will come from the *Base Diet*-Low-Calorie, and the when, you will eat will come from the *Remixx Diet*-Intermittent Fasting.

SLIM DOWN LEVEL UP FORMULA #1

Low Calorie Diets = Lower Insulin Levels

+

Intermittent Fasting Diet = Reduced Insulin Resistance

=

Successful Weight Loss

Recap: With this formula, by following a Low-Calorie Diet of your choosing, you will take care of the first part of the equation to losing weight. The second part will be addressed when you add in a Remixx Diet of Intermittent Fasting. This is where you will use the magic of lowering your insulin levels and insulin resistance. This is one of the ways your on-going weight loss battle can be won.

SLIM DOWN LEVEL UP FORMULA #2

LOW-CARB + LOW-CALORIE DIETS

The second *Slim Down Level Up Formula* combination can be utilized when you do not want to have Intermittent Fasting as a Base or Remixx Diet. Instead of using fasting in the mix, it combines the power of using **Low-Carb and Low-Calorie Diets** together. The *Base Diet* = Low-Calorie, will lower your insulin levels. Which you know is one piece of the puzzle needed to lose weight.

The Remixx Diet = Low-Carb, mixed with Low-Calorie Diets, can be an effective combination when used together. Why? By combining the two, you can reduce the amount of carbohydrates your body uses as its primary fuel/energy. How do carbohydrates work and provide energy? They are broken down into simple sugar molecules by a digestive process. When the supply is limited, it is beneficial for weight loss, because by being on a Low-Carb Diet (20-40 net carbs daily), the body can go into Ketosis.

Like being in a fasted state, Ketosis is the point where the body is using its fat as the primary source of fuel. It allows the body to burn belly fat as well. Being in this state can also decrease hunger and increase the metabolism. It is another recipe, you can use for weight loss success.

In the New England Journal of Medicine, individuals participating in a study of the benefits of a Low-Carb Diet, lost more weight than those on a Low-Fat Diet. In the article, it states,

"Get the best results from your diet by choosing foods that are low in carbs and (low) in calories." (23)

Recap: When you use a Low-Calorie Diet mixed with a Low-Carb Diet, it can be effective in addressing the two key elements of losing weight, insulin levels and insulin resistance. Combining the two can help you push your body into ketosis and help it stay there as well. If you decide to use this formula, be sure to cut your eating off 2-3 hours before bedtime. This will allow your body to experience a mini fast to increase your weight loss and reduce late night snacking.

Beyond losing weight there are other key benefits to the body in using a Low-Carb Diet.

"A low carb diet has been linked to several health benefits...Including weight loss, and improved blood sugar control and cardiovascular risk factors." (24)

SLIM/DOWN LEVEL UP FORMULA #2

Low Calorie Diets = Lower Insulin Levels

+

Low Carb Diets = **Ketosis** = Reduced Insulin Resistance

=

Successful Weight Loss

SLIM DOWN LEVEL UP FORMULA #3

KETO+ INTERMITTENT FASTING + LOW CALORIE DIETS

The third *Slim Down Level Up Formula* combination is **Keto with Intermittent Fasting and Low-Calorie Diets**. The Keto Diet is primarily a high fat, low carb formula, used to lose weight. It consists of consuming 75% of your daily caloric budget as fat. Combining it with a Low-Calorie Diet can also be helpful if you need help with portion control. It can be used as a guide to create the calorie deficit needed to lose weight. As well as help with controlling insulin levels.

Similar to the Low-Carb Diet, the Ketogenic (Keto), Diet works by pushing the body into ketosis by reducing the overall carb intake to 20 net carbs or less. Same premise as what can happen when using the other two formulas; this helps the body burn fat as its primary fuel, instead of using carbs. Combining it with Intermittent Fasting can help the body get into and stay in ketosis easier. It also addresses the piece of the puzzle that helps with controlling insulin resistance. This is another formula you can use to reach your goal.

SLIM DOWN LEVEL UP FORMULA #3

Low Calorie Diets = Lower Insulin Levels

+

Keto Diet + Intermittent Fasting = Ketosis Faster=Reduced Insulin Resistance

=

Successful Weight Loss

Recap: The power of using any of the three *Slim Down Level Up Formulas* can eliminate your body's natural instinct, to want to resist you being on a diet and losing weight. In Chapter 2, we talked about when you reduce your calories, on any diet, your body will eventually work against you and slow your metabolism down. It is inevitable, and the reason why eventually, the diet stops working. The way you can counteract that is by incorporating one of the formulas to address the slowed metabolism and the increased hunger that will occur. Either one of the formulas will lower your insulin levels and reduce your insulin resistance, so you can continue losing weight. Unlocking the missing piece. And in the process, it will help to shift your body's set weight down, allowing less resistance to your new weight. It is specifically easier to achieve this when you add fasting to your diet routine.

Even if you have never thought about using Intermittent Fasting or thought it was too hard, by adding it to your diet regimen, even a few days a week, it can be effective. Allowing your body to be pushed into ketosis, sporadically, can help it to burn fat. Ketosis is a very predictable way to target the fat stores that otherwise can remain unused.

Using fasting to lose weight does more than help us burn stored body fat. There are other health benefits to adding it to your combinations. For example, cancer is a terrible disease that affects many people every year and, unfortunately, as we read earlier, takes over 9 million lives annually worldwide. More research is being conducted that shows fasting having several beneficial effects on the metabolism that may lead to reduced risk of cancer. (25)

Side Note: Later in the book, we will go over additional benefits and food options with using the Intermittent Fasting, Low-Calorie, Low-Carb and Keto Diet. We will discuss more examples, testimonies and research on the power of how you can combine different diets together. As, well as various ways the formulas can help you lose weight. For instance, before moving on to the next chapter, let us take a quick look at two examples of combining and using different eating styles together. They both start out using a *Base Diet* and a *Remixx Diet*. But add in and mix up their food choices from other diets.

BUSY BEATRIS

Beatris wants to lose 55 pounds and decides to start a diet. Her *Base Diet* is Keto, and her *Remixx Diet* is Intermittent Fasting.

- She has been losing weight successfully since starting and has gotten a handle on the food options she can enjoy. However, she does not cook much lately because she has a very hectic schedule.

- Having meals already prepared with the nutrition information would be helpful to her, to make sure she is staying within her correct daily body budget numbers for the day.

- She looks, into the South Beach and Weight Watchers Diet meal options. She finds out she does not have to join either program to purchase their foods or to try some of the recipes, she found on their websites, and on Pinterest and Google.

- She discovers they both offer a variety of Keto friendly, low-carb items to choose from.

- While searching online for more food options, she discovers *Home Chef*, a food delivery service that offers freshly made premeasured meal kits that are also Keto friendly.

- Having those options ready in her freezer was helpful to her on those busy hectic days when cooking at home was not a reality. It was a cost savings to her weekly grocery bill as well.

VARIETY VALERIE

Valerie wants to lose 75 pounds and decides to start a diet:

- She uses a *Base Diet* of Weight Watchers, a *Remixx Diet* of Intermittent Fasting and combines it with a *Bonus* Low-Carb Diet.

- Weight loss is happening, and she is enjoying some of the food and recipes.

- The recipes she has made thus far were tasty and easy to follow. However, she has been following the diet for a few months now and wants to try some different foods.

- She heard about the South Beach Diet from a friend and decides to try some of their food options. And discovers a whole list of new, low-carb favorites to use while continuing to lose weight. She becomes even more excited when she realizes they can deliver the meals to her home.

- She also finds out about a food delivery service online called *Blue Apron* that offers freshly made premeasured meals for about $10 each and can accommodate several dietary needs. She especially liked they had Weight Watchers friendly meals and low-calorie options to choose from. They also delivered her meals to her home. It was a huge help in saving her money and meal prep time. Plus, it provided the variety in food she was looking for.

Beatris and Valerie experimented with different diets and food options as a way, to help with losing weight. As mentioned in Chapter 8, your long-term weight loss is going to be about having a variety of food choices available. So, that you can create your own personal **Diet Buffet.** That will take some experimenting on your part, as you figure out what food options you like best.

I implore you to not give up on the first try of a different food type or the first recipe you explore with. While I was experimenting, I had a few not so pleasant tasting meals. A soy-burger disaster, a terrible chicken with rice dish, and a steak that tasted like leather. But I did not let it stop me from continuing to try other food options. What I did was either learn to cook it another way, tried a different brand or ate at a different restaurant. All brands are not created equal, and you will find you prefer some over the others. Or one recipe over another.

Similar to what Valerie and Beatris utilized, in the coming chapters you will find a list of resources of home delivery meal kit websites. Offering a variety of freshly prepared, premeasured meals that are calorie, fat grams, and carb conscious. As well as plant-based, gluten, dairy, and soy free meals.

Options like these can be an affordable weight loss choice for you, some as little as $8.00 a meal. They can provide you a convenient alternative to cooking or ordering out. The bonus is they can keep you on track, while losing weight.

Here are a few examples of some of the types of food from different meal kit delivery services I have tried before:

- Steak Peppercorn with Sautéed Carrots & French Green Beans

- Homestyle Chicken with Butternut Mac & Cheese

- Smothered & Stuffed Meatloaf with Potato Wedges

- Honey Glazed Pork Chops with Roasted Brussels Sprouts & Ranch Seasoned Potatoes

- Pan Seared Tilapia Piccata with Broccolini & Linguine Pasta

- Honey Poppyseed Salmon Salad

Side Note: After we go over all the different diets, eating options, meal plans, snack ideas, etc. you may decide not to utilize some of them throughout your weight loss journey. That is more than okay. They will be there if, and when you decide to use some of their options. What I have learned over the years is successful dieting is not a one size fits all. Knowing which parts of the different eating styles you can use and how it can benefit your weight loss journey will be key. This will give you an edge over *traditional dieters* because most do not think about or explore the food and recipes from other diets. Especially, to use in conjunction with their weight loss plans.

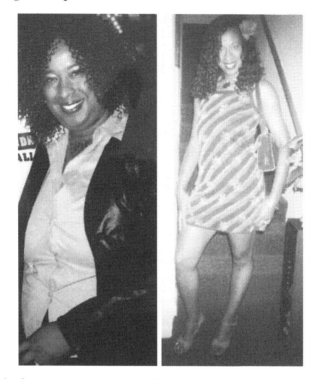

The before picture on the left where I am busting through my shirt, I remember being one of the last pictures I took before I completely started avoiding the camara. On the right was the after picture of me at 143 pounds. In it, you can see I had the bobble-head thing going on, I mentioned earlier in Chapter 5. It was when I went full-blown extreme weight loss crazed and had stopped listening to my body and got too skinny. Before finally, realizing what was a happy, healthy weight for me to be at.

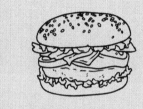

PART FOUR
EAT THE
CHEESEBURGER &
CHOCOLATE CAKE

10
DAILY BODY BUDGET CHARTS

We have now looked at the three *Slim Down Level Up Formulas,* which means, you are on track for your transformation to soon start. We saw some testimonies using a series of different Low-Calorie and Low-Carb Diets together, to maximize weight loss. We even read about some of the types of food choices and which of the diets the food came from. However, how much food were they eating? Based on your weight loss needs, what would be considered low-calories and low-carbs, for you? And while using the formulas, what is your daily body budget to lose weight?

There are two **Daily Body Budget Charts** available for you to refer to, when starting on the *6-Week Program.* As, well as in the next chapter, a three tier, **Low-Carb Chart.** All three charts are designed to help keep you within a set budget. The calculations in the charts are the same ones I followed to lose my weight.

The first one you will see is the *Conservative Weight Loss Daily Body Budget Chart.* If you want to start losing weight at a more conservative pace and do not want to reduce your calories and fat grams, too low to get started, this chart is for you. The set numbers in the chart will still create the desired calorie deficit to lose weight but it is more of a gradual decrease in your overall daily intake.

The second is the *Aggressive Weight Loss Daily Body Budget Chart*. If you want to jumpstart and accelerate your weight loss with lower calories and fat grams, this chart is for you. The calculations of the calories and fat grams in this chart are designed to be more aggressive with your weight loss goals. If you are over 50, and/or not active, I recommend you start with using the numbers in the Aggressive Chart for better results because, as we age or are less active, our metabolism tends to slow down.

Both Body Budget Charts, if followed, can help you lose weight and assist you with using your daily food budget wisely. The fat grams are included and are just as important as the calories to follow because they can help you make better food choices with your overall budget.

I want to stress the importance of following all the numbers that are listed in the charts. Including the ones, we will talk about in the next chapter, net carbs. What I have discovered while losing weight and sticking to my daily body budget numbers is, I can have enough calories to *afford* a certain food item, but not have enough fat grams or net carbs. Which would often guide me to make better use of my remaining body budget.

For example, if you are on a daily budget of 1,800 calories, 60 fat grams, and 20-50 net carbs, what would be the better option to spend part of your daily budget on for lunch?

1. 1 Cheeseburger Deluxe, 16 oz sparkling water=530 calories, 30 fat grams (44 net carbs)

2. 4 oz Grilled Chicken Breast, ½ cup of cauliflower rice, 1 cup of mixed vegetables, 16 oz sparkling water=421 calories, 11 fat grams (9 net carbs)

If the goal is to lose weight by eating healthier food and to make us feel fuller longer, then the obvious choice in this situation would be the second option. It gets more bang for the buck and uses the daily calories, fat grams and net carbs smarter.

However, let us pause for a moment because I want to make sure I am clear about the spending of the daily body budget. I am not saying to never choose option one. That is not realistic, and **there may be times when you just want the cheeseburger. Eat the cheeseburger!** And if you are like me, sometimes it will mean you want the cheeseburger and the chocolate cake. That is okay as well (In the next chapter we will talk about how to eat out successfully and still lose weight).

The key to losing weight long-term is all about balance and accepting you will eat *non-diet* food some days (I don't like to use those words, non-diet food, but you know what I mean). I did not eat all healthy food the entire time I was losing weight.

Back then, I was pre-diabetic, had high blood pressure and high cholesterol as mentioned earlier in the book. So, I often paid attention to those factors when deciding what to eat. I ate the types of food that would help me continue losing weight and help me fight the diagnosis at the same time. I followed the 80 Whole/20 Soul, Rule. I aimed for 80% of the time, my food choices were on the healthier side.

However, there were occasions within the 20% time frame when I fed my soul, and I did eat the cheeseburger, and the chocolate cake and you can, too. As long as you keep three things in mind when deciding to:

1. Budget for it, 2. With the cheeseburger example, acknowledge that 30 fat grams would be half of your daily budget, and 3. The net carbs spent is almost five times option 2.

Point is, on days like that, when you would use a larger part of your fat grams and net carbs on a splurge meal, you would just make better use of your remaining budget and choose healthier options. Simple, right? No stress. No need to add stress while losing weight; you will be dealing with enough as you are processing the shift with your food choices.

You can eat pretty much anything if you budget for it. However, all calories are not the same, and that is why paying attention to the fat grams and net carbs will help you make better use of your budget on things like lean meats, fruits, vegetables, and whole grains.

Keep in mind, things like cheeseburgers, cake, ice cream, chocolate, white bread, rice, candy, chips, soda, are the *sometimes* items we can enjoy. I highly recommend you do not put them in the never category. By doing so, you can potentially set yourself up to fail.

For example, I have always loved Twinkies, and when I started losing weight years ago, I said I would not eat them again, ever. Of course, that did not happen, and when I first got my hands on a box of them, I ate 7! All within about ten minutes and drank a soda with it. Then as I sat there with all the empty wrappers on my lap, I stared at the other 3 in the box thinking about eating them, too. It was terrible! I had such a sugar rush and felt miserable afterwards.

When we completely remove items from our diet, it can cause us to binge. I do not believe in telling you to completely delete the foods you enjoy. Rather, decrease the amount and the frequency of the consumption of them. I can tell you now, when I do have a Twinkie, I only have one because I know it is my sometimes food and not the forbidden treat anymore.

Calories and fat grams matter when it comes to losing weight. If you have not done it in the past, going forward, make knowing your calories and fat grams budget a top priority when you set out on your new journey. The *6-Week Program* is designed around you sticking to these numbers so you can be successful. When dieting, even on a Keto Diet, if you only focus on the caloric numbers and not the fat grams, especially the types of fat, your food decisions may not always be the best choice for you.

Here is an estimate of how I calculated the Body Budget Charts for you as it relates to the calories and fat grams. To lose weight, taking in roughly between 8-10 calories per pound of weight you are, is ideal and can create the desired weight loss calorie deficit. The other key number, as I stated, is to track the fat grams. To calculate that number, take your calorie budget divided by 30 and that number will be your fat grams daily allowance.

Example: Your Current Weight is 200 Pounds

Weight x 8=1,600 calories divided by 30 = 53 fat grams	Lowest Daily Intake
Weight x 9=1,800 calories divided by 30 = 60 fat grams	Medium Daily Intake
Weight x 10=2,000 calories divided by 30 = 66 fat grams	Maximum Daily Intake

Side Note: As you are losing weight, it is important to check back with the charts to reduce your daily numbers to accommodate for the new weight loss. To keep your scale heading in the right direction, be sure to stick to your numbers as closely as possible on most days.

Important Tip: Make time to weigh yourself prior to starting, to confirm you are taking in the correct calories and fat grams. As I mentioned in Chapter 5, I highly recommend you weigh yourself only on *Wednesdays*. It can be physically and emotionally beneficial. If, for some reason, you splurged on the weekend with your eating, you have a few extra days to get back on track and make healthier choices. Which can reset your scale back in the right direction and encourage you to continue making better choices more days than not.

Bonus Charts: To give you some ideas of the key benefits to making healthier food choices with your daily budget, following the Body Budget Charts, are a variety of fruits and vegetables, you can refer to while on your journey. It is beneficial to incorporate more fruits and vegetables in your diet especially, to help you lose weight. However, the best part, as you will see in the different charts, is, all the natural healing, protective properties and, the ways in which they can contribute to your overall health. (26)

CONSERVATIVE WEIGHT LOSS DAILY BODY BUDGET CHART

Weight	Calories	Fat Grams
300 LBS	2,400-2,500	80-83
280 LBS	2,300-2,400	76-80
260 LBS	2,000-2,200	66-73
240 LBS	1,800-2,000	60-66
220 LBS	1,600-1,800	53-60
200 LBS	1,500-1,600	50-53
180 LBS	1,400-1,500	46-50
160 LBS	1,300-1,400	43-46
140 LBS	1,200-1,300	40-43

*If you are under 50 and/or active, you can use this chart to start with while using the *6-Week Program*. If, while losing weight, you hit a plateau or want to accelerate your weight loss at any point, you can switch to following the numbers in the Aggressive Chart on the next page.

AGGRESSIVE WEIGHT LOSS DAILY BODY BUDGET CHART

Weight	Calories	Fat Grams
300 LBS	1,500-1,600	50-53
280 LBS	1,500-1,600	50-53
260 LBS	1,400-1,500	46-50
240 LBS	1.400-1,500	46-50
220 LBS	1,300-1,400	43-46
200 LBS	1,300-1,400	43-46
180 LBS	1,200-1,300	40-43
160 LBS	1,200-1,300	40-43
140 LBS	1,100-1,200	36-40

*If you are over 50 and/or less active, as stated, I recommend you follow the numbers in the Aggressive Chart when first starting the program due to the chances of having a slower metabolism and not burning as many calories daily.

SOME KEY BENEFITS TO EATING FRUIT-Part 1

Benefits of Banana	Benefits of Apple	Benefits of Pomegranate	Benefits of Mango	Benefits of Watermelon
*Stabilizes Blood Sugar Levels *Aids in Digestion *Reduces Bad Cholesterol Levels *Fights Cancer *Great for the Eyes	*Boosts Digestive System *Controls Diabetes *Good for the Heart *Promotes Weight Loss *Improves Cognitive Functioning	*Treats Anemia *Cures Stomach Disorders *Prevents Arthritis *Improves Memory *Strengthens the Immune System	*Prevents Cancer Occurrence *Fights Heat Stroke *Great for Pregnant Mothers *Treats Kidney Stones	*Enables Hydration of the Body *Regulates Blood Pressure Levels *Prevents Macular Degeneration (loss of vision) *Promotes Weight Loss
Benefits of Grapes	Benefits of Avocado	Benefits of Papaya	Benefits of Oranges	Benefits of Pineapple
*Regulates Blood Pressure *Reduces Problems with Constipation *Treats Asthma *Strengthens Bones *Prevents Cavities	*Promotes a Healthy Heart *Protects Liver *Good for the Eyes *Encourages Longevity *Heals Wounds Faster	*Boosts Digestive System *Eases Menstrual Pain *Fights Inflammation *Prevents Diabetes *Protection Against Skin Damage	*Alkalizes the Body *Fights Various Infections, Mainly Viral Ones *Good for Brain Health *Has Anti-Cancer Properties *Prevents Constipation	*Protects the Heart *Relieves Asthma *Lowers Cancer Risks *Improves Bone Health *Improves the Digestive System

153

SOME KEY BENEFITS TO EATING FRUIT-Part 2

Benefits of Grapefruit	Benefits of Guava	Benefits of Cherries	Benefits of Berries
*Improves Vision *Helps to Get Rid of Respiratory Problems *Lowers Bad Cholesterol Levels *Eliminates Gum Problems *Cures Arthritis	*Cleanses the Body *Improves Thyroid Health *Eliminates Stomach Problems *Treats Cough and Cold *Treats Scurvy	*Prevents Gout (inflammatory arthritis) *Promotes Healthy Sleep *Helps to Shed Excess Belly Fat *Maintains the pH Level of the Body *Reduces Muscle Pain	*Regulates Blood Glucose and Insulin Levels *Reduces Inflammation *Fights Oxidative Stress (imbalance of free radicals in the body) *Good for the Brain *Protects the Heart
Benefits of Apricot	Benefits of Kiwi	Benefits of Lime	Benefits of Peach
*Strengthens the Bones *Cures Fever *Can Relieve Earache (apricot oil) *Treats Anemia *Increases Stamina	*Aids in the Digestive Process *Fights Sleep Disorders *Boosts Immunity *Protection from DNA Damage *Good for the Eyes	*Promotes Weight Loss *Heals Peptic Ulcers *Treats Gout *Prevents Piles *Treats Cystitis or Urinary Tract Infections	*Good for Digestion *Strengthens the Nervous System *Detoxifies the Body *Improves Cellular Health *Treats Blood Stasis (stagnant blood not circulating properly)

SOME KEY BENEFITS TO EATING VEGETABLES-
Part 1

Benefits of Carrots	Benefits of Spinach	Benefits of Cabbage	Benefits of Beans	Benefits of Radishes
*Boosts Cardiovascular Health *Anti-Cancer Effects *Controls Diabetes *Teeth Health *Good for Your Eyes	*Improves Brain Function *Strengthens Muscles *Promotes Healthy Metabolism *Helps in Bone Mineralization *Prevents Ulcers	*Boosts Digestive System *Soothes Inflammation *Lowers High Blood Pressure *Promotes Weight Loss *Detoxifier	*Protects the Liver *Improves Gut Health *Prevents Scurvy (vitamin C deficiency) *Treats Jaundice (Yellowing of the eyes and skin) *Good for the Brain	*Treats Urinary Disorders *Prevents Hemorrhoids *Protects Kidneys *Prevents Leucoderma (Vitiligo-skin disorder) *Treats Fever
Benefits of Broccoli	**Benefits of Squash**	**Benefits of Sweet Potatoes**	**Benefits to Kale**	**Benefits of Eggplant**
*Good to Strengthen Bones *Cures Allergies *Improves Eyes *Treats Diabetes *Good for the Heart	*Colon Health *Reduce PMS Symptoms *Improves Muscle Contraction and Stimulates Nerve Impulses *Reduces Asthma Problems	*Treats Bronchitis *Prevents Dehydration *Heals Stress and Relaxation Elements	*Possess Anti-Cancerous Elements *Combats Depression *Good for Brain Development *Good for Your Heart *Strengthens the Immune System	*Controls High Cholesterol Levels *Prevents Anemia *Birth Defect Prevention *Good for Throat Problems *Treats Stomach Issues

155

SOME KEY BENEFITS OF EATING VEGETABLES-Part 2

Benefits of Cauliflower	Benefits of Peas	Benefits of Lettuce	Benefits of Calabash	Benefits of Turnips
*Treats Nervous Disorders	*Repairs Broken Tissues	*Possess Anti-Cancerous Elements	*Cooling System	*Good for the Lungs
*Balances Hormones	*Improves Vision	*Combats Depression	*Reduces Stress	*Prevents Atherosclerosis (plaque buildup inside the arteries)
*Prevents Stroke	*Prevents Alzheimer	*Good for Brain Development	*Treats Sleep Disorders	*Cures Asthma
*Heals Colitis (irritation of the colon)	*Treats Celiac Disease (autoimmune disorder/ triggered by gluten)	*Good for Your Heart	*Promotes Healthy Weight Loss	*Stronger Bones
*Reduces Hypertension	*Anti-Aging Properties	*Strengthens the Immune System	*Treats Urinary Disorders	*Improves Blood Circulation

11
LOW-CARB CHARTS

This chapter brings us to the third chart to utilize while losing weight, as it relates to what range your daily food budget should stay within. It is the three tier, **Low-Carb Chart.** Whether you follow either of the three *Slim Down Level Up Formulas*, lowering your daily carb intake can help you lose weight and can cause your body to burn stored fat.

The first is **Liberal Low-Carbs,** and this option is if you want to lower your carb intake, however, not by a drastic amount to get started. Staying within these numbers can help you lose weight and are the ideal range to be in, when you transition into maintenance mode, after reaching your goal. The range is provided as a guide, and you do not have to use all of the daily intake each day. Some days, based on your food choices, you may use less.

The second option is **Moderate Low-Carbs,** and this is if you would like to reduce your overall carb intake to a semi-aggressive lower amount. Staying within this range can help you lose weight by selecting more whole foods and less processed products.

The third option is the **Ketogenic Low-Carbs.** This is if you want to start out being more aggressive with reducing your daily intake, to push your body into ketosis using this method. Any of the three tier options can be used in conjunction with the calorie, and fat gram numbers in the previous chapter to guide you on your journey in reaching your goal weight.

The three-tier, **Low-Carb Chart** is for total *net carbs* for the day. To calculate the net carbs, you would take total carbs and minus the dietary fiber in the item. For example, if the food choice has total carbohydrates at 18 grams and the dietary fiber is 5 grams, total net carbs for that item would be 13 net carbs. (You can use fitness apps to help you with these calculations also).

LOW-CARB-CHART

Formula: Total Carbohydrates – Dietary Fiber = Net Carbs

Tier 1: Liberal Low-Carbs = 50-100 Net Carbs Intake Daily
Tier 2: Moderate Low-Carbs = 20-50 Net Carbs Intake Daily
Tier 3: Ketogenic Low-Carbs = 20 or less Net Carbs Intake Daily

Regardless of which one of the formulas you follow, it is a good idea to know which fruits and vegetables are low in carbs, so that you can make better use of your daily budget. To give you a few ideas, below you will see Low-Carb vegetables and fruits examples. Keep these types of choices in mind when you decide on your meals and snacks for the day.

NET CARBS IN SOME FRUITS AND VEGETABLES

FRUITS

*Watermelon 7	*Berries 10	*Cantaloupe 7	*Avocado 2	*Honeydew 7
*Peaches 8	*Apples 12	*Orange 9	*Pineapple 12	*Grapes 16
*Kiwi 12	*Plum 10	*Banana 20	*Coconut 6	*Strawberries 6

*=Net Carbs/Serving Size=3 oz

VEGETABLES

*Cucumber 3	*Celery 2	*Spinach 1	*Tomato 3	*Potato 15
*Bell Peppers: Green 3, Red 4, Yellow 5	*Leeks 12	*Brussel Sprouts 5	*Cauliflower 3	*Sweet Potato 17
*Iceberg Lettuce 2	*Broccoli 4	*Zucchini 3	*Shallots 14	*Asparagus 2
*White Mushrooms 4	*Carrots 7	*Onion 8	*Cabbage 3	*Green Beans 4

*=Net Carbs/Serving Size=3 oz

Also, it is important to take in adequate sources of fiber while losing weight. Especially, if you decide to fast, to avoid being constipated. Therefore, in this chapter, fiber charts are also provided as a reference.

DAILY RECOMMENDED FIBER INTAKE

There are a few examples in the charts of ways to take in adequate amounts of fiber daily. Women should try to eat at least 21 to 25 grams of fiber a day, while men should aim for 30 to 38 grams a day. (27)

Here is a look at how much dietary fiber is found in some common foods. When buying packaged foods, check the Nutrition Facts Label for fiber content. It can vary among different brands.

FIBER REFERENCE CHARTS

Fruits	Serving size	Total fiber (grams)*
Raspberries	1 cup	8.0
Pear	1 medium	5.5
Apple, with skin	1 medium	4.5
Banana	1 medium	3.0
Orange	1 medium	3.0
Strawberries	1 cup	3.0

Vegetables	Serving size	Total fiber (grams)*
Green peas, boiled	1 cup	9.0
Broccoli, boiled	1 cup chopped	5.0
Turnip greens, boiled	1 cup	5.0
Brussels sprouts, boiled	1 cup	4.0
Potato, with skin, baked	1 medium	4.0
Sweet corn, boiled	1 cup	3.5
Cauliflower, raw	1 cup chopped	2.0
Carrot, raw	1 medium	1.5

FIBER REFERENCE CHARTS

Grains	Serving size	Total fiber (grams)*
Spaghetti, whole-wheat, cooked	1 cup	6.0
Barley, pearled, cooked	1 cup	6.0
Bran flakes	3/4 cup	5.5
Quinoa, cooked	1 cup	5.0
Oat bran muffin	1 medium	5.0
Oatmeal, instant, cooked	1 cup	5.0
Popcorn, air-popped	3 cups	3.5
Brown rice, cooked	1 cup	3.5
Bread, whole-wheat	1 slice	2.0
Bread, rye	1 slice	2.0

Legumes, nuts and seeds	Serving size	Total fiber (grams)*
Split peas, boiled	1 cup	16.0
Lentils, boiled	1 cup	15.5
Black beans, boiled	1 cup	15.0
Baked beans, canned	1 cup	10.0
Chia seeds	1 ounce	10.0
Almonds	1 ounce (23 nuts)	3.5
Pistachios	1 ounce (49 nuts)	3.0
Sunflower kernels	1 ounce	3.0

*Rounded to nearest 0.5 gram.

PART FIVE
THE 4 STEP WEIGHT LOSS FOOD SHIFT

12

STEP 1-2 EATING OUT/MRE KITS

Raise your hand if you would like more convenient, time-saving options, and less stress when it comes to planning and cooking meals? Oh, and if you would especially like those things while losing weight? (Just so you know, I have both my hands raised in the air). I want you to picture this: You are ready to lose weight. You understand the power of combining different diets together and have selected which one of the *Slim Down Level Up Formulas* you will start with. You also know your daily food intake, from referring to the charts in the book. You have made the decision in your mind and are determined to win this time. However, who is cooking your food? What kind of snacks are you eating? And are you ready to make the *Weight Loss Food Shift?* Confused? I was too when I started losing weight years ago. I started without making the shift in my food choices and then wondered why the weight stopped coming off.

I mean, technically, I knew why the weight stopped coming off because my food habits had not completely shifted yet. **Let's be honest, it is so easy to be overweight and find cheap, convenient, delicious food options, almost everywhere**. The way the fast-food, takeout, super-size, all-you-can-eat world of food is set up, you would have to drive around with blinders on to not be tempted to stop and get something to eat. In a five-mile radius near my home, for example, I have access to no less than thirty-five fast food, take-out, high-fat, food restaurants. Which would mean a pre-weight loss food shift, was filled with some of those options on more days than not. Unfortunately, as most of us already know, food convenience can come at a price. Consuming multiple items from fast-food dollar menus or the $5.00 fill up combos may cost us less in our pockets, but it has been adding more to our hips.

Here is what a *convenient* normal day of eating for me would look like. It involved a few fast-food items, some overly processed snacks and a deep fried or sauteed in bacon grease or butter type of a meal at home. My plate would have a meat with two to three side dishes, no less. Usually, fried chicken, ribs, or smothered pork chops, mash potatoes, baked macaroni and cheese or fried rice. That is not even including the desserts. Every now and again, my family would eat a healthier salad and some baked chicken with me. Which, somehow, often ended up being packed with extra fats and calories. Especially after adding bacon bits and croutons to the salad and putting cheese on the chicken. My son liked it that way. (Honestly, that was how I used to like it, too).

What is the Weight Loss Food Shift? It can be one of the key reasons why people fail at losing weight, because often they do not understand the importance of making the *shift*. Most of us are creatures of habit and are comfortable cooking and eating the same things daily. We buy the same types of meat, make the same meals, and frequently visit the same restaurants. It was what I used to do for a very, long time. I had my signature seven to eight meals I knew how to make. Those were the ones I often turned to and cooked for my family. I also had programmed in my phone (saved under favorites), four to five takeout restaurants near my home and job (I ordered so much from one of them, I was on a first name basis with most of the employees, and I had some of the menu item numbers memorized).

The problem was, those eating, and cooking habits were what contributed to my weight gain in the first place and continuing to practice them was not helping me. At that time, familiarity and convenience were what dictated what I was eating. As it does for a lot of people. For example, instead of cooking a healthy meal, have you stopped off at a fast-food restaurant on your way home because it was easy? Ordered take-out or a pizza because you had gotten tied up at work or with the kids and did not have time to grocery shop or meal prep? Threw together a quick last-minute meal not even thinking about the calories, fat grams or carbs? Turned to your signature, go-to unhealthy snacks in the pantry only because they were in the house? Been there, done that and then some.

When we are dieting, even if we cut our calories and switch to a low-carb diet, clearly, we are going to eat something. Food choices will always be a big part of our lives. What will we eat and who will do the cooking are constant daily questions that will always remain. When we do not make the *weight loss food shift*, we can revert right back to cooking unhealthy meals at home, pulling up to the fast-food restaurants and ordering takeout that is familiar to us. I have done it in the past, and it happened up until it finally clicked. Which meant every time before that, I sabotaged my weight loss goals because I had not completely shifted. The good thing is, the tips and tools in this book will not allow that to be the case, in your situation because there are buffers, we are going to put in place.

As I said in the beginning of the book, you are going to be able to *dominate* losing weight. By grocery shopping for healthier items, eating out successfully, learning to cook more low-calorie meals and having a variety of food options available to order.

I have a question for you: Do you like to grocery shop or meal prep and cook and clean up everyday? Or, as my earlier question asked, would you prefer convenient, time saving, less stressful meal options? If your answer is yes, I have a few steps you can take on ways to make your *weight loss food shift* easier. They can help change the trajectory on how you decide to eat while losing and maintaining weight.

Imagine it is dinner time and not having to meal prep, pre-measure, cook, and clean up for the majority, of the meals you eat. Imagine having a list of healthier snack ideas you can choose from when you're craving something salty or sweet. Or better yet, imagine if those same meals and snacks helped you to lose weight. They would take the guesswork out of if you are eating the correct number of calories, fat grams and net carbs. And what if some of those items could be delivered directly to your door and stored away to use at a later date? Especially on days when you do not feel like cooking or need a quick bite to eat. Oh, and what if you could get some of them for less than what you would pay for a fast-food meal? Lastly, what if they had options even your family could enjoy, would that make losing weight easier? The good news is, you do not have to imagine it, because it is real. You want convenience, it is here. You want to stop ordering the weight loss sabotaging fast-food and takeout combos you keep spending $12.00-$15.00 on? It is here. You want to make fewer trips to the grocery store, spend less time in the kitchen, washing, chopping, and prepping to cook dinner? It is here. You want to spend less time stressing about measuring and counting to see if your portion sizes and snacks are correct? It is here.

Years ago, having tasty alternatives to eating healthier meals and snacks was hard to find and usually were expensive. Not anymore, we are fortunate to be living in a time with massive, convenient weight loss food options to choose from.

When it comes to who will be cooking our food, and what kind of snacks we will be eating, we have the choice to decide. The good part, it does not have to involve a lot of work or guilt for eating something that is not helping us reach our weight loss goals.

Hands down, your success in losing and maintaining weight will be linked to the food you eat. Whether it is fast-food, takeout, snacks, cooking at home or eating at restaurants, the food matters. In the next section, we will go over how the *Weight Loss Food Shift* can position and prepare you for being food successful. These are the same steps I took on my journey, which empowered me to be able to lose my weight.

They are broken down into four steps. **Step 1**: Is about the ways, you can still lose weight eating at fast-food places and restaurants and save more of your money. **Step 2**: Is the building of your *Food Arsenal*. This is significant because it applies to the times when you are at work, home, and eating with family and friends.

Step 3: Includes tips on cooking successfully at home, shopping in the grocery store, portion sizes, recipes, and tools to make life easier in the kitchen. Lastly, **Step 4:** Is a variety of food options from meal delivery kit services, to provide convenience, and ease while you are losing weight.

STEP 1 OF THE WEIGHT LOSS FOOD SHIFT:

EATING OUT

Here we go, **Step 1**, the good stuff, eating out. At, some point, on your weight loss journey, this can be a reality, that can happen. Whether it be takeout, fast-food, or restaurants. No worries if you decide to because there are a few ways you can effectively eat out, enjoy the food, and not interfere with reaching your goal weight.

My number one tip to eating out successfully while losing weight is to remove the words "combo" and "meal" from your vocabulary. Driving up and ordering your food by a number ("Let me get a #3, large with no pickles, and a Coke") is not going to help you with reaching your goal weight. I am not saying you cannot still eat at those places, because you can. However, the *shift* is going to require a little different technique when ordering your food and to take note of the nutritional contents of your choices.

When eating out, by not ordering the combo, or the meal, it is not only going to be a savings in your wallet, but also a savings on your hips. Let me explain. The examples we will look at in the next section will show breakfast, lunch and dinner options and the nutritional information. They are from, a few popular, fast-food and dine-in restaurants. I also included the cost of the food. (28) No judgement, some of the restaurants listed are the ones I used to frequently visit and were on a first name basis with some of the staff. If you take a look at the calories, fat grams and net carbs of the meals in each example, you will see at first glance, they could cost a majority of a person's daily body budget, if not all in one meal. See if you can spot any meals you may have ordered previously. Each example comes with a daily body budget, so you can see what would be the better of the choices to make.

Why is This Important to Know? Seeing the numbers in black and white can help you gain an understanding of why the *weight loss food shift* is an important step to take. If you are going to be successful with losing weight and position yourself to maintain it as well, seeing where to spend and how not to spend your daily body budget can be beneficial.

The reason I included the cost is, because later in the book, when we get to the food from the meal delivery services, it can seem expensive at first glance. It was for me when I first looked, into ordering from them. I thought, wait a minute, $60.00 for six prepackaged meals is a lot and so was, $110.00 for twelve meals. That was until I broke down the cost per meal, which was between $9.00-$10.00 a meal. When I compared those prices to my everyday spending at local takeout and fast-food restaurants, I realized there was not much of a difference.

For instance, in the upcoming examples, take note of several of the items on the menus and their prices. Based on the calculations of the meals I ordered from the delivery services, the healthier options I chose, cost less or, in some instances, about the same of what I paid for an unhealthy meal. Not to mention the savings on not eating the excess calories if I decided to eat a fast-food or take-out meal instead.

A part of your *weight loss food shift* will be to use your actual money and your daily body budget wisely to help you lose weight and save money at the same time. **When eating out, the question is not so much about the things you cannot have on the menu, but rather, what can your body budget afford?** As you know, when starting the *6-Week Program*, you will have your daily body budget numbers of calories, fat grams and net carbs, for the day to spend on your food intake. As you look at the examples think of the ways your weight loss food shift will change how you order when eating out.

For the first example, on the next page it is, McDonald's, and your Daily Body Budget is: 1800 calories, 56-60 fat grams and 50-100 net carbs. Compare the Grilled Chicken Club Sandwich with the Big Mac and see how the calories and net carbs are almost the same! The grilled chicken option on the menu may not always be the healthiest choice when you are deciding on what to eat. With the *weight loss food shift,* if you did decide to eat from this type of menu, look at how much of your daily budget you will save by not ordering the combo, and holding the French Fries, hash browns, and the drinks. *Holding the bun and just eating the meat, (Keto), or only eating one half of the bun, (Low-Carb), can save you even more calories and lower your carb intake.

McDonald's

> * $2.99 **Hot and Spicy Chicken Biscuit**
> 410 Calories, 20 Fat Grams, 39 Net Carbs
> * $4.80 -**2 Sausage Burritos**
> Burritos: 380 Calories, 16 Fat Grams, 26 Net Carbs
> Hash Browns:150 Calories, 9 Fat Grams, 15 Net Carbs
> 10 oz OJ: 140 Calories, 0 Fat Grams, 30 Net Carbs
> * $5.49 **Hot Cakes and Sausage**
> 520 Calories, 24 Fat Grams, 58 Net Carbs
> * $5.36 **Southwest Chicken Salad**
> Salad: 450 Calories, 22 Fat Grams, 35 Net Carbs
> * $7.16 **Grilled Chicken Club Sandwich Meal** (Large)
> Sandwich: 510 Calories, 10 Fat Grams, 41 Net Carbs
> Fries: 490 Calories, 24 Fat Grams, 63 Net Carbs
> 40 oz Drink: 420 Calories, 0 Fat Grams, 55 Net Carbs
> * $7.27 **10-Piece Nugget Meal (**Large)
> Nuggets: 470 Calories, 30 Fat Grams, 28 Net Carbs
> Fries: 490 Calories, 24 Fat Grams, 63 Net Carbs
> 40 oz Drink: 420 Calories, 0 Fat Grams, 55 Net Carbs
> * $7.16 **McWrap Chicken Bacon Wrap Meal** (Large)
> Sandwich: 630 Calories, 32 Fat Grams, 53 Net Carbs
> Fries: 490 Calories, 24 Fat Grams, 63 Net Carbs
> 40 oz Drink: 420 Calories, 0 Fat Grams, 55 Net Carbs
> * $6.71 **Big Mac Meal** (Large)
> Sandwich: 530 Calories, 30 Fat Grams, 44 Net Carbs
> Fries: 490 Calories, 24 Fat Grams, 63 Net Carbs
> 40 oz Drink: 420 Calories, 0 Fat Grams, 55 Net Carbs

Weight Loss Tip: Burger wraps? Yes. In a Ziplock bag, I sometimes carry a couple of low-carb wraps in my purse on the days I know I will order a Bunless burger. I put the meat, cheese, lettuce, tomato, and onions in the wrap. I also eat one of my snacks I carry with me and drink plenty of water. By doing this, it saves money, as, well as I still get to eat out, and it does not spend a lot of my daily body budget.

For the Burger King example, your Daily Body Budget is: 1600 calories, 50-53 fat grams, 40-50 net carbs. Would you order from this menu? Compare the Whopper with the Impossible Whopper (plant-based burger) and see the calories, fat grams and the net carbs in both. The Impossible Whopper is higher in fat and carbs than the Whopper. Plant-Based foods may not always be the best choice for your daily body budget on the menu when eating out. As with the first example, with the *shift*, if you decide to eat from this menu, look at how much of your daily budget you will save by not ordering the combo and holding the French Fries, hash browns, and the drinks.

Burger King

* $5.36 **Croissan'wich with Egg Cheese Ham Meal** (Medium)
Sandwich: 330 Calories, 16 Fat Grams, 29 Net Carbs
Hash Browns: 480 Calories, 33 Fat Grams, 45 Net Carbs
10 oz OJ: 140 Calories, 0 Fat Grams, 30 Net Carbs
* $5.36 **Biscuit with Egg Cheese Bacon Meal**
Biscuit: 380 Calories, 23 Fat Grams, 29 Net Carbs
Hash Browns: 480 Calories, 33 Fat Grams, 45 Net Carbs
10 oz OJ: 140 Calories, 0 Fat Grams, 30 Net Carbs
* $7.72 **Impossible Crossiant Meal** (Medium)
Sandwich: 491 Calories, 29 Fat Grams, 34 Net Carbs
Hash Browns: 480 Calories, 33 Fat Grams, 45 Net Carbs
10 oz OJ: 140 Calories, 0 Fat Grams, 30 Net Carbs
* $7.27 **Whopper Meal** (Large)
Burger: 678 Calories, 37 Fat Grams, 48 Net Carbs
Fries: 430 Calories, 19 Fat Grams, 57 Net Carbs
40 oz Drink: 420 Calories, 0 Fat Grams, 55 Net Carbs
* $8.39 **Crispy Chicken Sandwich Meal** (Large)
Sandwich: 670 Calories, 41 Fat Grams, 51 Net Carbs

Fries: 430 Calories, 19 Fat Grams, 57 Net Carbs
40 oz Drink: 420 Calories, 0 Fat Grams, 55 Net Carbs
* $7.16 **Big Fish Meal** (Large)
Sandwich: 510 Calories, 28 Fat Grams, 48 Net Carbs
Fries: 430 Calories, 19 Fat Grams, 57 Net Carbs
40 oz Drink: 420 Calories, 0 Fat Grams, 55 Net Carbs
* $6.71 **10-Piece Chicken Nugget Meal** (Large)
Nuggets: 430 Calories, 27 Fat Grams, 24 Net Carbs
Fries: 430 Calories, 19 Fat Grams, 57 Net Carbs
40 oz Drink: 420 Calories, 0 Fat Grams, 55 Net Carbs
* $9.16 **Impossible Whopper Meal** (Large)
Sandwich: 628 Calories, 34 Fat Grams, 54 Net Carbs
Fries: 430 Calories, 19 Fat Grams, 57 Net Carbs
40 oz Drink: 420 Calories, 0 Fat Grams, 55 Net Carbs

For the Arby's example, your Daily Body Budget is: 1700 calories, 53-56 fat grams, 20-50 net carbs. Have you eaten any of these items before? When you compare the Creamy Mediterranean Chicken Wrap to the Classic Roast Beef Sandwich, you will see how the Chicken Wrap is higher in calories, fat grams and the carbs are almost the same. When eating out, do not let the name of the meal fool you into thinking it will always be the healthier of the choices. As we will discuss later in the book, the Mediterranean Diet is one of the eating styles you can use to help you lose weight. However, just because a dish has the name in it does not mean it is the best choice. You can check the nutritional facts information on most fast-food and dine-in restaurants' websites. Or you can also go to calorieking.com and nutritionix.com for free and look up the information there.

Arby's

* $6.37 **Classic Roast Beef Sandwich Meal**
Sandwich: 450 Calories, 20 Fat Grams, 43 Net Carbs
Fries: 250 Calories, 13 Fat Grams, 26 Net Carbs
Drink: 400 Calories, 0 Fat Grams, 44 Net Carbs
* $8.61 **SmokeHouse Brisket Sandwich**
600 Calories, 35 Fat Grams, 39 Net Carbs
Drink: 400 Calories 0 Fat Grams, 44 Net Carbs
* $8.50 **Roast Turkey Ranch Bacon Meal**

630 Calories, 32 Fat Grams, 40 Net Carbs
Fries: 250 Calories, 13 Fat Grams, 26 Net Carbs
Drink: 400 Calories, 0 Fat Grams, 44 Net Carbs
* $7.27 **Crispy Chicken Sandwich Meal**
510 Calories, 25 Fat Grams, 44 Net Carbs
Fries: 250 Calories, 13 Fat Grams, 26 Net Carbs
Drink: 400 Calories, 0 Fat Grams, 44 Net Carbs
* $7.87 **Creamy Mediterranean Chicken Wrap Meal**
550 Calories, 30 Fat Grams, 38 Net Carbs
Fries: 250 Calories, 13 Fat Grams, 26 Net Carbs
Drink: 400 Calories, 0 Fat Grams, 44 Net Carbs

Side Note: If you are someone who normally drinks soda, weaning yourself off, over time will be beneficial to your overall success. As you can see from the examples, the soda can be just as many calories as the entrée. I do not know about you, but when I was losing weight, I preferred to eat, my calories, rather than drink them (minus the times when I had liquid meals). A big benefit to following the *Slim Down Level Up Formulas* is, you can use your daily body budget wisely and can eat or drink almost anything. However, to get the biggest bang for the buck and to not completely delete an item out of your diet, you can work on a decreasing plan. For instance, if removing soda from your diet is not a realistic goal for you to *maintain*, then you can reduce your intake each week, and drink more water until you arrive at a point to where drinking soda is a sometimes item. Just keep in mind if you continue to drink sodas, you use a large part of your daily body budget that could otherwise be spent on actual foods.

Your Daily Body Budget for the Chick-Fil-A example on the next page is: 1900 calories, 60-63 fat grams, 40-50 net carbs. Compare the Asian Cobb Chicken Salad to the Chick Fil-A Sandwich and you will notice the salad is higher than the sandwich in calories, fat grams and carbs. When eating out, it is a good idea to check the nutritional information on the items you are looking at, to make sure it is the better of the choices and how much of your daily budget you are spending on the entrée. Based on all the items listed, the better of the choices would be the 12-Piece Grilled Chicken Nuggets, because they are only 200 calories, 5 fat grams and

2 net carbs (not the combo, just the nuggets). They do offer side salads and with any of their salads, you can opt for grilled chicken instead of the fried.

Chick-Fil-A

* $5.92- **4-Piece Chick-n-Mini's Combo**
Mini's: 350 Calories, 14 Fat Grams, 40 Net Carbs
Hash Browns: 240 Calories, 16 Fat Grams, 23 Net Carbs
OJ: 160 Calories, 0 Fat Grams, 23 Net Carbs
* $5.54 **Bacon Egg Cheese Biscuit**
420 Calories, 21 Fat Grams, 41 Net Carbs, OJ: 160 Calories, 0 Fat, 38 Net Carbs
* $5.43 **Breakfast Burrito**
Burritos: 680 Calories, 38 Fat Grams, 50 Net Carbs
Hash Browns: 420 Calories, 21 Fat Grams, 41Net Carbs
* $6.33 **Chicken Egg Cheese Bagel**
Bagel: 480 Calories, 18 Fat Grams, 51 Net Carbs
Hash Browns: 240 Calories, 16 Fat Grams, 23 Net Carbs
OJ: 160 Calories, 0 Fat Grams, 23 Net Carbs
* $6.65 **Chick-Fil-A Sandwich Combo**
Sandwich: 440 Calories, 17 Fat Grams, 40 Net Carbs
French Fries: 420 Calories, 24 Fat Grams, 41 Net Carbs
Drink: Lemonade 220 Calories, 0 Fat Grams, 58 Net Carbs
* $9.62 - **12- Piece Grilled Chicken Nugget Combo**
Nuggets: 200 Calories, 5 Fat Grams, 2 Net Carbs
Fries: 420 Calories, 24 Fat Grams, 41 Net Carbs
Drink: Dr Pepper 390 Calories, 0 Fat Grams, 48 Net Carbs
* $9.13 **Grilled Chicken Cool Wrap Combo**
Wrap: 350 Calories, 28 Fat Grams, 42 Net Carbs
Fries: 420 Calories, 24 Fat Grams, 41 Net Carbs
Drink: Coke 420 Calories, 0 Fat Grams, 39 Net Carbs
* $8.05 **Asian Cobb Chicken Salad**
540 Calories, 29 Fat Grams, 27 Net Carbs

Weight Loss Tip: When I was losing weight, one of the things that was helpful to me, was whenever I ate something, I drank 16-20 ounces of water (a little before, during and after eating). This helped me save, money and calories by not ordering the drink when eating out and, it made me feel fuller eating less calories. Incorporating more water, into your diet, if it isn't already, can be a wonderful way to help you reach your weight loss goals.

For the Chipotle example, your Daily Body Budget is: 1500 calories, 46-50 fat grams, 20-50 net carbs. This is one of those menus that can be a little tricky when you hear the name of the items. Because I think most people may think the chicken would be the better choice. Compare the Keto Salad Bowl to the Chicken Bowl and look at the calories, fat grams and net carbs. This is an example of why I like being exposed to food from different diets. These two dishes are similar in fat grams; however, the Keto Salad Bowl is 150 calories less and 39 net carbs less than the Chicken Bowl! That can be a huge savings on your daily body budget numbers. When eating out, be open, to looking at the different styles of food from all the diets you will learn in this book, because it may help you spend less of your body budget. While still being able to eat tasty foods. If you decide to eat from this type of a menu, they do offer options where you can add or delete items to your bowls, tacos and burritos that can lower the calories, fat grams and net carbs.

Chipotle

> * $7.50 **Steak Burrito**
> 825 Calories, 36 Fat Grams, 88 Net Carbs
> * $6.50 **Vegetarian Burrito**
> 715 Calories, 16 Fat Grams, 82 Net Carbs
> * $7.50 **Chicken Bowl**
> 685 Calories, 35 Fat Grams, 56 Net Carbs
> * $7.50 **Steak Tacos**
> 3 Tacos: 1085 Calories, 49 Fat Grams, 92 Net Carbs
> * $9.25 **Paleo Salad Bowl**
> 460 Calories, 29 Fat Grams, 20 Net Carbs
> * $9.25 **Keto Salad Bowl**
> 535 Calories, 36 Fat Grams, 17 Net Carbs

FOOD FACT ALERT: The fast-food, takeout and restaurant industry has profited heavily from our food addictions and struggles with being overweight and obese. **In 2015, globally, they generated $570 Billion dollars from people eating out. Of which, $200 Billion dollars came from the eating habits of Americans. That was a huge jump in revenue compared to what the United States spent in 1970, which was $6 Billion dollars.** (29) Over the years, the *convenient* food industry has made it so easy to have a weight problem by constantly serving larger portions of food. Instead of contributing to helping us lose weight, they keep adding things like 'double, triple, ultimate, extreme' items, with extra-large portion sizes to their menus. Some have gotten better and have added healthier items to choose. But the bulk of the menus are the real money makers, and I do not see them reducing their portion sizes any time soon. When you make the *weight loss food shift,* they are not going to like that you will be spending less of your money on their meals, entrées, and overall eating less. The fact is, the financial savings of your choices will stay in your wallet and the true savings, of bettering your health by eating healthier foods instead, will be priceless.

Your Daily Body Budget for the Popeyes example is: 1400 calories, 42-46 fat grams, 20-50 net carbs. This example is not a comparison as much as it is about looking at the amount of your daily body budget, that would be spent on some of their menu items. This is a situation where even if you hold the French Fries and the drink, the entrée is still high on the calories, fat grams and net carbs scale. If you choose to order something from their menu, you can do two things to help with reducing the amount of your body budget you will spend. One, order the entrée only, and two, eat only half of it. You could share the rest with family or a friend. **I am not big on throwing food out or being wasteful. So, on the days you decide to eat something from a menu like this, planning to have someone to share your food with can be helpful. If not, you may decide to throw the rest away, so you are not tempted to keep eating it. If you do eat the other part of the entrée, just remember it falls in the category of a sometimes food. And it is okay. Just like we talked about in Chapter 10, just make better choices at the next meal or the next day. By making the *weight loss food shift,* you are already saving money and spending less of your daily body budget, because you are not ordering the combo or the meal regularly.

Popeyes

> * $7.69 **Classic Chicken Sandwich Combo**
> Sandwich: 699 Calories, 42 Fat Grams, 48 Net Carbs
> Fries: 268 Calories, 14 Fat Grams, 30 Net Carbs

Drink-22 oz: 270 Calories, 0 Fat Grams, 73 Net Carbs
* $7.99 – **3-Piece Dinner Combo** (2 thighs and a leg)
600 Calories, 51 Fat Grams, 17 Net Carbs
Fries: 268 Calories, 14 Fat Grams, 30 Net Carbs
Drink-22 oz: 270 Calories, 0 Fat Grams, 73 Net Carbs
* $6.99 **1/4 Pound Shrimp Combo**
390 Calories, 25 Fat Grams, 24 Net Carbs
Fries: 268 Calories, 14 Fat Grams, 30 Net Carbs
Drink-22 oz: 270 Calories, 0 Fat Grams, 73 Net Carbs
* $9.29 – **5-Piece Tender Combo**
741 Calories, 34 Fat Grams, 45 Net Carbs
Fries: 268 Calories, 14 Fat Grams, 30 Net Carbs
Drink-22 oz: 270 Calories, 0 Fat Grams, 73 Net Carbs

For the Buffalo Wild Wings and Firehouse Subs examples, your Daily Body Budget is: 1800 calories, 50-56 fat grams, 50-100 net carbs. These two food places are listed and can represent other wing places and sub shops you may have visited or will visit on your weight loss journey. In this case, knowing what the nutritional information is, can help you make a better choice. It can also allow you the opportunity to decide if eating half of an entrée you want, would fit into your body budget. With the *shift*, you will save money and make others happy if you share your meals with them. For example, instead of having the ten wings, you could give five to a friend and maybe have the other five with a side salad.

Buffalo Wild Wings

* $10.99 **Traditional 10 Wings**
720 Calories, 41 Fat Grams, 30 Net Carbs
* $10.49- **5-Piece Crispy Tenders**
820 Calories, 40 Fat Grams, 53 Net Carbs
* $11.29 **All American Cheeseburger**
820 Calories, 53 Fat Grams, 35 Net Carbs
* $10.79 **Southwest Philly Cheesesteak**
680 Calories, 27 Fat Grams, 56 Net Carbs
* $9.29 **Buffalo Ranch Chicken Wrap**
780 Calories, 44 Fat Grams, 66 Net Carbs

> * $11.29 **Chicken Caesar Salad**
> 780 Calories, 59 Fat Grams, 25 Net Carbs

Firehouse Subs

> * $8.69 **Firehouse Steak and Cheese (Medium)**
> 830 Calories, 51 Fat Grams, 49 Net Carbs
> * $9.49 **Smokehouse Beef and Cheddar (Medium)**
> 890 Calories, 59 Fat Grams, 57 Net Carbs
> * $8.79 **Turkey Bacon Ranch (Medium)**
> 830 Calories, 48 Fat Grams, 57 Net Carbs
> * $8.39 **Corn Beef Brisket (Medium)**
> 740 Calories, 39 Fat Grams, 50 Net Carbs
> * $8.79 **Grilled Chicken Breast (Medium)**
> 720 Calories, 36 Fat Grams, 52 Net Carbs

Weight Loss Tip: When eating out, you can look at ordering from the kid's menu or if it applies, from the senior's menu, as they usually cost less, and the portion sizes are smaller.

The next example IHOP; is one of those dine-in restaurants where I used to hurt myself with the amount of food I would eat. After looking up the nutritional information, I realized, I was constantly choosing the heaviest meals to eat. It was no wonder how I got to be over 300 pounds! Look, at the numbers of the Country Fried Steak and Eggs, the BBQ Bacon Cheeseburger, and the Breakfast Sampler. This type of dine-in restaurant can be a little tough when it comes to making the *shift*. Even if you cut the portions in half, some of the meals will still be too high and could use up a lot of your daily budget. If you choose to go, look for the better options on the menu, cut the portions in half, and make your trips there, *special sometimes* outings (not weekly visits like I used to).

IHOP

> * **$6.79 Pancakes (3)**
> 430 Calories, 17 Fat Grams, 53 Net Carbs
> * **$8.99 The Big Steak Omelette**
> 1040 Calories, 69 Fat Grams, 34 Net Carbs
> * **$8.99 Chicken Fajita Omelette**

910 Calories, 57 Fat Grams, 22 Net Carbs
* $7.99 **Country Fried Steak & Eggs**
1360 Calories, 87 Fat Grams, 98 Net Carbs
* $8.49 **Breakfast Sampler**
850 Calories, 54 Fat Grams, 56 Net Carbs
* $6.79 **Strawberry Banana French Toast**
840 Calories, 31 Fat Grams, 112 Net Carbs
* $6.99 **BBQ Bacon Cheeseburger**
950 Calories, 54 Fat Grams, 72 Net Carbs
* $7.99 **Philly Cheese Steak Super Stacker**
800 Calories, 40 Fat Grams, 56 Net Carbs
* $6.49 **Turkey Sandwich**
550 Calories, 27 Fat Grams, 31 Net Carbs
* $12.99 **T-Bone Steak (10oz)** with potatoes and corn
890 Calories, 38 Fat Grams, 42 Net Carbs
* $9.99 **Grilled Tilapia Hollandaise**
825 Calories, 33 Fat Grams, 39 Net Carbs with potatoes and corn
* $8.99 **Chicken Spinach Salad**
1160 Calories, 79 Fat Grams, 30 Net Carbs

Side Note: Craving French Fries? During your weight loss journey if you are craving some fries, you can do one of two things to satisfy your tastebuds, save money and not spend a large part of your daily body budget. One, you can order a kids' meal, as stated, their portions are usually smaller and cost less. You can eat the fries but do not have the soft drink that comes with the meal. Or two, you can just have an order of fries, therefore creating a meatless meal. If it is one of those splurge situations and you want the combo, eat the combo. Just remember to make better choices the remaining part of the day or the next day to get back on track with eating healthier meals.

These last two examples, Olive Garden and Red Lobster, can be comparable to other Italian or Seafood restaurants when it comes to the types of food you may decide to choose from, while losing weight. You can use the cut the portion in half technique when ordering or order from the kid's or seniors menu to help with keeping your daily body budget in check. However, the key point to make with these types of restaurants is, to take note of the nutritional information with the breadsticks and biscuits that come *free* with any meal. They can add up quickly and probably should be avoided or limited because they can use up a lot of your daily budget. (Confession Time: My old eating habits, before the shift, was so out of control. Besides eating the whole meal at places like these, I used to eat 6-8 breadsticks, or 5-6 biscuits! Look at the calories, fat grams and net carbs for each one).

Olive Garden

*$18.79 **Chicken and Shrimp Carbonara**
1390 Calories, 94 Fat Grams, 71 Net Carbs
*$16.99 **Shrimp Alfredo**
1370 Calories, 90 Fat Grams, 91 Net Carbs
*$13.29 **Eggplant Parmigiana**
1060 Calories, 54 Fat Grams, 102 Net Carbs
*$17.99 **Tour of Italy (Chicken Parmigiana, Lasagna, Fettuccine Alfredo)**
1680 Calories, 104 Fat Grams, 96 Net Carbs
*Each Breadstick is: 140 Calories, 2.5 Fat Grams, 25 Net Carbs

Red Lobster

*$9.79 **Parrot Isle Jumbo Shrimp**
960 Calories, 61 Fat Grams, 69 Net Carbs
*$12.99 **Maple Glaze Chicken**
470 Calories, 7 Fat Grams, 46 Net Carbs
*$6.79 **Lobster Bisque** (Bowl)
600 Calories, 28 Fat Grams, 23 Net Carbs
*$14.29 **Classic Caesar Salad with Salmon**
830 Calories, 52 Fat Grams, 13 Net Carbs
*$18.49 **Seaside Shrimp Trio**
1560 Calories, 66 Fat Grams, 94 Net Carbs
*$25.99 **Bar Harbour Lobster Bake**
1150 Calories, 72 Fat Grams, 64 Net Carbs
*$12.99 **Hand battered Fish and Chips**
980 Calories, 48 fat Grams, 68 Net Carbs
*Each Biscuit: 160 Calories, 10 Fat Grams, 16 Net Carbs

Side Note: For these two examples, your Daily Body Budget is: 1700 calories, 53-56 fat grams and 20-50 net carbs. Take a look at my three, previously, all-time favorite menu items, Shrimp and Chicken Carbonara, the Tour of Italy, and the Seaside Shrimp Trio. If you were to order either of those and eat the whole meal, it would cost almost your entire day's budget and that isn't even adding in the breadsticks or biscuits, let alone a soft drink or a cocktail!

Not that you can't eat at places like these because you can. However, eating half of the portion and drinking water as, well, as limiting your breadsticks or biscuits consumption, will be how you can manage outings like these successfully.

Eating out with friends and family can be fun and is a reality. But when you are deciding to make healthier eating choices in your life, making the shift can be a little intimating, as to what you should eat. If you are going to eat out at a restaurant or at the homes of family or friends, follow this rule, **"Whenever in doubt, (or eating out) take half of it out."** I am a big believer in this saying because when eating out, you may not be able to get an exact amount of the calories, fat grams and net carbs. Life is going to happen during and after you reach your goal weight. Having multiple food options available and knowing which foods you can choose, will encourage you to stick to your long-term plan, of eating healthier. With making the *shift*, it is something you can adapt to and still be able to enjoy good tasting foods.

Recap: When eating out, if you see something on the menu you would like to enjoy, order it. When the food comes to the table, ask your server for a to-go box and remove half of the portion off of your plate, right away, and set it to the side. Or offer some to your friends or family. By doing this, you can avoid being wasteful and not overeating. If sharing your food with someone is not an option, depending on what it is, you can have something to eat for lunch the next day with the other portion.

Best Tips on How to Eat Healthy at Restaurants

1. Order Water or Unsweet Tea

2. Hold the Butter and Oils

3. Be Cautious of Salad Dressings (ask for it on the side and dip salad into it)

4. Avoid the Breadsticks/Biscuits and Butter (even if it comes free with the meal-or limit your consumption)

5. Plan Ahead for What You Want to Order (look up nutritional information prior)

6. At Buffets, Keep to the One Plate, One Trip Rule (only one time up to the buffet/one meal)

7. Plan to Take Leftovers Home (whenever eating out, take half of it out)

STEP 2 OF THE WEIGHT LOSS FOOD SHIFT:
WEIGHT LOSS MRE'S

This brings us to **Step 2** in the *weight loss food shift* equation. It is a very, important step in making the shift easier. It is time to make your Weight Loss MRE Kits. Let me explain.

In the military, from what I know, the importance of having the right equipment and being well prepared is essential. Not having to think about what you will eat or drink is also important. Especially in battle. Having what you need when you need it, is key. This is why soldiers are given compact food packages called MRE's. (30) Which stands for Meals Ready (to) Eat. So, they do not have to worry about where their next meal is coming from. If you have never seen one, picture a rectangle vacuum sealed package about 12" long, 8" wide and 3" high. Filled with essential meal items packed with nutrients. They are light weight and easy to store and can be taken anywhere.

Your *weight loss food shift,* and your ability to stand up in the ring and fight to dominate losing weight, is a battle we are getting you prepared to face. You have already begun positioning yourself to add to your *Food Arsenal* with successful ways to eat out. We will also discuss additional food and meal options and how to make it easier for you with cooking your own meals at home. All, of these steps will be centered around you, being able to have the convenience and access to a variety of food while losing weight.

Therefore, we cannot leave out your Weight Loss MRE Kits. They are too important to your success.

TO SNACK OR NOT TO SNACK WHILE DIETING?

Depending on which weight loss book you read, or who you ask, this question can pose different responses. I believe snacking is more than okay if you, 1. Budget for it, 2. Make sure it is inside of your eating window if you are fasting, and 3. That it is not late at night, past your, eating cut off time. The key is to plan for what you will be snacking on, and it does not only include fruits and vegetables either.

Making the *weight loss food shift* does not mean to completely do away with your cravings and ignore them altogether when they happen. That is not realistic nor is it a good idea because as we discussed earlier in the book, that can lead to binge eating. While losing weight you, may have cravings for something salty, sweet, or crunchy. What will you eat when this happens?

There are so many snack options to choose from in the grocery store. A good rule of thumb I have used when snacking is to follow the **140/4 Rule**. Which is to primarily choose snacks that are no more than 140 calories and 4 fat grams each. When I snack, what I usually do is budget for two snacks in between each meal. They, are there, if and when I need them. While fasting, it usually equates to once a day of snacking inside of my eating window.

There is a clause in the snacking deal I made with myself. First, I drink 16-20 ounces of water while snacking (that includes before, during and after the snacks). Second, I can choose a packaged snack as one of my choices, but if I do, I will make the second snack some type of fruit or vegetable to either compliment or go with my first snack.

Third, if I do not go with the first type of combination, then I can choose to combine my calories and fat grams and use them on one item. So, instead of the 140/4 Rule for each snack, I would combine the two and use up to 280 calories and 8 fat grams on my one selection. In short, it is either two snacks that fall under the rule or one snack with the combined amount of the two.

Here are examples of using both options: For my first snack example, because I am craving something salty, I choose to have a pack of 100-calorie mini pretzels. My second snack would be ½ cup of strawberries, because I am also craving something sweet. Both snacks are under the 140/4 Rule and satisfied both my sweet and salty cravings.

The key thing to point out in this type of example is, to select and budget for the first snack and then, based on that choice, to combine it with either fresh fruits or vegetables. One of the main reasons I used this technique is because of how much the net carbs can be in the packaged items selected. What I mean by that is, I spent 21 net carbs on the mini pretzels, of my 50-100 net carbs max daily budget. The ½ cup of strawberries was 30 calories and 6 net carbs. In total, my two snacks equaled 130 calories, 0 fat grams and 27 net carbs. This is, why, in Chapter 10, I talked about using all *three* numbers on the daily body budget charts: calories, fat grams, and net carbs, so that the food choices you make are healthier, more well-rounded ones (with a few splurge items in there, too).

For instance, for my second snack example, instead of two snacks, I choose to combine my budget and splurge on a 3-pack of Chips Ahoy Cookies. Which is 160 calories, 8 fat grams and 22 net carbs (it has 11 grams of sugar). **Yes, I chose that as my option because, in my world, where I live and diet, eating cheeseburgers, chocolate cake, as, well as, cookies is allowed.**

You are probably thinking wow, these examples are not traditional diet food talk, and they include processed packaged foods. Aren't I supposed to stay away from those while losing weight?

That is why I purposefully used those types of examples to make a point. Most diets preach and tell you to stay away from all processed foods. That is not realistic nor is it going to be a reality you can maintain. I have known quite a few dieters in my life, and unfortunately, I remember several of them, telling me they started a diet, rushed out and only shopped at whole food stores. Threw everything away in their pantry and refrigerator and said they would never buy packaged foods again. Making someone think those are the steps required to lose weight is why people fail at dieting. It can be too structured and limited in food choices. Especially choices that do not fit into everyday real-life experiences.

I have a secret to tell you. I lost weight eating some processed foods, but by following my daily body budget numbers, the reduction in how much I was eating, compensated for my choices. That is because the daily budget is what is key, above all.

For example, have you ever heard the story about the Twinkie Diet? In 2010, there was a nutrition Professor from Kansas State University, who wanted to show his students that it did not matter what they ate. (31) As long as they reduced their calories to create a calorie deficit, they could lose some weight. He conducted his own experiment using this theory and reduced his daily caloric intake to 1,800 calories. The thing was, to prove his point even further, he used about two-thirds of the 1,800 calories eating food found at convenience stores. Like Twinkies, Little Debbie's, Doritos, donuts, and a host of other snacks. He took a multivitamin and drank a protein shake once a day. At the end of the two-month experiment, he lost 27 pounds and lowered his LDL, the bad cholesterol. Making the point, it is not so much about where the calories are coming from, as it is, about *how many* are being consumed. (Just for the record, I am not recommending you try this diet, nor was it, I was trying to duplicate it when I had my Twinkie binge eating session I mentioned in Chapter 10).

You are probably going to eat some processed foods while making the *weight loss food shift*. Contrary to what you may have been told, it is okay. The goal is to get you to start reducing the amount, of processed foods you eat and replace the majority, of your diet with more whole foods, lean meats, and even meatless options. But do not put pressure on yourself to say it has to be an all or nothing event and it needs to happen overnight. However, in the first two weeks of the program, you will remove eating mostly processed foods to help jumpstart your weight loss. But you will not remove them completely from your diet while losing weight (think decrease not delete).

The truth is, as we just saw from the Twinkie Diet experiment, you can *technically* eat anything. That is, if your budget can afford the cost of the items. When we look at, the food from structured diets, meal kit services, cooking recipes at home, and with continuing to talk about your Weight Loss MRE Kits, they will all play significant roles on your, journey. Because they will provide healthy well-rounded ways, you can decide to spend your daily body budget.

One of the tips I used when making the *weight loss food shift* that was helpful to me was, to start looking at eating and making food choices like shopping for clothes or shoes. I may see something I like and want it, but because of the price tag, I may have to shop on the clearance rack and choose something else instead. That is not a bad thing, because my second choice can be just as good as the first one but cost me less. This is not to say I have never had the more expensive item because there were times when I did. I would either plan for it, or if I went over budget enjoying it, I just put my eating right back in line with making better choices, for the rest of the day and started fresh the next day. (If the splurge happened before dinnertime, what I would normally do is have a liquid/smoothie-dinner instead of my regular meal, to try and balance out my day, and I would not stress about it).

That is because I finally learned to stop slashing my other three tires when I had one flat. You may have heard that analogy as it relates to binge eating. For example, I went to a birthday party one day when I was dieting, and because I *splurged* by having a large piece of chocolate cake and ice cream, I felt bad and started stressing over it. Instead of stopping there and just getting back on track, I went ahead and had two slices of pizza, too. Oh, and a bag of chips as well.

If, while on your journey, you splurge, do not stress about it, or beat yourself up. Just remember the saying, **"Never miss eating a healthy meal more than once." Get right back on track and make the very next meal or food choice a healthier one.**

In the next section, you will see a list of recommended MRE Kits, you can create, as a way to help you prepare for your journey. Especially for when the situations and the needs come up for them. Besides creating the previously mentioned salty, sweet, and crunchy kits, there are a few more you can benefit from while losing weight.

For example, storing a kit at the homes of family and friends you frequently visit can be helpful. Especially during the *shift*, for the times when you want to have an alternative food option, to help keep your budget on track. This was helpful to me when losing weight, because the last thing I was going to find in some of my friends' refrigerators was something healthy to eat. I was not judging them for their food choices, because they used to be my food choices. However, to make the shift easier and to be less tempted to join in and eat the typical snacks or food I used to eat, I kept a few items at their homes for the times when I would need them (Weight Loss MRE Kits can be smaller meals/smoothies/snack options).

For the times, when I went to eat with family or friends and was not sure of the calories, fat grams, and net carbs, I just followed the eating out rule. "Whenever in doubt, take half of it out." What I would also do is fix my food on a smaller plate, or if a smaller plate was not available I would just keep my meal in the center of a regular size plate. Being mindful not to fill my plate up. I would enjoy the company, the food and drink my water and not focus on how much I had just eaten. Remember, life is about balance, follow the 80/20 Rule. As, long as it's not an everyday occurrence of not knowing how much you are eating, it will be okay. You will be fine and still be able to create your calorie deficit for the week.

The other Weight Loss MRE's on the list fall in line with the same philosophy of having kits available for when you need them. Like in the car and at work. Especially at work. I do not know about your work environment situation. However, I can tell you, having MRE Kits at work with me, when I was dieting years ago, was priceless. Have you ever heard of the call center 20-pound spread? It is a statement that says it is inevitable, you will gain at least 20 pounds when working in those types of environments. It is a real thing. The temptation to avoid it, can be hard. For example, when I worked in a call center, every other day it was somebody's birthday cake in the breakroom for all employees to eat. Or if it wasn't someone sitting close by me eating some delicious smelling food, it would either be working lunch Wednesday or potluck Friday. Food was everywhere. Trying to lose weight in that environment was not easy. Especially because the vending machine kept talking to me on my way to the bathroom. It happened several times throughout my shift.

Again, I am not saying I did not join in and eat some of the things with my co-workers. Or that I did not get something out of the snack machine. You know the type of world I live and diet in, so, of course, you know I did. However, I did not make it a recurring event, because it would have hindered my weight loss success.

The last one of the kits I am going to stress the importance on you creating is the Weight Loss MRE Kit for the *morning after* or the *late-night* diet reset. What? Let me explain. Holidays, Special Events, Birthdays and the hanging out partying just because it's Friday Night Events, may take place while you are losing weight. For instance, when I went from 304 pounds down to 143 pounds, in those 15 months, I attended a lot of different events. Some of them involved drinking alcohol too. Unfortunately for me, when that happens, food is usually the only thing on my mind. Most times, greasy and salty food.

What would happen is after some of those events, I would either stop off somewhere and get one or two of my go-to combo meals or go home and cook a not so healthy meal. So, a big part of my *weight loss food shift* involved me having, on standby, some make-ahead meals in the freezer. The kind I could quickly and easily heat up in the microwave. Having kits was helpful in those situations because even though I was eating late at night, at least my food choices were healthier and not packed with excess calories, fat grams or carbs.

The same concept helped me on the occasions when I overate at, the Holidays or Special Events. You ever overeat at Thanksgiving or Christmas dinner? How about at a friend's wedding or birthday party? Or were there times, when you were too tired to cook but needed to eat something that did not include ordering out? No worries, because by having your Weight Loss MRE Kits, (with prepackaged healthier meal options, for the day of or the day after the

STEP 1-2 EATING OUT/MRE KITS

events), you can reset your body budget back in order. Whether it is with preselected meals, smoothies, or snacks. Here are my eleven key words to losing weight:

Create Your MRE Kits, They Will Come In Handy One Day.
WEIGHT LOSS MRE KITS TO MAKE

1. Salty Foods MRE Kit	5. Secret Stash MRE Kit for the car
2. Sweet Foods MRE Kit	6. After/Holidays/Events MRE Kit
3. Crunchy Foods MRE Kit	7. Traveling MRE Kit
4. Secret Stash MRE Kit at work	8. Diet Reset MRE Kit

THE SNACKS

To help you get started with snack ideas and options to build your Weight Loss MRE Snack/Meal Kits, in the next section, multiple lists of a variety of choices for you to use are provided. There are snack ideas under 100 calories, under 200 calories and a list of healthy snack combinations. The key things to look at, when you are choosing your snacks, are the serving size and the calories, fat grams and carbs, listed on the nutrition food labels (if you need to pay attention to sodium and sugar, those numbers are listed also).

After you create your kits and start on the *6-Week Program*, you will have a clearer picture of how, even with eating some packaged foods, and eating out, you can look forward to four things that can happen when following the program:

1. You will use the power of combining different diets together to address the two key factors for weight loss.

2. You will create the desired calorie deficit to lose weight by following the Daily Body Budget Charts.

3. You are going to eat a variety of different foods, some of which may be processed, and you can still lose weight.

4. Over time, you will work towards making the majority, of your diet healthier, with lean meats, whole grains and by incorporating more fruits and vegetables.

36 SNACKS UNDER 100 CALORIES

1. Mini Pretzels (100 calorie packs)

2. Nonfat Yogurt: 6 oz

3. Banana: 1 Small

4. Dark Chocolate: 3 squares (1 oz)

5. Graham Crackers & Peanut Butter

6. Air Popped Popcorn: 3 cups

7. String Cheese (1-2 depending on brand)

8. Laughing Cow Cheese Wedge (each wedge is about 35-45 calories)

9. Turkey Pepperoni (17 slices is about 70 calories)

10. Sherbet: ½ cup of your Favorite Flavor

11. Baked Potato with Salsa (1 small baked potato (2-3oz) with 1 tablespoon salsa)

12. 2-4 Mini Fun Size Candy Bars (check label for correct quantity amount)

13. Seasoned Whole Wheat or Multi- Grain Crackers (about 8-10 crackers)

14. Frozen Banana Dipped in Melted Dark Chocolate (1 small banana and 1 square of dark chocolate melted)

15. 1 Low-Calorie Slice of Bread, Toasted with Sugar-Free Fruit Spread

16. Baby Carrots with Greek Yogurt Ranch Dip (mix 1 cup Greek yogurt with ranch seasoning mix to create a fat-free delicious dip)

17. Chocolate Milk (8 oz skim milk with 1 tablespoon sugar free chocolate syrup)

18. Baby-Bel Cheese Wheel

19. Sugar Free Fudgesicle

20. Small Baked Sweet Potato

21. ½ Toasted English Muffin with Sugar-Free Fruit Spread

22. Turkey Hot Dog (no bun)

23. 8 oz Soft Drink (your favorite flavor -sometimes)

24. Dry cereal: ½ - ¾ cup of your favorite flavor

25. Small Latte with Skim Milk

26. Baked or Grilled Salmon (2 oz with no oil/margarine/butter. Bake or grill with capers, dill, and garlic)

27. ¼ cup of Tuna (canned in water drained with 1 teaspoon of spicy mustard)

28. Nutella: 1 tablespoon

29. Cottage Cheese with Fresh Fruit (1 cup fat-free)

30. Roasted Tomato Slice with Low-Fat Mozzarella (1 small tomato sliced with 2 tablespoons of cheese, with a sprinkle of your favorite Italian seasonings on top)

31. Instant or Overnight Oats (plain – add sugar substitute & cinnamon for flavor)

32. 8 oz V8 (or other tomato juice blend)

33. Hard-Boiled Egg (1 egg with salt & pepper is only 80 calories)

34. Egg White Scramble (2 egg whites, with spinach & diced tomato)

35. Hummus & Vegetables (3 tablespoons of hummus are about 80 calories. You can use carrots, celery, broccoli, etc. for dipping and account for intake accordingly)

36. Low-Fat/Low-Sodium Canned Soup (you can find brands that carry soups under 100 calories per serving of 1- ½ cups)

Inspirational Quote Time

"You will never change your life until you change something you do daily. The secret to your success is found in your daily routine."

John C. Maxwell

30 SNACKS UNDER 100 CALORIES

1 Apple	Nonfat Greek Yogurt	20 Pistachios	2 Cup Melon (diced)	1 ¼ String Cheese
1 Cup Cheerios	1 Cup Strawberries	1 Boiled Egg	3 Cups Air- Popped Popcorn	A frozen Yogurt Bar
Small Latte w/ Skim Milk	1 Cup Sugar Snap Peas	2 Flavored Rice Cakes	Almond (15 pieces)	½ Cup Cottage Cheese
1 Cup Blueberry	1 Orange	½ Cup Oatmeal	2 Egg Whites & 1 Low-Carb Tortilla Wrap	2 Tbsp Hummus & 5 Celery Sticks
28 Grapes	20 Roasted Peanuts	1 Small Banana	4 Medium Carrots	4 Slices of Turkey Breast
1/2 an Avocado	1 Sweet Potato	1/2 Cup of Edamame	33 Cherry Tomatoes	1 Tablespoon of Peanut Butter

16 AMAZING FAT LOSS FOODS*

Strawberries	Watermelon	Peach	Cucumber
34 calories	35 calories	35 calories	15 calories
Honeydew	Blueberries	Pear	Red pepper
59 calories	48 calories	44 calories	33 calories
Orange	Pineapple	Broccoli	Black Cherries
47 calories	50 calories	33 calories	55 calories
Blackberries	Raspberries	Lettuce	Melon
40 calories	44 calories	13 calories	35 calories

*Serving Size=3 oz

SNACK COMBINATIONS UNDER 200 CALORIES

- 1 Apple+1 Slice Reduced Fat Provolone Cheese+0.4 oz. Dark Chocolate=196 calories

- 12 Almonds+7 Small Strawberries+1 cup Dark Chocolate Almond Milk=199 calories

- 1/2 Whole Wheat Bagel+1 tbsp. Low Fat Cream Cheese+1/2 tbsp. Apricot Preserves=179 calories

- 5 Melba Toast Crackers+1 Sliced Tomato+1/4 Cup Fresh Basil Leaves+0.5 oz. Gouda Cheese=164 Calories

- 1 Granola Bar

- 1 Small Pita Pocket, 4" diameter + 1 tbsp. Cashew Butter + 1/4 Cup Blackberries=199 calories

- 27 Cheez-it Crackers

- 2 Celery Stalks+ 1tbsp. Natural Peanut Butter+ 2 tbsp. Raisins=166 calories

- 28 Rold Gold Tiny Twists Pretzels

- 1 Cup Grapefruit Juice+ 10 Pistachios+1 Cup Cubed Cantaloupe=188 calories

SWEET SNACK IDEAS UNDER 200 CALORIES

*1 Skinny Cow Milk Chocolate Wafers *3 Chips Ahoy Chocolate Chip Cookies
*1 Nutri Grain Bar *3 Keebler Deluxe Grahams *4 Mini Fun Size Kit Kat's
*1 Frozen Fruit Bar/Popsicle *2 Mini Fun Size Twix *1/2 cup Frozen Yogurt
*1 Drake's Devil Dog Food Cake *1/2 cup Sherbet *3 Oreo Cookies

*You can also check for a variety of "100 Calorie" and "200 Calorie" pre-packaged snacks in your local grocery store or online. When you do, pay attention to the fat grams and net carbs also when making your selections. Remember to incorporate the **140/4 Rule** and have fun choosing snacks that are low-calorie and the kind you will enjoy.

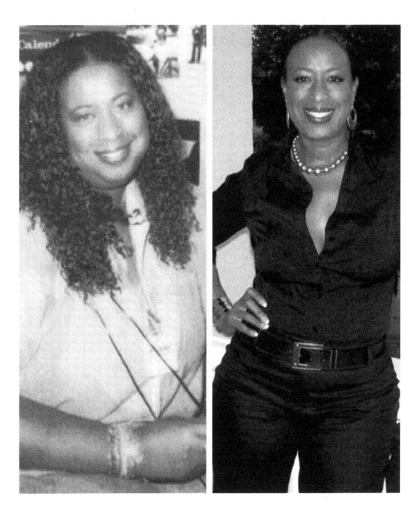

The picture on the left (300 pounds) was during the time when I worked at the call center and had just started losing weight. As I stated earlier, at work, food was always in abundance. Luckily, for me, the picture on the right (143 pounds) was thanks to the power of using the Slim Down Level Up Formulas and having my Weight Loss MRE's with me everywhere I went. Especially at work.

13

STEP 3-4 COOKING/FOOD DELIVERY KITS

STEP 3 OF THE WEIGHT LOSS FOOD SHIFT:
WHO IS COOKING YOUR FOOD?

Up next is **Step 3**, which is for the at-home do-it-yourself chef who wants to start cooking healthier weight loss-friendly meals. Is that going to be you? The good thing is, nowadays, when it comes to cooking, there are a lot of easy to follow, step by step recipes with simple ingredients you can use to lose weight.

Let's be honest again, sister to sister, woman to woman, girlfriend to girlfriend, if you can cook, and have been cooking for years, are some of your go-to recipes not so weight loss-friendly? I will go first, none of mine were, and it was the reason why this part of the *weight loss food shift* needed to take place in my house. Especially if I was going to be successful. I did not grow up learning to cook weight loss meals, they were comfort meals. Even going into adulthood, when I cooked, the only thing on my mind was how to make those same comfort meals even more delicious. Not less fattening.

Let me give you an example of one of my go-to recipes that was, for sure, one of the culprits helping me to pack on the pounds over the years. Here is what my famous, *five-meat baked beans* consisted of. It started out good with having just the baked beans,

193

placed in an oversized aluminum pan. However, this is where it would get interesting, and the comfort part would come in. First, I fried up a whole pack of bacon, put the grease and the strips to the side. Then, cut up and sauteed two different kinds of sausage, one spicy, one regular, and added in ½ pound of small chucks of ham. Then in a separate pan, I fried a pound of ground beef. Once all the meat was ready, that is when, the fun would really begin. I would add white sugar, brown sugar, butter, tons of maple syrup, and a few spices. Baked it in the oven for about 30 minutes and then served it over a bed of white rice. You do not even want to know the calories and fat grams on that recipe.

The point is, my weight loss food shift involved learning to cook food differently than what I was so used to doing. I learned new ways to still make comfort foods I enjoyed but were not so fattening. I still make my baked beans, but with just ground turkey meat, turkey bacon and sausage, with herbs and spices and a little butter. It was a tradeoff, but I was able to make it taste good and for only a third of the fat grams and calories that was in my original recipe.

The *weight loss food shift* in the kitchen is essential to you losing weight. What are you going to cook? How many ounces of food will you eat, and will you measure portion sizes when you make your plate? Who is keeping track of your food intake? Do you have weight-loss friendly recipes ready to use? And are you using cooking instruments to help reduce your time in the kitchen and make cooking easier?

These are the questions that can be easily answered when there is a plan in place. A plan that can simplify you making the shift and creating a new normal in your cooking regimen.

Let us address each one of the questions with tips and resources to set you on a path to making the weight loss food shift easier.

What Are You Going to Cook?

Heading to the grocery store can be a mission within itself. Having a plan and a list as to what you will buy and cook for the week is always a good idea. It can reduce the number of extra items thrown in the cart that may go to waste if you do not cook them.

A well-balanced diet includes a variety of proteins, carbohydrates, and vegetables.

Depending on which diet eating style you choose to follow, your options in the grocery store can be endless when you know what to look for. Here is a reference sheet you can refer to when planning your meals at home. You can select items from each column and plan a delicious meal for you and your family. Quantity sizes will depend on how many servings you will make.

WEIGHT LOSS MEALS REFERENCE SHEET

PROTEIN + CARBOHYDRATES + VEGETABLES		
Chicken	White rice	Broccoli
Ground Turkey	Brown rice	Eggplant
Lean Beef	Cauliflower Rice	Bell Peppers
Shrimp	White/Red Potato	Mushrooms
Tuna	Oats	Carrots
Steak	Beans	Asparagus
Greek Yogurt	Lentils	Cabbage
Salmon	Quinoa	Zucchini
Tofu	Sweet Potato	Cauliflower
Bison	Buckwheat	Brussels Sprouts
Duck	Barley	Okra
Pork Chops	Broccoli Rice	Squash
Prawns	Pasta	Tomatoes
Turkey	Couscous	Collard Greens

How Many Ounces of Food Will You Eat and Will You Measure Your Portion Sizes?

These two questions are significant in making the *weight loss food shift*. Understanding the basics of measuring your food by sight will be helpful. You may order or already have a food measuring tool in your home, to use. However, for those times when you eat out with family and friends and make your own plate, it is a good idea to recognize portions. Provided on the next page is a portion size reference chart you can use when cooking, making your plate at home or eating out. It uses commonly recognizable items, so you have something visual to reference when measuring your portions.

FOOD PORTIONS REFERENCE SHEET

1 CUP = BASEBALL **½ CUP**= LIGHTBULB
1 OZ OR 2 TBSP= GOLF BALL **1 TSP**= POKER CHIP
1 OZ LUNCH MEAT= COMPACT DISC
3 OZ MUFFIN OR BISCUIT = HOCKEY PUCK
1 ½ OZ CHEESE= 3 DICE **1 BREAD SLICE**=CASSETTE TAPE*

*If you're too young to remember cassette tapes you can Google it and see what it looks like

GRAINS	FRUITS & VEGETABLES	MEAT, FISH & NUTS
1cup of Cereal= Baseball	1 Medium Fruit= Baseball	3 oz Lean Meat = Deck of Cards
1 Pancake= Compact Disc	½ cup Grapes=about 16 Grapes	3 oz Fish= Checkbook
½ cup Cooked Rice= Lightbulb	1cup Strawberries= 12 Berries	3 oz Tofu= Deck of Cards
½ cup Cooked Pasta= Lightbulb	1cup Salad Greens= baseball	2 tbsp Peanut Butter= Golf Ball
Baked Potato=Computer Mouse	1cup Carrots= 12 Baby Carrots	2 tbsp Hummus= Golf Ball
1Bagel= 6 oz Can of Tuna	1cup Cooked Vegetables= Baseball	¼ cup Almonds= 23 Almonds

Side Note: Getting control of portion sizes can be easy to misjudge visually when first starting out. It was a little challenging for me initially when fixing my plate because, of the extra-large portions I had gotten used to over the years. In the next section is an easy reference sheet that helped me figure out what my new *weight loss food shift* plate should look like. It may be helpful to you too.

PORTION SIZE YOUR PLATE FOR WEIGHT LOSS

- **½ Plate with Vegetables:** Fill half of your plate with a variety of different vegetables or salad to add more low-calorie dense foods to help you feel fuller longer

- **¼ Plate with Proteins:** Fill a quarter of your plate with low-fat proteins. This can be a better choice for your health and can help reduce belly fat. Look for recipes that include to bake, broil, or grill the meats and add in a variety of herbs and spices to bring out the flavors

- **¼ Plate with Starches:** Fill a quarter of your plate with whole grain starches which can also make you feel fuller longer. Vegetables like yams, potatoes and corn are high in starch and when making your plate, they should go in this spot.

Besides the previously mentioned measuring techniques, you naturally already have one of the best portion control tools ever made, with you. Your hands. Believe it or not, the correct size portions we all need can be dictated by the size of our hands. Here is another reference tool you can use when making your plate and cooking. The open palm of your hand is good for measuring your proteins, your cupped palm is a good measure for your carbs portions, fats is your thumb size (above where it bends) and your vegetables are the size of your closed fist.

Open Palm	Cupped Palm	Thumb Size	Closed Fist
Proteins	**Carbs**	**Fats**	**Vegetables**
Chicken	Rice	Avocado	Broccoli
Fish	Pasta	Eggs	Spinach
Beef	Oats	Whole Cheese	Zucchini
Turkey	Bread	Nuts	Green Beans
Pork	Beans	Butter	Carrots
Tofu	Lentils	Oils	Cauliflower
Salmon	Fruit	Seeds	Asparagus

Who is Keeping Track of Your Food Intake?

Do you want to not worry about writing down or remembering what you ate for the day? Making sure you are in your daily body budget numbers to lose weight and be able to track your activities? If you have not used or heard of fitness tracking apps, they can be a wonderful addition to your weight loss tool bag. Using fitness apps can help you keep track of cutting calories, ensuring you are eating more protein or keep track of your reduced carb intake. They can also be a great tool for shopping in the grocery store and coming up with recipes. In the next section are five free apps I have used and recommend you check out, to see if you would like to use either one of them when you start the *6 Week Program*.

CALORIE/ FITNESS TRACKER APPS

MyFitnessPal! It is a great app to use in helping you keep track of your weight loss goals. Whether you want to lose weight, or change your lifestyle habits, it will provide you the assistance you need. On the main App page, with the information provided, you will see a variety of resources available for you to use:

- Over six million food items in their database to help with calculating your daily intake

- Barcode capabilities with over four million barcodes to logging different foods

- Calorie counter to calculate your food, meals, and recipes

- Tracks calories, fat grams, protein, carbs, sugar, fiber, and cholesterol to name a few

- Food diary log

- Fitness and Steps tracker

- And over 350 exercises to choose from

It is user-friendly in helping you with figuring out your recommended daily caloric intake. To assist you with calculating and tracking how many calories you have consumed daily. It can show how many calories you have remaining for the day as well. This

STEP 3-4 COOKING/FOOD DELIVERY KITS

App provides an exercise log, which tracks how many calories you burned by being active. It is free to download and use, but they do offer a premium subscription.

Lose It! Is a calorie counting app that can be used in helping you lose weight and reach your goals. This app can take a lot of the guesswork out of whether, or not you are creating the desired calorie deficit to lose weight. It provides an easy-to-use food diary and exercise log to assist you on your fitness journey. On the main App page, you will see a variety of options to choose from to track your food, weight, and activities. Some of the other features are:

- Barcode scanning capabilities in helping to track the foods you eat

- Tracks calories, macros, proteins, water, carbs, sugar, to name a few

- Meal planning

- Food log

- Over 27 million searchable foods in their database

- Fitness apps syncing capabilities

- Workout guides and fitness challenges to stay motivated

- Tracks body measurements, sleep cycle and more

Tracking calories is an effective way to be accountable and successful while losing weight. The app offers a personalized approach to assisting you with calculating your daily food needs. Using your weight, height, fitness goals and age, they provide a recommended daily caloric intake. As well as offering a variety of themes to choose from as a way to speak to your personality. The app is free to download and use, but they do offer a premium subscription.

FatSecret! Also referred to as "Calorie Counter by FatSecret." It is an easy-to-use calorie counter app you can utlize in assisting you on your weight loss journey. It can help with providing weekly and monthly caloric intake calculations so you can see your progress along the way. On the main App page, you are provided a variety of features:

- Barcode scanning capabilities

- Easy to use food diary

- Diet calendar to track calories consumed and burned

- Health App, Apple Watch and Fitbit exercise tracking integration

- Weight tracker

- Exercise diary

- Recipes and meal ideas

Tracking apps like this one can be very, helpful in being accountable to yourself. But they also offer a large supportive community you can connect with, to share success stories, support, recipes, and tips. The homepage provides a display showing total caloric intake and the breakdown of protein, fat grams and carbs. They also have a cool feature called Challenges. Users can create or participate in dietary challenges in a closed group. To motivate, encourage and support one another. On their website, they provide information and tips, as well as articles on a variety of different topics. The app is free to download and use, but they do offer a premium subscription.

Cron-o-meter! Is a wonderful app to use to lose weight and reach your fitness goals. Their food diary is user-friendly and easy to follow. What makes them unique is they provide tracking and support for those who are following a Keto, Paleo, Vegan or have a restrictive diet set by their doctor, nutritionist, or dietitian. And based on which diet you are following, the recommended macronutrients will be specific to your selection. On the main App page, you can see a variety of key features available:

- Barcode scanning capabilities

- Tracks calories, protein, carbs, cholesterol and more

- Exercise log

- Custom food and recipes

- Tracks food from restaurants

- Integrates with Apple Watch, Fitbit, Garmin, Withings, Polar and more

- Syncs with Keto-Mojo ketone & glucose meter & Biosense keto breath monitor

- Intermittent Fasting support with a fasting timer

- Provides a Keto calculator

Using this kind of app can be helpful by providing more in-depth data about your health. Besides calories, it tracks up to 82 macronutrients, logs your BMI (Body Mass Index) and your BMR (Basel Metabolic Rate). Which can be helpful if you are following a specific diet and would benefit from tracking those numbers. According to the information on the main App page, it is used and preferred by healthcare professionals and can be synced to the Apple Health App. The app is free to download and use, but they do offer a premium subscription.

SparkPeople! It is an app designed to track your calories and fitness activities to help you lose weight. They provide tools to use whether you are following a Low-Calorie, Atkins, Low-Fat, Weight Watchers, the DASH Diet, or another diet. On the main App page, you will see a list of features available to use:

- Barcode scanning capabilities

- Food tracker

- Meal Planner

- Tracks calories, carbs, protein, fat grams, fiber, cholesterol, and more

- Exercise demos

- Health and Fitness articles provided

- Syncs with Fitbit, MapMyFitness, Misfit, Runkeeper, Garmin, HealthKit & more

Using this app can be useful when trying to lose or maintain weight. They offer over 600,000 recipes to choose from and have created a support community for members to motivate and encourage one another while losing weight. As a member, you can gain access to their vast library of healthy-living fitness videos and exercise planning tools. The app is free to download and use, but they do offer a premium subscription.

Do You Have Weight Loss-Friendly Recipes to Use?

As discussed, having access to a variety of tasty-weight-loss-foods can be essential on your journey. Provided in this section is a list of over 2,000 *free* recipes, tips, and resources, combined, that you can use to lose weight. There is a total of 75 different websites I have used and found awesome recipes and tools. They include a variety of breakfast, lunch, and dinner ideas. Like, soup, salad, smoothie and sandwich recipes with dessert and snack options you can turn to when you need ideas on, what to cook and eat at home. There are even some make ahead, and freeze meal recipes included.

Most of the websites have step by step instructions on how to make the meals, which can be helpful if you're a less experienced at home chef. Some even provide alternate ways the dish can be made to satisfy certain dietary requirements. Like exchanging the meat option, and removing dairy, nuts or soy.

They are free websites, like I said, but some of them have a host of advertisements to weed through before you get to the recipes. Here is a tip to navigate them easily: if you do not need the full instructions on how to make the meal, you can scroll about halfway down the page and get to the good part, the recipe. This is also where you can find, if it is available, the nutritional information to know the daily intake and serving size of the meal. Many of the recipes are in a printable format you can save for later use.

Side Note: When I was making the *shift*, once a week, I would work on building up my recipe stash of weight loss meals. Some of which I was able to find on different websites. I would print out my favorite ones and put them in a folder or screenshot them on my phone to use later. On those days when I could not think of what to cook, the recipes came in handy.

On the websites you will find, Low-Calorie, Low-Carb, Keto, Paleo, Vegan, Mediterranean, and Weight Watchers recipes, snack ideas and tips on meal prepping and more. Weed through all the pop-ups and advertising, and you will find a treasure trove of delicious options to choose from. Here is a snapshot of what you will see.

- 30 Breakfast Recipes Under 300 Calories

- 7 Late Night Snacks When Losing Weight

- 15 One-Pot Vegan Meals Anyone Can Eat

- 12 Healthy Desserts Under 100 Calories

- 21 Weight Loss Smoothies

- 59 Make Ahead and Freeze Meals

- 100 Weight Loss Recipes

- 26 Weight Watchers Lunches

IMPORTANT TIP

I highly recommend you do not scroll through the recipes and websites if you are hungry, in your fasting window timeframe, or it is past your cut off time to eat in the evenings. Seeing the images can make you want to eat immediately and probably is not a good idea because it can cause you to snack unnecessarily. One of the best times to search for new recipes and snack ideas is after you have eaten.

OVER 2,000 RECIPES, SNACKS, TIPS & TOOLS YOU
CAN USE TO LOSE WEIGHT:

1. 14 day Weight Watchers Meal Plan: https://skinnyms. com/two-week-weight-watchers-weight-loss-challenge/ website: SkinnyMs.com

2. Low Carb Recipes: https://tasteandsee.com/category/recipes/low-carb-recipes/ it's on website tasteandsee.com

3. 25 Easy Keto Snack Ideas: https://oliviawyles.com/25-genius-quick-easy-2-minute-keto-snack-ideas/   website: oliviawyles.com

4. 85 Keto Dinners in 30 Minutes or Less: https://www. eatwell101.com/quick-keto-dinner-recipes?pp=1   website: eatwell101.com

5. Easy Vegan Recipes: https://www.kathysvegankitchen. com/cruchwrap-supreme/?utm_source=pinterest&utm_medium=social&utm_campaign=grow-social-pro website: kathysvegankitchen.com

6. Healthy Low-Calorie Recipes: https://dishingouthealth. com/category/recipes/ website: dishingouthealth.com

7. Vegan Dinner Recipes: https://runningonrealfood.com/ category/recipes/entrees website: runningrealfood.com

8. Vegetarian Recipes: https://cozypeachkitchen.com/recipes/# website: cozypeachkitchen.com

9. 30 Low-Calorie Weight Loss Meals: https://wholelottayum. com/healthy-meal-prep-ideas-for-weight-loss/website: wholelottayum.com

10. 56 Delicious Weight Loss Meals Under 500 Calories: https://www.trimmedandtoned.com/56-unbelievably-delicious-weight-loss-dinner-recipes-500-calories/   website: trimmedandtoned.com

11. Over 100 Weight Loss Recipes: https://www.jessicagavin. com/recipe-index/ at website jessicagavin.com

12. Vegan Dishes: https://veggiesociety.com/recipes/ website: veggiesociety.com

13. 25 Easy Weight Watchers Meals: https://blastaloud.com/weight-watchers-recipes-smartpoints/ website: blastaloud.com

14. 20 Tasty Keto Desserts: https://blastaloud.com/low-carb-keto-desserts/ website: blastaloud.com

15. 30 Weight Watchers Dinner Recipes: https://skinnyms.com/weight-watchers-recipes-for-dinner/ website: skinnyms.com

16. 15 One Pot Easy Vegan Meals Anyone Can Eat: https://www.purewow.com/food/vegan-one-pot-meals?amphtml=true website: purewow.com

17. 15 One Pot Healthy Under 350 Calorie Recipes: https://sweetcsdesigns.com/recipes/#feastmobilemenu website: sweetsdesigns.com

18. 11 One Pot Healthy Recipes: https://xokatierosario.com/11-one-pot-healthy-meals-for-minimal-clean-up/ website: xokatierosario.com

19. 9 Delicious Keto/Low Calorie Weight Loss Salad Recipes: https://ketodietrule.com/keto-salad-recipes/ website: ketodietrule.com

20. 12 Amazing Vegan Salads That Aren't Boring: https://veganheaven.org/all-recipes/vegan-salad-recipes/ website: veganheaven.com

21. 200 Tasty Healthy Salad Recipes: https://www.prudentpennypincher.com/cheap-and-easy-salad recipes/?utm_medium=social&utm_source=pinterest&utm_campaign=tailwind_tribes&utm_content=tribes&utm_term=642502038_25023330_200128 website: prudentpennypincher.com

22. 15 Vegan Desserts: https://veganhuggs.com/category/recipes/dessert-food/ website: veganhuggs.com

23. 33 Weight Watchers Desserts: https://kellystilwell.com/20-delicious-weight-watchers-desserts/ website: kellystillwell.com

24. 12 Healthy Desserts Under 100 Calories: https://www.merakilane.com/healthy-desserts-under-100-calories-12-recipes-to-indulge-in/ website: merakilane.com

25. 100 Healthy Desserts Under 100 Calories: https://www.purewow.com/food/100-calorie-desserts website: purewow.com

26. 30 Keto Desserts: https://www.cushyspa.com/keto-dessert/ website: crushyspa.com

27. Keto Candy Recipes. https://oliviawyles.com/8-keto-candy-copycats-satisfy-cravings/ website: oliviawyles.com

28. 25 Snacks for Weight Loss: https://www.fitwirr.com/health/healthy-snacks-weight-loss/?utm_source=pinterest&utm_medium=social website: fitwirr.com

29. 20 Store Brought Healthy Snacks: https://www.momskitchenhandbook.com/shopping-and-household-tips/how-to-shop-smart-in-the-snack-aisle/ website: momskitchenhandbook.com

30. 22 Low Carb Weight Loss Snacks: https://medmd.org/22-low-carb-snack-ideas-for-weight-loss/amp/ website: webmd.org

31. 25 Healthy Snacks for Weight Loss: https://www.seemamago.com/25-healthy-snacks-for-weight-loss/website: seemamago.com

32. 45 Snack Ideas to Lose Weight: https://tealnotes.com/healthy-snack-ideas-to-lose-weight/ website: tealnotes.com

33. 7 Late Night Snacks When Losing Weight: https://nutritiontwins.com/top-late-night-snacks-picks-weight-loss/ website: nutritiontwins.com

34. 30 Weight Loss Breakfast Recipes: https://www.fitwirr.com/health/healthy-breakfast-challenge/?utm_source=pinterest&utm_medium=social website: fitwirr.com

35. 20 Weight Loss Smoothie Recipes: https://onewholesomelife.com/smoothies-for-weight-loss/ website: onewholesomelife.com

36. 30 Breakfast Recipes Under 300 Calories: https://www.merakilane.com/30-breakfasts-under-300-calories-to-kick-start-your-day/ website: merakilane.com

37. 16 Keto Breakfast Recipes for Weight Loss: https://www.ketodietyum.com/keto-breakfast-recipes/ website: ketodietyum.com

38. 15 Keto Breakfast Recipes: https://www.hotbeautyhealth.com/food/keto-breakfasts-ready-in-5-minutes-or-less/ website: hotbeautyhealth.com

39. Keto Weight Loss Smoothies: https://www.ketodietyum.com/keto-smoothie-recipes/ website: ketodietyum.com

40. 5 Delicious Keto Smoothies: http://www.dailydietdish.com/low-carb-keto-smoothies/ website: dailydietdish.com

41. Vegan Smoothies: https://thefitchen.com/3-prep-ahead smoothies/ website: thefitchen.com

42. 21 Weight Loss Smoothies: https://www.ambitiouskitchen.com/21-healthy-smoothie-recipes-for-breakfast-energy/#more-12414 website: ambitiouskitchen.com

43. 31 Vegan Smoothies: https://www.fooduzzi.com/2016/01/healthy-vegan-smoothie-recipes-for-the-new-year/#_a5y_p=4820223 website: fooduzzi.com

44. 40 Vegan Breakfast Recipes: https://www.vegannie.com/breakfast-brunch/40-amazing-vegan-gluten-free-breakfast-recipes/ website: vegannie.com

45. 100 Healthy Weight Loss Tips: https://www.shinesheets.com/100-healthy-actions-that-help-you-get-fit/?utm_medium=social&utm_source=pinterest&utm_campaign=tailwind_smartloop&utm_content=smartloop&utm_term=43514380 website: shinesheets.com

46. Make Ahead and Freeze Meals: https://pinchofyum.com/freezer-meals website: pinchofyum.com

47. 59 Freeze Ahead Meals: https://sweetpeasandsaffron.com/healthy-freezer-meal-prep-dinners-for-new-moms/ website: sweetpeasandsaffron.com

48. Freeze Ahead Meals: https://www.organizeyourselfskinny.com/freezer-casseroles/ website: organizeyourselfskinny.com

49. 14 Healthy Freeze Ahead Crockpot Recipes: https://www.blessthismessplease.com/healthy-freezer-to-slow-cooker-recipes/ website: blessthismessplease.com

50. 15 Easy Make Ahead Freezer Meals: https://happymoneysaver.com/easy-freezer-meals/ website: happymoneysaver.com

51. 70 Healthy Make Ahead Freezer Meals: https://thrivinghomeblog.com/70-healthy-freezer-meals/ website: thrivinghomeblog.com

52. 20 Easy Quick Make Ahead Meals for Busy Women and Moms: https://justbrightideas.com/freezer-meals-for-new-moms/ website: justbrightideas.com

53. 40 Vegan Snacks: https://moonandspoonandyum.com/plant-based-snacks/ website: moonandspoonandyum.com

54. 20 Vegan Snacks: https://www.simplyquinoa.com/20-savory-vegan-snack-recipes/ website: simplyquinoa.com

55. 14 Vegan Breakfast Recipes. https://tasty.co/article/jesseszewczyk/high-protein-vegan-breakfasts website: tasty.co

56. 25 Vegan Snack Ideas. https://www.karissasvegankitchen.com/vegan-snack-ideas/ website: karissasvegankitchen.com

57. Vegan Meal Prep: https://veganfamilytravels.com/vegan-meal-prep-ideas/ website: veganfamilytravels.com

58. 21 Keto Meal Prep Recipes: https://ketofoody.com/keto-meal-prep-recipes/?utm_medium=social&utm_source=pinterest&utm_campaign=tailwind_tribes&utm_content=tribes&utm_term=978024958_44012146_549430 Website ketofoody.com

59. 30 Keto Meal Prep Ideas: https://wholelottayum.com/10-keto-lunch-meal-prep-ideas/ website: wholelottayum.com

60. 20 Keto Meal Prep: https://www.cushyspa.com/keto-meal-prep-ideas/ website: cushyspa.com

61. 25 Weight Watchers Packable Meals: https://www.merakilane.com/25-packable-weight-watchers-lunch-recipes-with-points/ website: merakilane.com

62. 26 Weight Watchers Lunches: https://www.hotbeauty-health.com/food/the-best-weight-watchers-lunches-with-smart-points/ website: hotbeautyhealth.com

63. 17 Frozen Weight Watchers Foods: https://simple-nour-ished-living.com/weight-watchers-frozen-foods-favorites/ website: simplenourishedliving.com

64. 25 Low Point Weight Watchers Snacks: https://point-edkitchen.com/best-low-point-snacks-weight-watchers/ website: pointedkitchen.com

65. Food Calculator for Cooking at Home: www.nutritionix.com

66. 60 Weight Watchers Desserts: https://mealplanningmom-mies.com/60-weight-watchers-friendly-desserts/ website: mealplanningmommies.com

67. 7 Day Vegan Meal Plan: https://runningonrealfood.com/one-week-vegan-meal-plan/ website: runningonrealfood.com

68. 7 Day Keto Meal Plan for Weight Loss: https://www.fit-wirr.com/health/keto-diet-menu/?utm_source=pinter-est&utm_medium=social website: fitwirr.com

69. Free Style Weight Watchers Meal Plan: https://www.mid-lifehealthyliving.com/weight-watchers-meal-plan-freestyle-meal-plan/ website: midlifehealthyliving.com

70. 175 Weight Watchers Recipes; https://www.midlifeheal-thyliving.com/weight-watchers-meal-plan-freestyle-meal-plan/ website: midlifehealthyliving.com

71. 100 Weight Watchers 0 Points Meals: https://www.prudentpennypincher.com/zero-point-weight-watch-ers-meals/?utm_medium=social&utm_source=pin-terest&utm_campaign=tailwind_tribes&utm_con-

tent=tribes&utm_term=726187268_29375836_109845
website: prudentpennypincher.com

72. 30 Days Pantry Staples Meal Plans: https://www.pru-dentpennypincher.com/free-1-month-pantry-meal-plan/ website: prudentpennypincher.com

73. 30 Make Ahead Weight Watchers Lunch Ideas: https://deedeedoes.com/31-fantastic-satisfying-weight-watch-ers-freestyle-0-point-lunch-recipes/ website: deedeedoes.com

74. Ultimate Guide to Intermittent Fasting: https://blog.pi-quetea.com/intermittent-fasting-schedule/amp/?utm_source=pinterest&utm_medium=social website: blog.pi-quetea.com

75. 100 Keto-Vegan Recipes: https://www.vegannie.com/recipes/dairy-free/100-amazing-keto-vegan-recipes-for-weight-loss/ website: www.vegannie.com

*Health Tip: When choosing your recipes, find ways to incorporate some of the items listed below for additional improved health. You can also refer to the more detailed list of fruits and vegetables and their benefits in Chapter 10.

FEED YOUR WHOLE BODY

BRAIN – Salmon, Tuna, Sardines, Walnuts	**LUNGS** – Broccoli, Brussels Sprouts
HAIR – Green Vegetables, Beans, Salmon	**BONES** – Oranges, Celery, Milk
EYES – Eggs, Corn, Carrots	**BOWELS** – Prunes, Yogurt
MUSCLE – Bananas, Red Meat, Fish, Eggs	**HEART** – Tomatoes, Potatoes
SKIN – Blueberries, Salmon, Green Tea	

Are You Using Cooking Instruments to Make Your Life Easier in the Kitchen?

This brings us to the last question in **Step 3** of the *Weight Loss Food Shift*. You now have ideas on grocery store shopping and a sample meal lists to reference. You have a host of websites with recipes, tips, and ideas to choose from, but what are you going to prepare the food in? Besides popping a pan in the oven or cooking food on the stove and in the microwave, what other instruments are you using in the kitchen that can make your life easier?

I will share with you the four that changed my life when it came to cooking healthier and made it more convenient. They reduced my stress levels as well as the time I spent standing up in the kitchen. You may already have some of the items, but if you do not, try to work on budgeting these items into your, must haves *weight loss food shift* list. (Some of the websites on the reference lists, we just went over, have recipes for preparing your meals using one or more of the four items I will mention).

The first is a good ole' fashioned **Crockpot**. They can make meal planning a breeze for you and even if you are a new chef, it can make you feel at ease when preparing meals. What I loved the most about using one is, while I was losing weight, I could throw everything in the pot before leaving for work or to run around with my family and not have to worry about it.

Whenever I got back home, dinner was done. Clean up was so easy, and I found tons of recipes and cookbooks. The recipes were specifically catered to making mealtime easier and healthier. The Crockpots come in a variety of sizes and brands, and you can find one for about $25.00-$45.00.

Second on my list is equivalent to taking a Crockpot to the next level. It is an **Instant-Pot.** Unlike the Crockpot, where you usually have only two settings of high and low, an Instant-Pot has several features to use for cooking. For example, the one I use has seven different options to cook meals. To name a few, I have made rice, soups, beef stew, sauteed vegetables, oatmeal, chili, and chicken with potatoes. The fact that I can throw the entire recipe ingredients in there, set the timer and forget about it, is so convenient.

An added, bonus with using this cooking tool is, if you are not experienced in the kitchen, they have set times and temperatures already programmed into the machine. Like the Crockpot, they come in different sizes and brands. You can get one for about $50.00-$60.00.

The third item on my list is one of my all-time favorites and a new addition to my kitchen tools: an, **Air Fryer.** It was a gift from my brother-in-law, and I could not have thanked him enough. (I was hesitant in using it at first because I thought, "Who air fries, food?"). Luckily for me my, *Fried Chicken Fridays* was back and was no longer a thing of the past! You can air fry almost anything in them.

The best part, the food comes out crispy and juicy, but is not packed with the grease that comes with traditional fried chicken. When the food is done cooking, you see the amount of grease that collects in the tray pan below the food. Seeing it can make you feel even better about the cooking style you chose. All that grease is less fat and calories going into your body. Like the Instant-Pot, an Air Fryer comes with a variety of cooking options.

The Air Fryer I use has nine different cooking features available. Besides cooking my fried chicken in it, I have made Cornish Game Hens, fried zucchini, chicken and shrimp skewers, steak and even made my son some French Fries and chicken nuggets using it.

The preset times and temperatures are very convenient to use, and the machine and the trays can be easy to clean. They come in different sizes and brands; you can find a smaller one for about $50.00 and the larger ones are about $100.00.

The fourth and final one on the list is a good smoothie making **Blender.** The *6-Week Program* calls for you to have liquid meals on a set number of days because they will assist you with losing weight. You can buy premade smoothies from different places. However, if you are going to make your own, by having a good blender on standby, you can whip together delicious fruit and vegetable smoothies for breakfast or dinner. You can get one for about $25.00-$50.00.

Either one of these four suggestions can make your life easier in the kitchen and help with making the weight loss food shift smoother. Convenience is the key word in helping you transition into a new way of cooking and eating.

WEIGHT LOSS TIP TIME

Did you know at the first sign of gas, or an upset stomach, you can use one of the best at home remedies for acidity? Either you, can eat a few basil leaves or boil 3-4 of them in a cup of water and let it simmer for a few minutes. Sip on it frequently. It can help calm your stomach, especially if you are introducing more fruits and vegetables into your diet and as your body is adjusting to the change in your eating habits. Here are a few additional tips that might be helpful to you on your journey.

TOP 10 TEAS TO DRINK AND WHY

1. Chai Tea: Enhances immune system, fights inflammation, and colds

2. White Tea: Beneficial for, reducing stress, weight loss and detoxification

3. Green Tea: Treats, bloating, allergies, acne, promotes weight loss

4. Matcha Tea: Burns belly fat, immunity booster, and detoxifier

5. Peppermint Tea: Remedy for bloating, nausea, PMS, and bad breath

6. Chamomile Tea: Beneficial for, sleep, headaches, anxiety, and bloating

7. Ginger Tea: Reduces bloating, colds, upset stomach and sore throats

8. Hibiscus Tea: Best for high blood pressure, respiratory diseases

9. Black Tea: Treats anxiety, headaches and is good for weight loss

10. Oolong Tea: Promotes weight loss and boosts metabolism

STEP 4 OF THE WEIGHT LOSS FOOD SHIFT:
MEAL DELIVERY FOOD KITS

Last up in the weight loss food shift is **Step 4**: Meal Delivery Food Kits. We have talked about eating out successfully, making your Weight Loss MRE Kits and cooking at home. This final option is also about convenience. While losing weight, if you are not going to sign up or order food from any of the structured diet programs, like Nutrisystem or the South Beach Diet, and do not want to worry about eating out or cooking, this option may be perfect for you.

In this section, we will look at a variety of meal delivery services and their food kits, that you can order and use while losing weight. Many of which can accommodate almost any dietary restriction or eating style of choice. For example, meals that are Keto, Vegan, Low-Calorie and Low-Carb, gluten, nut and dairy free friendly.

Using meal kit services as one of your *weight loss food shift* options can be an easy way to save time, reduce your food stress and can save you money.

The food kit services have come a long way with the quality and taste of their food since starting out a few years ago. Many of them even offer a wide variety of menu options that change weekly. This is to help you not get bored with the food. When I discovered meals like these existed, it was so convenient for me because, at the time, I was the only one dieting in my household. It was hard to prepare a separate meal for myself that was not high in calories, fat grams and net carbs. However, ordering meals that were about $9.00 each gave me the opportunity to eat a healthy meal with my family, kept my portions in check and did not break the bank. At the same time, I also won my husband and son over because eventually they noticed all the delicious options I was enjoying. When they did, they started eating them, too. Which made my meals a little cheaper because most of the meal kit services have it set up so the more meals you order, the cost of each meal goes down. It was a win-win situation for me because it meant less time grocery shopping, meal prepping and cooking in the kitchen. As well as a cost savings to my family with limited food waste of uneaten meals and not spending extra money eating out.

In this section, you will find a list of twenty food delivery options you can choose from, most of which you will be able to order online. The whole point of you ordering and using premeasured, packaged meals is, for the convenience while dieting and losing weight. When you start following the *6-Week Program*, you will already have enough going on in your life that will require your attention.

You may be a busy woman, mom, entrepreneur, or just in general busy, and have a lot on your plate (no pun intended). Using these types of services and options and not having to meal prep and cook, let alone do the dishes and everything else that goes with meal planning, can be worth it within itself. Some of the options will involve very little cooking, and others you would just simply heat up. Using these types of services can help make the *weight loss food shift* a more streamlined process for you.

Side Note: You may not like all the food you order from the meal delivery food kit services. It took me ordering from four different ones before I figured out which ones, I preferred the most. You may need to experiment with a few different ones also until you decide which one is best for your dietary needs and food preferences. Just as I mentioned earlier in the book, all food brands and companies are not created equal.

Full Disclosure: With some of the meals, I added a little hot sauce and some extra seasonings to make it more specific to my tastebuds. Keep in mind, if you do add to the meals, make sure you track the calories, fat grams and net carbs.

One last little point to make is, if you are like me, and you decide to order from these services, it can be a little surprising to see the small portion sizes when you open the meals (actually, some are larger than others). The reality is, they will be the correct portion sizes *needed* for you to lose weight. However, I do understand if your eyes are in shock when you do receive the packages.

In the beginning of this chapter, we went over portion sizes because it will be a big part of you getting control of your daily intake and shifting, to eating smaller meals. To help with visually making less food look like more, you can always transfer the meal

215

to a small plate. Like a salad size plate or lunch plate. Initially, after eating the smaller meals, you may still be hungry. Same thing happened to me and what I would do is, drink more water, and have some type of steamed or sauteed vegetables or a piece of fruit to help *fill* me up. I took those steps because during my shift, I had to learn to eat to be satisfied, not stuffed.

Years ago, I had gotten so used to, jokingly getting up from the table saying I had to unbutton my pants to breathe, because I had eaten so much. Or after eating at an all-you-can-eat, buffet, or at a family get-together, I was so stuffed and needed to be rolled to the car. Taking control of my eating played a huge role in my ability to lose and maintain weight, as it can for you also. Because when you get a handle on your portions and make the *weight loss food shift*, it will be the key to helping you reach your weight loss goals.

In each of the meal delivery food kit services listed, you will find a little about each company, their prices, where to find them and some of their menu options. The good thing about many of them: after your first order, there is no commitment to place additional orders. Some offer the option to order as little as 1 to 4 meals at a time and list ways you can cancel or skip future orders.

Meal Planning Tip: Even if you do not order from the different food services listed, you can find some useful information on their websites. Most have the recipes, ingredients, and instructions on how to make each meal. If nothing else, you can use them for your weekly meal planning ideas.

20 FOOD DELIVERY MEAL KIT SERVICES

SNAP KITCHEN

What do they offer? **Snap Kitchen** offers a variety of delicious meals which require no prep. Their meals arrive in a container and are ready to be heated and served. Most require about 20 minutes or less in the oven or they can also go in the microwave. They have a variety of breakfast, lunch, dinner, and snack options to choose from. Which can be catered to a set calorie budget from 1,200 to 1,800 calories. Or for those needing a higher caloric intake, they offer flexible build your-own-meal kits. You can choose meals either high in protein, Keto-friendly, Paleo, dairy-free for vegetarians and several other food options. For example, they have a Turkey Cobb Salad, which is 240 calories, 16 fat grams and 7 net carbs. Chicken Piccata, which is a Keto, Whole30 and Paleo friendly meal. It is 350 calories, 21 fat grams and 14 net carbs. As a bonus, all, of their meals are gluten-free. They also have a variety of smoothies and soups and salads that are low in calories and carbs. Popular menu items include: Chimichurri Beef, Almond Crusted Salmon, Chicken Burrito Bowl with Avocado Salsa, Almond Butter Pancakes, and the Breakfast Platter which comes with pork sausage, scrambled eggs, and cheesy cauliflower. **Cost:** Depending on which meal plan you select, you can expect to pay about $29-$39 a day. That would include three meals and two snacks. Roughly about $8.00-$10 a meal. Check for special coupons and pricing when you place your first order. **Availability:** Currently, they are shipping to most of Texas, Oklahoma, Arkansas, Louisiana, Kansas, New Mexico, Pennsylvania, Connecticut, New Jersey, Maryland, Delaware, New York, Massachusetts, Virginia, and West Virginia. However, on their website, you can find out additional new service areas as they become available.

Website: Snapkitchen.com

FRESHLY

What do they offer? **Freshly** offers a variety of delicious meals which require no cooking. Their meals arrive in microwave safe containers and are ready to be heated and served. They are not frozen, so most can be heated up in less than five minutes. They have a variety of lunch and dinner options to choose from. Which can be catered to a set caloric budget, and they have over twenty different meals under 500 calories. They also offer low carb and dairy-free products as well. This would be a good choice if you have food allergies, because their meals are made in a peanut and gluten free facility. Their meals are freshly prepared and have a shelf-life of 4-5 days. However, they can be frozen and eaten at a, later date. They rotate over thirty different meal options bi-weekly. Some popular meal items are: Sicilian Style Chicken Parmesan with Broccoli, Homestyle Chicken with Butternut Mac & Cheese, Steak Peppercorn with Sautéed Carrots & French Green Beans. **Cost:** Depending on which option you choose, they have meal plans that include 4, 6, 10 or 12 meals. Ordering the 12-meal option comes out to about $102.00 a week. Which would equate to roughly $8.50 a meal. Check for special coupons and pricing when you place your first order. **Availability:** They currently ship Nationwide, excluding Alaska and Hawaii. **Website:** Freshly.com

EAT FIT LIFE FOODS

What do they offer? **Eat Fit Life Foods** offers a variety of delicious meals which require no cooking. Their meals arrive in vacuum sealed packages and can be stored in the refrigerator for up to ten days or stored in the freezer for up to six months. They can be heated in the microwave, stove top or oven and then served. They have a variety of breakfast, lunch and dinner options and offer meals that are Keto, Vegan, Paleo, Low-Carb, Plant-Based, Vegetarian and Whole30 friendly. As a bonus, they can accommodate dietary preferences of gluten and dairy free meals. They offer three sizes to choose from when selecting your meals. Small, medium, and large, and the meals range from 250-600 calories. Some of the menu items are: Pumpkin French Toast with Chicken Bacon, Pecan Crushed Chicken with Maple Pecan Sweet Potato Mash and Roasted Green Beans with Carrots, Butternut Turkey Breast with Low-Carb Cauliflower Mashed Potatoes with a side of Cranberry Chutney. **Cost:** Depending on which plan you choose, they have ten medium meals for about $115.00 and twelve medium meals for $124.00. Which comes out to roughly $10.00-$11.00 a meal. Check for special coupons and pricing when you place your first order. **Availability:** Shipping to Florida and Georgia. Check on their website to see if they have added additional shipping locations. **Website:**Eatfitlifefoods.com

SUNBASKET

What do they offer? **Sunbasket** offers a variety of delicious meals which require some cooking. They take the guesswork out for you of measuring and the how-to of preparing the food. Step by step instructions on how to cook the food in an easy-to-follow format is provided. They have a variety of breakfast, lunch, dinner, and snack options to choose from and even offer kid-friendly meals. They provide organic produce, antibiotic-free meat, with no added hormones. The seafood they use is fresh caught in the wild. They have a variety of food options for Paleo, Vegan, Vegetarian, Pescatarian, Mediterranean, gluten-free, lean & clean, and diabetes friendly meals. They even give you the option of mixing and matching recipes from the different eating styles. Some of their menu items are: Gingered Steak Stir-Fry with Steamed Vegetables, One Pot Chicken and Spanish Rice, Black Angus Ribeye Steaks, Lyonnaise Potatoes, and Horseradish Mayo. **Cost:** Depending on which plan you choose, they have options for two to four meals a week or the family plan with four recipes and total servings up to sixteen. The cost is about $90.00 a week for two meals for four people. Roughly $11.00 a person for a meal. They offer other plans with more options with less cost per meal. Check for special coupons and pricing when you place your first order. **Availability:** Shipping Nationwide, excluding Alaska, Hawaii, Montana, and parts of New Mexico. **Website:** Sunbasket.com

BLUE APRON

What do they offer? **Blue Apron** offers a variety of delicious meals which require some cooking. Step by step instructions with the recipes on how to cook the food in an easy-to-follow format is provided. They have the recipes easily accessible on their website as well. They have a variety of lunch and dinner options to choose from. As an added, bonus, for those losing weight, they partnered up with Weight Watchers to offer a variety of meals that easily align with their points system. For non-meat eaters, they do offer options in their two-person plan and have added Beyond Meat boxes. Designed so you can make your own plant-based burgers at home. Some of their menu items include: Stir-Fry Tofu and Vegetables, Glazed Pork Meatloaf with Mash Potatoes and Bok Choy, General Tao's Chicken with Rice and Shishito Peppers, and Seared Steaks with Lemon Caper Butter with Oven Fries. **Cost:** Depending on which plan you choose, they have options for three meals for two people for about $60.00 a week for six meals. Which comes out to $10.00 a meal. Check for special coupons and pricing when you place your first order. **Availability:** Shipping Nationwide. **Website:** Blueapron.com

HOME CHEF

What do they offer? **Home Chef** offers a variety of meals that can be ready to serve in less than thirty minutes. They provide lunch and dinner options that can accommodate low calorie, carb conscious, meat eaters, vegetarians, non-dairy lovers, and options without nuts, soy, or wheat. As an added, bonus, they offer five-minute lunches and fifteen-minute meals you can pop right in the oven, in one of their oven safe tins. If you are a planner and like knowing what you will eat ahead of time, you will like that their menus are set five weeks ahead. Giving you ample time to make necessary choices on what you will eat. Some of their menu items include: Scallop Rockefeller Risotto with Spinach and Crispy Fried Onions, Chicken Cordon Bleu and Chive Crema with Wild Rice, Roasted Butternut Squash Fish Cake, Caesar Salad with Remoulade and Almonds, Teriyaki Steak and Peppers with Peanuts and Jasmine Rice and Crispy Potato- Crusted Buffalo Chicken with Cheesy Ranch Cauliflower.
Cost: Depending on which plan you choose, meals are about $7.00 a person and can be customized for an additional fee. They offer a variety of different plans to choose from on their website. Usually, delivery is free for orders over $49.00 and can cost $10.00 for anything less. Check for special coupons and pricing when you place your first order.
Availability: Shipping Nationwide. **Website:** Homechef.com

VEESTRO

What does it offer? **Veestro** offers a variety of delicious meals which require no cooking. Their meals arrive in a container and are ready to be heated and served. They have a variety of breakfast, lunch, and dinner options to choose from. Which can be catered to a set calorie budget as low as 1,200 calories. They offer 100% plant-based meals where you can select ten to thirty meals per week and can tailor your meals to suit your dietary needs. They offer high-protein meals, gluten, nut, and soy free options and even have a weight loss tab on their website directing you to the low-calorie choices. Some of their menu items are: Pasta Bolognese, Red Curry Tofu, Enchilada Casserole, Spanish Torta, and Breakfast Burritos. **Cost:** Depending on which plan you choose, they have five and seven-day plans with three meals a day, which comes out to about $10.00-$11.00 a meal. They have other plan options available on their website. Check for special coupons and pricing when you place your first order. **Availability:** Shipping Nationwide, excluding Alaska and Hawaii.
Website: Veestro.com

FACTOR

What do they offer? **Factor** offers a variety of delicious meals which require no cooking. Their meals arrive in a container, and all you have, to do is pop them in the microwave and serve. They have a variety of breakfast, lunch, and dinner options, as well as soups, snacks, and energy juices to choose from. They offer meals that are Keto, Paleo, Low-Carb, Plant-Based, Vegetarian and High-Protein friendly. Some of their menu items are: BBQ Brisket Roast, Pork Tenderloin with Green Peppercorn Sauce, Shrimp Alfredo, Blackened Salmon with Vegetables and Breakfast Enchilada Bake. They switch up their menu weekly to provide you a variety of different options. **Cost:** Depending on which plan you choose and how many meals you want a week, the cost ranges from $11.00 to $15.00 a meal. Plans start at about $60 per week and are for four meals a person. Other plan options are available on their website. Check for special coupons and pricing when you place your first order. **Availability:** Shipping Nationwide, excluding Alaska and Hawaii. **Website:** Factor75.com

YUMBLE

What do they offer? **Yumble** is one of the food-delivery services I wanted to add to the list because it can be a perfect option for busy dieting moms who want healthier meals prepared and ready to eat for her kids too. Having meals delivered to you is one thing while dieting, not having to prep and cook a separate meal for your kids can be a bonus. Yumble's meals are designed for kids between the ages of 1 to 12 years old. The prepackaged meals come precooked and only require reheating and then serving. Some of their options on the menu can even satisfy a picky eater. They offer gluten, dairy, and soy free options as well as a variety of vegetarian dishes. Some of their menu items are, Meatball Mac n Cheese, Chicken Marinara and Alfredo, Classic Cheese Ravioli, BBQ Chicken with Cornbread, Sesame Ginger Veggie Stir Fry and Chicken Nuggets with Mac n Cheese. You can check the nutritional fact sheet on each meal on their website to see the benefits each provides. A bonus is the boxes the meals come in, include activities like table topics and sticker sheets to encourage engagement at mealtime. **Cost:** Depending which plan you choose, they offer six meals for $24.00 a week per child and $48.00 a week for twelve meals. Which costs about $4.00 a meal. They have other plans available on their website. Check for special coupons and pricing when you place your first order. **Availability:** Shipping to most of the East Coast, Texas, and parts of the West Coast and Midwest. You can enter your zip code on the website to see delivery options. **Website:** Yumblekids.com

FRESH DIRECT

What do they offer? **Fresh Direct** was another one I wanted to make sure I added to the list, because not only do they offer meal delivery kits, but they also are a grocery delivery service company. Where you can have your meals, groceries and a host of other things delivered right to your front door. They offer a variety of packaged meals, some of which can be heated and ready to eat in under four minutes. They have options for Low-Calorie, Vegan, No Added Sugar, Vegetarian, Low-Sodium, High-Fiber, and meals under 500 calories. Many can be prepared in less than twenty minutes. Some of their meal items are: Lemon Herb- Shrimp with Saffron Cauliflower Rice and Asparagus, Sweet Potato Shepherd's Pie, Beef Bolognese, Mango Greek Yogurt and Granola, Baked Ziti and Lobster Ravioli. **Cost:** Depending on what you choose to order, they have A la Carte Entrées and some of their meals are around $10 and up for one serving. Each meal kit serves two people. **Availability:** Shipping only in the Northeast and some Southeast areas. You can check on their website to see if they deliver in your area. Check for special coupons and pricing when you place your first order. **Website:** Freshdirect.com

SPLENDID SPOON

What do they offer? **Splendid Spoon** offers a variety of delicious ready-made smoothies, soups, noodle, and grain bowls. They can be perfect options for an easy and quick breakfast or lunch. Their smoothies are packed with plenty of nutrients, and compared to some other smoothies, I have tried, they are relatively low in sugar. They offer their food options in categories like Heal, Energize and Refresh, based on your preferences. They also have gluten and dairy free options as well as no added sugars and low-sodium products. Splendid Spoon has a full day, soup cleanse add-on feature to "reset" your system. Some of their menu items are Mango Guava Smoothie, Roasted Cauliflower Bowl, Creamy Butternut Squash Noodles, Mint Chip Smoothie with Almond Butter, Vegetable Bolognese Bowl, and Pumpkin Spice Smoothie. **Cost:** Depending on which package you choose, they offer a breakfast/lunch plan that has five smoothies and five veggie packed soups or grain bowls for roughly $95.00. Their breakfast, lunch and reset plan has five smoothies, five bowls and five light soups for $135.00. Which comes out to roughly $9.00 a meal. Check for special coupons and pricing when you place your first order. It is a subscription; however, you can cancel any time after your first order. **Availability:** They currently ship Nationwide, excluding Alaska and Hawaii. **Website:** Splendidspoon.com

DAILY HARVEST

What do they offer? **Daily Harvest** offers a variety of smoothies, chia bowls, soups, and flatbread options to choose from. They also have organic, gluten and dairy free, plant-based options. Their smoothies, like their other food options, have everything included all in one cup. The smoothies can be quickly prepared by mixing all the ingredients in a blender. Afterwards, the contents can be poured back into the cup and enjoyed. Some of their menu items are: Cauliflower and Leek Stew, Chocolate Blueberry Smoothie, Pumpkin and Chai Oat Bowl, Artichoke and Spinach Flatbread, and Strawberry and Peach Smoothie. **Cost:** Depending on which items you choose, you are looking at roughly $6 to $8 per cup/per item. Check for special coupons and pricing when you place your first order. **Availability:** Shipping Nationwide. **Website:** Dailyharvest.com

HELLO FRESH

What do they offer? **Hello Fresh** offers a variety of delicious meals which require some cooking. They take the guesswork out for you of measuring and the how-to of preparing the food. Step by step instructions on how to cook the food in an easy-to-follow format is provided. They even list their dishes on a range of difficulty from one to three, so you can decide which meals are the easiest to prepare. They have a variety of lunch and dinner options to choose from. They offer meals that are low-calorie, vegetarian, and family friendly and they come in convenient packages that can be easily stored in the refrigerator. They offer the option to remove meat or seafood from the recipes and have a weight loss friendly Fit Meals feature, which allows you to choose three of their nutrient dense recipes of the week. Quick Meal options are available and can be ready in thirty minutes or less. Some of their menu items are: Pork Sausage over Autumn Pilaf, Old Bay Buttered Up Chicken with Mashed Potatoes and Roasted Veggies, Garlic Butter Shrimp, Peppercorn Crusted Beef Tenderloin with Mashed Sweet Potatoes and Asparagus, and Tilapia with Scallion Sriracha Pesto and Ginger Rice with Green Beans. **Cost:** Depending on which of their plans you choose, it will be roughly about $60.00 a week for three meals for two people or $96.00 a week for three meals for four people. Which comes out to about $8.00-$10.00 a serving. Check for special coupons and pricing when you place your first order. They have other plan options available on their website. **Availability:** Shipping Nationwide. **Website:** Hellofresh.com

GREEN CHEF

What do they offer? **Green Chef** offers a variety of meals that can be ready to serve in less than thirty minutes. They provide lunch and dinner options that are specifically geared towards the Keto, Paleo, Vegan, Vegetarian, and gluten-free diets. They also offer meal kits with meat and a variety of color-coded recipes that are easy to follow. Some of their menu items are: Moroccan Cauliflower and Cuban Tofu with Chimichurri, Teriyaki Chicken Rice Bowls, Creamy Beef with Mushrooms, Spaghetti Squash Noodles and Cheesy French Onion Cauliflower with Sauteed Mushrooms. **Cost:** Depending on which plan you choose, they have three meals for two people at about $79.00 and two meals for four people at $95.00. Which is about $11.00-$13.00 a serving. Check for special coupons and pricing when you place your first order. They have other plan options available on their website. **Availability:** Shipping Nationwide. **Website:** Greenchef.com

FRESH AND EASY

What do they offer? **Fresh and Easy** offers a variety of delicious meals which require some cooking. Their aim is to offer additional convenience with meals arriving already sliced and diced and ready to be heated in their oven-safe trays. They also have a variety of salads that only require tossing together before serving. If you are looking for a quick dinner, they do provide fifteen-minute meal kits. As, well as for outdoor cooking, they have kits that can be assembled in a grill-safe bag and prepared directly on the grill. They have low-calorie and low-carb options available on their menu and can accommodate vegetarian diets as well. Their menu options change weekly, and every Monday they send you an email with over twenty different options to choose from, so planning can be made easier. They have family-meal kits available also. **Cost:** Depending on which plan you choose, they have three meals for two people for roughly $60.00 a week or three meals for four people for $119.00. Check for special coupons and pricing when you place your first order. They have other plan options available on their website. **Availability:** Shipping Nationwide. **Website:** Freshandeasy.com

GOBBLE

What do they offer? **Gobble** offers a variety of delicious meals which require some cooking. Some of their menu items can be ready in fifteen minutes. Step by step instructions on how to cook the food in an easy-to-follow format is provided. They have a variety of breakfast, lunch, and dinner options to choose from. For the calorie and carb conscious, they offer a Lean and Clean plan with meals that include lean protein, healthy fats and are under 600 calories. They can accommodate gluten and dairy free requirements and have a list of vegetarian and kid-friendly options on the menu. Some of their food choices are: Seared Salmon with Kale, Pan Roasted Chicken with Broccoli, Chinese Five-Spice Tofu with Lime Coconut Vegetable Stew, Salisbury Steak with Potatoes Colcannon and Brussel Sprouts and Artisanal Belgium Waffles with Mixed Berry Compote and Cinnamon Brown Sugar Butter. **Cost:** Depending on which one of the plans you choose, they have three meals for two people for roughly $79.00 and three meals for four people for roughly $150.00. Which comes out to about $12.00-$13.00 a serving. Check for special coupons and pricing when you place your first order. They have other plan options available on their website. **Availability:** Shipping Nationwide. **Website:** Gobble.com

PURPLE CARROT

What do they offer? **Purple Carrot** offers a variety of delicious meals which will require some cooking. They are a 100% Vegan based meal kit service company offering a variety of breakfast, lunch, and dinner options to choose from when planning meals. Some of their meals do take some time and skill to put together, but if you are ready to cook quality, homemade vegan dishes, they have plenty on their menu. Some menu items are: Mushroom Cheddar Black Bean Burger with Garlic Aioli and Carrot Fries, Coconut Lentil Soup, Hoisin Tofu Steaks with Sticky Rice and Spinach Poppy Seed Salad, Banana Chia Pudding, Overnight Oats with Apricot and Sesame Ginger Noodles with Stir-Fry Green Beans and Toasted Peanuts. **Cost:** Depending on which plan you choose, they offer three meals for two people at about $72.00 and three meals for four people at $119.00. Which is roughly $10.00-$12.00 a person. Check for special coupons and pricing when you place your first order. They have other plan options available on their website. **Availability:** Shipping Nationwide. **Website:** Purplecarrot.com

EVERY PLATE

What do they offer? **Every Plate** is on the list because they are one of the most affordable services, offering a variety of delicious family friendly meals, which require some cooking. Some of their meals can be ready in thirty minutes and come with step-by-step instructions in an easy-to-follow format. They have a variety of lunch, and dinner options to choose from. This service is more for if you are looking for alternative meal options for your family while you are losing weight. Their items are *not* low-carb, low calorie or clean and lean friendly, but they do provide a convenient way to have meals ready for your family that can cost about $5.00 a person. Some of their menu items are: Apricot Sriracha Pork Chops, Garlic Rosemary Chicken, Carne Asada Fajitas and Cowboy Skillet Pie. **Cost:** Depending on which plan you choose, they have three meals for two people at about $39.00 and three meals for four people at about $70.00. Which is roughly $5.00-$6.00 a person. Check for special coupons and pricing when you place your first order. They have other plan options available on their website. **Availability:** Shipping to most areas in the United States. You can put in your zip code on their website to check delivery options in your area. **Website:** Everyplate.com

HUNGRY ROOT

What do they offer? **Hungry Root** is more of a hybrid of a grocery store delivery service and a pre-seasoned, prepackaged healthy food and snacks, delivered to your door company. This is a good option if you like to cook but are looking for the flexibility and convenience of being less restrictive to set menus that traditional meal kit services offer. Based on your food preferences, they send weekly high-quality grocery items that can be easily prepared. They have vegan, meat lovers, gluten, dairy and soy free meals on their menu to choose from and offer bread, sauces, and dips. Some of their menu items are: Mushroom Chicken Meatballs, Cauliflower Sandwich Thins, Crunchy Carrot-Lentil Mix, Basil Zucchini White Bean Salad, Superfood Almond Butter and Portobello Meatless Meatballs. **Cost:** Depending on which plan you choose, they have small grocery delivery plans around $69.00. That would include groceries to make three to four meals for two people, plus snacks. Their large deliveries are about $130.00 which includes groceries to make five to six meals for two people plus snacks. They have other plan options available on their website. **Availability:** Shipping Nationwide. **Website:** Hungryroot.com

TRIFECTA NUTRITION

What do they offer? **Trifecta Nutrition** offers a variety of delicious meals which require no cooking. Their meals arrive in vacuum sealed packages and can be stored in the refrigerator for up to ten days or stored in the freezer for up to six months. They can be heated in the microwave, stove top or oven and then served. They have a variety of breakfast, lunch and dinner options and offer meals that are Keto, Vegan, Paleo, Low-Carb, Plant-Based, Vegetarian and High-Protein friendly. As a bonus, they can accommodate dietary preferences of gluten, dairy and soy free meals. Some of their menu items are: Keto Salmon with Lemon-Parmesan Salad, Matcha Green Tea Fat Bomb, Scrambled Eggs with Avocado, Mable Cinnamon Sweet Potato Waffles, Steak Kabobs and Mediterranean Quinoa Salad, Shrimp Ceviche with Rice, Protein-Packed Yogurt Parfait, and Teriyaki Beef and Rice Bowl. **Cost:** Depending on which plan you choose, they have about twenty-four- A La Carte Bundles that you can build your meals around based on your preferences. They calculate out to about $5.00 per serving. They also offer seven meals a week at roughly $108.00 and ten meals a week, at roughly $149.00. Which comes out to about $14.00-$15.00 a meal. They have other plan options available on their website. **Availability**: Shipping Nationwide. **Website**: Trifectanutrition.com

The twenty options are just a few of the ones available at your fingertips, you can use to help with making the weight loss food shift a lot easier. You can also do a Google search in your area to see if there are local options close to your home that also offer meal kits.

Why Use Meal Kit Delivery Services?

- For Convenience-less grocery shopping, meal prepping and cooking
- Cost savings
- Quick and Easy
- Takes the guesswork out of what you will eat
- Can help you lose more weight by staying on track with your daily intake
- The variety of food options are vast and can expose you to new, delicious meals
- You can order ahead for yourself and your family

- Helps to make the *weight loss food shift* a lot easier

Being able to check off your to-do list by having a variety of go-to food services and choices can make your life a lot easier. It can also make losing weight a cost savings in your wallet by limiting the amount of unnecessary items picked up when grocery shopping.

This option can also help remove the worry of not having time to cook and eliminates the need to order take-out or reach for an unhealthy meal or snack.

Another Food Kit Option: Amazon sells weight loss, meal products called HMR. They provide a variety of prepackaged meals that are also portioned-controlled (you can think of it as nutritious weight loss microwaveable TV meals).

They have Keto, Vegetarian and Low-Calorie options to choose from which include meals, shakes, soups, and snacks. One of their options has 14 meals for about $55.00. Which comes out to less than $4.00 a meal. You can check their website for more options: Amazon.com.

**Most of the meal kits from the twenty services listed come in containers that can be reused to premeasure the future meals you will cook and store at home. Instead of throwing them away, you can keep some as an easy way to portion out your food and easily store in the freezer or refrigerator. Plus, you can use them to make and store your Weight Loss MRE Kits, to stash at work, at the homes of family and friends or to take them with you on the go.

The Keys: At this point in the book, we have gone over several significant keys to your success; how to avoid the diet trap, identifying your WHY, setting realistic weight loss goals, the Daily Body Budget Charts, and the importance of making the weight loss food shift. Now it is time to go over the meat and potatoes to losing weight. In the upcoming chapters you will discover the seven key *eating styles* you can choose to use, on your weight loss journey. But before moving on, let us take a second look and recap the three *Slim Down Level Up Formulas,* so you can think about, as you look at the seven diets, which ones you would like to use when you start the 6-Week Program.

SLIM DOWN LEVEL UP FORMULAS

Slim Down Level Up Formula #1: Intermittent Fasting + Any Low-Calorie Diet

Slim Down Level Up Formula #2: Any Low-Calorie + Low-Carb Diet

Slim Down Level Up Formula #3: Keto + Any Low-Calorie + Intermittent Fasting Diet

POSITIVE MOMENT BREAK

Pause and breathe. Take a few deep cleansing breaths. I want to tell you something. In case no one has told you today, you matter, you are amazing, I believe in you and you can handle anything! Keep holding on to what you know is coming soon, a transformation. A success story, of how you will be victorious in taking back control of your health and your life.

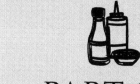

PART SIX
THE SECRET
SAUCE

14

3 MAGIC INGREDIENTS

Here we go! The secret sauce to your successful weight loss-*The Diets*. The, *what, when* and *how much* you are going to eat while losing and maintaining weight will be tied to which of the diets you decide to follow. We are going to look at the seven key eating styles I used to lose weight and how each one can help you reach your weight loss goals. They are all self-contained so they can be easily located and referred to later. What you will see is the basics of the different diets, their key benefits, food options, example meal plans and grocery shopping ideas, all to be able to assist you better when you start using the *6-Week Program*.

Should You Look at All the Diets? Yes. When you come out on the other side of the next two chapters, you will know which of the eating styles will work best for your lifestyle. To help you with making that decision, each of the diets are laid out to show you their effectiveness, food examples and additional success stories of how others combined the diets together to reach their goals.

First up in this chapter, will be the three key diets, Intermittent Fasting, Low-Calorie, and Low-Carb. We have briefly touched on them, but now we will take a more in-depth look at their benefits and examples. These were the *Base Diets* I used in helping me to lose weight.

Then, in Chapter 15, we will glance at the weight loss benefits of utilizing some of the *Remixx Diets* I used: the, Keto, Vegan, and Mediterranean Diet and the structured diet program, Weight Watchers. (Structured diet programs can be helpful if you need more support, premeasured options, meal plans and convenience).

While looking at the different diets, what you will discover is, the food options, recipes, and snack ideas, not only sound delicious but can aid in helping you lose weight faster. What you will also find in the two chapters, are various examples of different diet combinations, using all the eating styles mentioned in the book. They will be provided in a series of charts.

Side Note: Some of the diets and programs you may have used before and are familiar with the things they offer. As discussed earlier in the book, the best part about using the formulas is you will be able to take a diet that may not have worked so well for you in the past and now, combine it in various ways to make it work far better than ever before.

INTERMITTENT FASTING

"A little starvation can really do more for the average sick man than can the best medicine and the best doctors."
– Mark Twain

WHAT IS THE DIET?

Intermittent Fasting, (IF), for weight loss is something that has become a popular health trend in the last several years. Due to the fact, that while on a diet, determining *when* to eat is just as important as *what* to eat.

The key factor behind Intermittent Fasting is how it involves alternating between eating and not eating. Or you may also hear it referred to as feast and famine. It is about picking a specific shortened timeframe where you decide to eat. Then, when you are not eating for the prolonged periods of time, you push your body into the famine stage. The wonderful stage you are now familiar with, Ketosis. When you enter this stage, it will force your body to use its backup *stored fuel*, fat. I often refer to it as the, "Fasting's Fuel is Fat" stage of famine. It is one of my favorite *Base Diets* to use when losing weight.

Time restricting eating has so many health benefits to our bodies and metabolic health. Besides weight loss, it can aid in lowering inflammation, blood pressure and cholesterol and improving cognitive function. As mentioned earlier in chapter 3, it also helps with improving your insulin sensitivity.

What also happens when we fast is similar, to what happens when people get sick, and they have a forced fast. For example, normally, the last thing people want to do is eat when they are not feeling well. Instead, they mainly stay hydrated and rest while their body tries to recover from the illness and fight off infection.

When we fast, there is an activation of a self-healing process, called autophagy, that takes place. This is where the body recycles and removes old or damaged cell components. A cleaning out process which allows the body in so many, different ways to heal itself.

Intermittent Fasting is so much more than just deciding when you will eat. As we discussed in Chapter 2, the controlling of both insulin levels and insulin resistance are directly tied to weight loss. If you are overweight or obese, those key factors are contributing to your ability to gain and lose weight. The body's set weight (the weight your body has gotten the most comfortable at), is controlled by high insulin levels and persistence. Another way to say this is they are controlled from eating large amounts of food constantly throughout the day.

Therefore, reduction in food intake (Low-Calorie Diets) when losing weight can help reduce your insulin levels. Intermittent Fasting can help with lowering insulin resistance. The two can work together to help you lose weight by lowering your body's set weight. Allowing you to move past the initial dreaded plateau. Remember, another key benefit to fasting is, it also fights the faithful, hard to get rid of, visceral fat. Which, as you now know, I refer to as the dangerous fat. Carrying weight in the belly area pushes on major organs and can cause inflammation and can increase insulin resistance.

What Can You Expect When Fasting? When you decide to fast, within the first week, after your body has depleted your glucose stores and gets through the initial hunger pangs, it will switch over to using fat as its primary energy source. However, due to the lack of food, the effects can create a negative mood or irritability in some first-time fasters. Keep this in mind. This is, why it is recommended to meditate and pray during this time as, a way to rely on your faith and mental strength. It is also a good idea to not start a fast during a stressful week. Due to the possibility of you being short or impatient, or it is better known as being hangry. Hungry and angry mixed together because of the lack of food.

As you begin skipping more meals during your regular mealtime, you will be hungry. Even though fasting can decrease your appetite, you may be tempted to eat. Just know hunger comes in waves and will usually pass if you stay busy or focused on anything but eating. As time goes on, your body will adjust to receiving fewer calories. You will eventually feel less hungry, your mood will improve, and your energy levels will increase.

Fasting is not a new concept. The human body naturally adapted to fasting for centuries during the hunter/gatherer stages of mankind. Unlike today, they did not have the convenience of access to food all day long. They mainly spent the day hunting and gathering what they could and feasted on their finds at night. Even though they went for periods of time without food, they did not starve. But rather their bodies went into ketosis and used its' fat as fuel until they could get to their next meal. The science and benefits connected to when we fast are amazing. Fasting, compared to just receiving lower calories, helps to preserve muscle mass as well, especially when losing weight. (32) The human body knows how to survive and heal itself and will make the necessary adjustments to make sure we can still function, even when receiving less food.

If you do decide to use Intermittent Fasting, there are several schedules and methods you can choose from that can be modified to fit your needs. When first starting out, it is a good idea to *gradually* work yourself up to your desired fasting window. Because, initially, when hunger sets in, you can start to feel a reduction in your energy levels and need more time for your body to adjust. Drinking water, coffee, tea, or sparkling water can help with keeping you hydrated and reduce hunger (in Chapter 17, there is a list of approved drinks and protocols to incorporate when fasting, that you will be able to refer to).

CAN INTERMITTENT FASTING HELP YOU LOSE WEIGHT?

Absolutely! You can use Intermittent Fasting to lose weight by reducing your, eating window and pushing your body into ketosis. Allowing your body to rely on its back up fuel, fat and creating the desired fat burning weight loss phase. You can also reduce the number of meals you eat and your overall daily intake to create a calorie deficit. If you stick with the program, eat inside your scheduled window, monitor your caloric intake, coupled with eating more lean healthier foods, you can lose weight steadily.

However, fasting is not for everyone. Particularly if you are trying to lose weight but cannot imagine going *long* periods of time without food. But technically, you are already fasting and may not even realize it.

For example, if the last time you ate something was yesterday at 8 pm. And today, you did not eat breakfast until 8:30 am, you fasted for over 12 hours while preparing for bed and sleeping through the night.

What would be different if you "officially" started fasting is you would skip breakfast. Or push off eating it for 2 hours. Then cut off your, eating at night 2 hours earlier than you normally would. Making your eating window between 10 am –6 pm. Therefore, by default, utilizing the most-commonly used Intermittent Fasting method, the 16:8 Schedule. To lose weight, you would shorten your 12-hour eating window down to only 8 hours. That is one of the quickest ways to see your scale move in the right direction.

Unlike dieting, most people believe while using Intermittent Fasting there are *no* food restrictions and it is more of an eating pattern. As we saw from No Counting Carmen in Chapter 3, and from my excessive eating example, it may not always be helpful to utilize fasting without caloric parameters.

In the bigger picture, Intermittent Fasting is a style of eating that can and has been used to help people lose weight. Because they are limiting the time in which they eat down to a smaller window. However, if they eat unhealthy, high calorie dense meals during the shorter eating window, they are unlikely to see weight loss.

Therefore, if you decide to use Intermittent Fasting as your *Base Diet*, *Remixx Diet* or as an Enhancer-*Bonus Diet,* keep in mind, it is not a *free* for all. Even though you are eating in a shorter timeframe, for optimum weight loss, it is important to make healthier eating choices while fasting. Remember, you can always refer to Chapter 10, to see the Daily Body Budget Charts with the recommended caloric and fat grams based on your weight, age, activity level, and weight loss goals.

WEIGHT LOSS SUCCESS STORY TIME

Janet T.

"Using Intermittent Fasting and Low-Calorie foods has helped me to lower my blood pressure and lose 78 pounds. Watching my food intake, writing everything down and choosing a 16:8 fasting schedule has really changed my life." (33)

Janet was accountable and aware of her caloric intake, and it was a key tool in her successful weight loss story. This is where the power of combining different diets came into play. Combining Intermittent Fasting *and* a Low-Calorie Diet, helped with creating and keeping the needed calorie deficit. Fasting helped with burning fat and keeping her insulin resistance in check, so she could reach her weight loss goals.

In the next section you will see the five commonly used Intermittent Fasting Methods, and examples of how they can be used to help you lose weight.

INTERMITTENT FASTING METHODS

The 16:8 Method: This method of Intermittent Fasting is ideal for first time fasters and is one of the easier fasting schedules to follow, long-term. As with the previously mentioned example, it involves skipping or pushing back breakfast and eating in an 8-hour timeframe. For example, you may decide to eat between 11 am-7 pm, and fast the rest of the 16 hours. Within the 8-hour window, you may eat between two or three meals. Or decide to have four to five mini meals instead. As your body is adjusting to the new eating pattern, you will figure out what is the best 8-hour eating window for you, based on your schedule and lifestyle. Some examples of a 16:8 eating schedule are: **10:30-6:30 pm, 11-7 pm, 12:30-8:30 pm, or 1-9 pm**. During your fasting period, you can drink water, coffee, tea, and other non-caloric beverages. I like adding in fresh mint, lemons, or a dash of cinnamon. Drinking plenty of fluids can help with reducing hunger and keep you hydrated during the fasting period. This fasting method can also start with alternative times of, **12:12, 14:10, 15:9 and evolve to 18:6.**

16/8 Fasting Method Example

MIDNIGHT 7AM	DAY 1	DAY 2	DAY 3	DAY 4	DAY 5	DAY 6	DAY 7
	Fast	Fast	Fast	Fast	Fast	Fast	Fast
11 AM	FIRST MEAL	FIRST MEAL	FIRST MEAL	FIRST MEAL	FIRST MEAL	FIRST MEAL	FIRST MEAL
4 PM	Last Meal BY 7PM	Last Meal BY 7PM	Last Meal BY 7PM	Last Meal BY 7PM	Last Meal BY 7PM	Last Meal BY 7PM	Last Meal BY 7PM
7PM MIDNIGHT	Fast	Fast	Fast	Fast	Fast	Fast	Fast

The Eat Stop Eat/24 Hour Fast: This method of Intermittent Fasting is a wonderful *Enhancer* option to use in conjunction with the 16:8 method. It is a 24-hour fasting window, having only one meal a day. By using this method, it can keep your body in ketosis longer and burn more stored fat. It takes planning and some discipline and is not a recommended fasting schedule for first time fasters. If you follow this method, you would, eat dinner on one night, let's say at 7:30 pm, and then go the entire next day only having liquids until the same time the next night. Same fasting rules apply here, you can drink water, coffee, and other non-caloric beverages within your fasting window. This method is also referred to as, one meal a day or OMAD.

24-Hour Fast-OMAD- Eat Stop Eat Example

DAY 1	DAY 2	DAY 3	DAY 4	DAY 5	DAY 6	DAY 7
	Fast Day Only Liquids and OMAD			Fast Day Only Liquids and OMAD		

The 5:2 Method: This method of Intermittent Fasting is for you if you do not want to follow a smaller eating window 7 days a week but would like the benefits of fasting to lose weight. The **5:2 Method** gives you the flexibility to have five non-fasting days and two fasting days a week. On the non-fasting days, you do not have to skip breakfast or lunch and can eat throughout the day. However, as with any fasting schedule, be mindful of your food choices to create a calorie deficit to lose weight. For example, like sticking to a 1600 calorie budget on non-fasting days.

Even though you do not fast 7 days a week, there is a tradeoff with using this method. On the two fasting days (two-non-consecutive days), you will only eat between 500-600 calories total. You can choose to have the calories in two small meals or opt to eat all of them in one meal in the evening. Using the 500-600 calories wisely will be essential to your success on those two days. Whenever I used this method, I would eat prepacked food from the structured diet programs or meal delivery kit services, to ensure I was not taking in more than the desired calories. I also would eat low-calorie fresh fruits and vegetables, which was helpful and made me feel fuller longer.

An Example of Using the 5:2 Method:
Monday: Breakfast, Lunch & Dinner=1600 calories
Tuesday: Fasting Day=500-600 calories
Wednesday: Breakfast, Lunch & Dinner=1600 calories

Thursday: Breakfast, Lunch & Dinner=1600 calories
Friday: Fasting Day=500-600 calories
Saturday: Breakfast, Lunch & Dinner=1600 calories
Sunday: Breakfast, Lunch & Dinner=1600 calories

Side Note: The **5:2 Method** can be used as an *Extra or Bonus* with other fasting schedules to increase weight loss. You will see it as an option in the *6-Week Program*. If you are following the 16:8 Method, you can incorporate the two non-consecutive fasting days using the 500-600 calorie budget in your routine.

Example of Using a 4:3 Method: *Monday: Daily Intake *Tuesday: Daily Intake
*Wednesday: Fasting 500-600 calories *Thursday: Daily Intake
*Friday: Fasting 500-600 calories *Saturday: Daily Intake   ***Sunday: 500-600 calories**

4:3 Alternate Day Fasting Method: This method of Intermittent Fasting is similar to the 5:2 Method and can also be used if you do not want to fast 7 days a week. The **4:3 Method** gives you the flexibility to have four non-fasting days and *three* fasting days a week. On the non-fasting days, you do not skip breakfast or lunch and can eat throughout the day. However, as stated with using the 5:2 Method, be mindful of your food choices and how you are spending your daily body budget, to ensure you are creating a calorie deficit.

Like with using the 5:2 Method, on the three fasting days (three-non-consecutive days), you will only eat between 500-600 calories total. You can also choose to have the calories in two small meals or opt to eat all of them in one meal in the evening. Using the 500-600 calories wisely will be essential to your success on those three days. This is where having access to prepackaged meals can come into play and help you stay within the desired calories. Try incorporating low-calorie dense foods especially on those days, because they can make you feel full eating less calories (This fasting schedule can also be used as an *Extra or Bonus* with another schedule for added weight loss).

What Does 500-600 Calorie Meals Look Like?

Example 1:	Example 2:
1 Bowl of Oatmeal & 3 Berries=160 calories	Greek Yogurt with Nuts=150 calories
1 Medium Banana=100 calories	Cucumber/Tomato Salad=130 calories
Side Salad with Vinaigrette=160 calories	3 oz Baked Chicken Breast=155 calories
3 oz of Salmon=100 calories	1 cup of Carrots=50 calories
1 cup of Broccoli=30 calories	3 oz of Steamed Shrimp=85 calories
Total=550 calories	**Total=570 calories**

The Warrior Diet: This method of Intermittent Fasting schedule is not recommended for first time fasters. However, it can be done periodically as a detox or used with another fasting schedule as an *Extra or Bonus*. This method involves you eating the bulk of your day's calories in a four-hour window (feasting), and then fasting the other twenty hours (20:4 Method).

The goal of using this method would be to extend the 16:8 and 18:6 schedules by the additional hours. Reducing your, eating time-frame to a four-hour window. In that time, you can expect to eat one to two meals. And of course, during your fasting time, you can drink water, coffee, and other non-caloric beverages.

Unlike the Eat Stop Eat (OMAD), according to the creator of this method, Ori Hofmekler, you can consume small amounts of dairy products like yogurt and cheese inside of your 20-hour fasting window. As well as hard-boiled eggs and raw fruits and vegetables. Some people choose not to eat these items during that time but like having the option of being able to, if needed. Even though this method has a smaller eating window, it is still possible to overeat. To be successful while losing weight, be mindful of your caloric intake and the types of food you are eating.

Here is An Example of Eating Using the Warrior Diet

Breakfast	Lunch	Dinner
7am-12pm	12-5pm	5-9pm
Fast	Fast	Grilled Chicken Breasts
Water, Coffee	Water	Sauteed Vegetables
Tea	Tea	Steamed Garlic Shrimp
Hard-Boiled Eggs	Yogurt	Rice
Sparkling Water	Coffee	Sliced Avocado
Coffee	Water	Cup of Mixed Fruit

IS INTERMITTENT FASTING EASY TO FOLLOW?

When deciding to utilize Intermittent Fasting to lose weight, there is no need to feel overwhelmed when first starting. You can go slow and pick the schedule that will work best for your needs. Fasting is something you can do for life and doing it in a way, that fits your lifestyle is what will make you the most successful.

When first starting out, it is a good idea to put some planning and preparation in place. On how and when you will start your fast and with which schedule. If you are hesitant in starting out with a larger fasting window, you can reduce your eating window in small increments.

For example, if you normally eat in a 12 to 14-hour window and are aiming to use a 16:8 fasting schedule, reduce your eating window by 30 minutes every other day. By doing this in the first 7-14 days of starting your diet, you can gradually reach the desired fasting window. This technique will slowly push your body into getting used to going without food for longer periods of time. I recommend this format to all first-time fasters. This is, why it is a part of the *6-Week Program* when you use Formula #1 or #3. In case, you have not fasted before or if it has been a while since you last used Intermittent Fasting. My philosophy is, it is better to go slow and win the race than to go fast and never see the finish line.

After you start fasting, you will begin, to notice the more you do not eat, the more you can go without eating. Your body will switch over to utilizing stored fat as fuel and make the adjustment to receiving less calories. In the first two weeks, you can experience a decrease and then an increase in your energy levels. As well as an increase and then a decrease in hunger pangs.

Intermittent Fasting can be a little challenging at first, and you may have days and nights when you are hungry. I had several, before my body got used to going without food. But if you stick with it, in a short period of time, you can see results. When the scale moves and you experience the difference in how you look and feel, you can embrace the changes, knowing your decision to fast is increasing your overall health.

Also, if after reading this book you would like more information and tips on the benefits of using Intermittent Fasting, from a medical standpoint, besides the previously referenced book, The Obesity Code, I recommend The Power of Appetite Correction, by Dr. Bert Herring. In the book, Dr. Herring makes some key points about while using Intermittent Fasting to lose weight, there also needs to be a constant adjustment to which *schedule* will work best for you (I list a few other recommendations to read in the back of the book as well).

Each one of our bodies are different, and as he points out, using a 16:8 fasting schedule may work for one but not for another. Starting with one schedule does not mean that will be your "sweet spot" of where your body has enough energy, is not hungry, and you are burning the most, fat. Being open, to making adjustments to your fasting window while losing weight will be key to your success (varying Fasting Schedules are a part of the *Slim Down Level Up Formulas*).

Spontaneous Meal Skipping

Another option in the world of fasting, that can be used, if you choose not to follow either of the previously mentioned fasting schedules is, *Spontaneous Meal Skipping*. It is exactly as it sounds; you would randomly skip meals throughout the week. This is another way to reduce your food intake to create the desired calorie deficit and reap some of the benefits of fasting.

Spontaneous Meal Skipping Example

DAY 1	DAY 2	DAY 3	DAY 4	DAY 5	DAY 6	DAY 7
Breakfast	Skip Meal	Breakfast	Breakfast	Skip Meal	Breakfast	Breakfast
Lunch	Lunch	Lunch	Skip Meal	Lunch	Lunch	Lunch
Dinner	Dinner	Dinner	Dinner	Dinner	Skip Meal	Dinner

WHAT IS AN EATING EXAMPLE OF A FASTING DAY?

7am-11 am

Drink Coffee, Tea, Water, Sparkling Water

11am-7pm

Smoothie, Grilled Chicken Breast, Salad, Cup of Mixed Fruit, Mixed Vegetables

*Always refer to the Daily Body Budget Charts for your calories and fat grams

7pm-11pm

Drink Coffee, Tea, Water, Sparkling Water

11pm-7am

Sleep

SHOULD YOU EXERCISE WHILE FASTING?

Intermittent Fasting is only an eating pattern, and it does not mean you should not exercise. In fact, being physically active lowers your risk of heart disease and diabetes. It also, helps you get and keep the weight off and increases your energy levels. Most experts agree, getting at least 30-45 minutes of low to moderate intensity exercises, can be beneficial long-term for your health. Like brisk walking, bike riding, dancing, or swimming. Increasing your overall activity levels throughout the day contributes to your overall health. Aim for 8-10,000 steps a day.

Side Note: If after seeing all the dieting combinations, you decide to use Intermittent Fasting as your *Base Diet*, when following the *6-Week Program*, you will not add exercising to your weight loss routine until the beginning of week 2. The first 7 days will be all about your body adjusting to receiving fewer calories and making the changes to burning fat, as your primary fuel. It can be a lot to deal with when first starting a diet and focusing on your mental and physical preparedness will be the goal in Phase 1 of the program.

In that first week of the program, the time you would *normally* workout, use it to shop, meal prep and make necessary arrangements for cooking and/or signing up for meal plans.

When you do get started on the *6-Week Program*, always remember to drink plenty of water and non-caloric beverages while fasting. If, for some reason, while exercising or even if you are not exercising, if you feel faint, dizzy, or nauseous, stop and eat or drink something, as necessary. Do not ignore your body's signals being sent to you.

As, stated earlier, Intermittent Fasting is something you can do for life. Sis, listen, it is not going to be the end of the world, (and please do not beat yourself up) if you do not make it to your fasting schedule every day. Especially as you are first transitioning to the new lifestyle of eating. Be kind to your mind, take it one day and one pound at a time. Remember, this is about progress not perfection.

Take a look at the chart on the next page, and you will see various examples with the **Intermittent Fasting Diet,** we just learned about. The chart uses it as the *Base Diet* and combines it with a different *Remixx Diet*. Below the chart, is a snapshot of what two of the options would look like when combined. All the charts in this chapter and the next can be used as guides. After following the *6-Week Program,* you can choose to mix and match either diet eating style of your choosing.

INTERMITTENT FASTING BASE DIET EXAMPLES

BASE DIET	PLUS	REMIXX DIET
INTERMITTENT FASTING*		LOW-CALORIE
INTERMITTENT FASTING*		VEGAN
INTERMITTENT FASTING*		WEIGHT WATCHERS
INTERMITTENT FASTING*		KETO
INTERMITTENT FASTING*		MEDITERRANEAN
INTERMITTENT FASTING*		JENNY CRAIG
INTERMITTENT FASTING*		PALEO
INTERMITTENT FASTING*		SOUTH BEACH
INTERMITTENT FASTING*		LOW-CARB
INTERMITTENT FASTING*		NUTRISYSTEM

*You will be able to select a Fasting Method and Schedule from the Charts in Chapter 17.

You can also refer to Chapter 10 and 11 for your Calories, Fat Grams and Net Carbs prior to starting the program.

Examples:

1. Intermittent Fasting with a 5:2 Schedule using a Paleo Diet (Daily Body Budget is 1400-1500 Calories, 46-50 Fat Grams and Moderate Carb intake at 20-50 Net Carbs Max)

2. Intermittent Fasting with a 16:8 Schedule using South Beach/Keto food options (Daily Body Budget is 1600-1700 Calories, 53-57 Fat Grams and Ketogenic Low-Carbs of 20 or less Net Carbs Max)

Side Note: Combining either of the Remixx Diets listed on the previous page, with the Base Diet, Intermittent Fasting, takes losing weight to the next level for you. Based on your food preferences and the amount of weight you want to lose, you can use the food from more than one of the Remixx Diets while on your journey. The good part is, by the end of this book, you will have seen several options and will be able to choose how you want to lose your weight.

LOW-CALORIE DIET
WHAT IS THE DIET?

We briefly touched on low-calorie diets in Chapter 2. A Low-Calorie Diet usually involves eating more plant-based foods, as well as using meal replacements like shakes, protein bars, meatless dinners, or soups. Diets like these can help improve your insulin sensitivity, reduce inflammation, and provide better blood sugar control.

Most people, when following a Low-Calorie Diet, take in between 1200-1600 calories a day maximum. You can also see results by reducing your daily average intake by 500 calories. For example, a person taking in 2200 calories a day can reduce their daily intake down to 1700 calories for weight loss.

Doctors, nutritionists, and dietitians often prescribe a 1200 calorie program for rapid weight loss to their patients. It provides a significantly lower amount of calories, for the average person and creates the desired calorie deficit. A very low-calorie diet, VLCD, which is usually given under a professional's care, consists of taking in no more than 700-800 calories a day.

The key in using a Low-Calorie Diet is to eat more low-energy, (low-calories), dense foods to feel fuller longer. For example, foods like vegetables, fruits, nuts, seeds, fish, and eggs. Using a Low-Calorie Diet to lose weight is not so much about eating less, as it is about eating smarter. How you choose to spend your calories is just as important as how many you are taking in each day.

That is because all calories are *not equal*. We saw this when we looked at the Twinkie Diet experiment. Understanding this is essential in losing weight because it can help you pick healthier, more filling choices to use your calories wisely. Fortunately, there are plenty for you to choose from. For example, I discovered the Mediterranean and Paleo Diets have several food options available that are low-calorie and delicious. Similar to, some of the ones listed in Chapter 13 from the meal delivery kit services, Spanish Moroccan Fish and Slow Cooked Beef Stew with Mixed Vegetables.

CAN A LOW-CALORIE DIET HELP YOU LOSE WEIGHT?

Yes! You can use Low-Calorie Diets to lose and maintain weight. There arc several you can follow, using either prepackaged meal programs, or a combination of foods and recipes you enjoy and sticking to a low-calorie daily body budget. Keep in mind, most diets can work when you make healthy lifestyle choices in conjunction with the reduction in calories. Like increasing your daily activity, cooking more at home, reducing processed, refined foods, sodas, juices, and sugar from your diet.

Weight loss will vary from person to person depending on how low you reduce your caloric intake, whether, or not you combine it with another diet and your overall activity level. As we went over in Chapter 10, the *Daily Body Budget Charts,* have the recommended calories, and fat grams intake, based on your weight, age, and activity levels. The daily calculations are provided to help you lose weight without extreme restrictions. Low-Calorie Diets can help you achieve weight loss of up to 3 to 5 pounds per week when incorporated with healthier food choices and increased daily activity.

WEIGHT LOSS SUCCESS STORY TIME

Jeanette A.

"Tracking my intake motivated me to make healthy choices and stick to my calorie goals. I did Intermittent Fasting and used a calorie-counter app to lose 122 pounds." (34)

Two snaps in the air for her success with combining different diets together. Jeanette had been dieting for a while before she realized her counting calories was just as important as what she was spending them on. When she finally made the connection, her success was inevitable.

That is because when using a Low-Calorie Diet, it can be helpful when you use your calories on volume foods like vegetables, whole grains, and lean proteins. They provide the biggest bang for the buck and use a smaller amount of your daily calorie budget. It is also important when following a Low-Calorie Diet to incorporate healthy fats into your daily intake. They are necessary for cell growth and organ protection. Examples of healthy fats are nuts, seeds, and plant-based oils.

IS A LOW-CALORIE DIET EASY TO FOLLOW?

Yes! Low-Calorie Diets can be easy to follow if you utilize key tools to help you with keeping track of your overall intake. To ensure you are in fact on a low-calorie diet, it is important to know what your daily consumption is. You can use any of the free apps listed in Chapter 13 to keep a daily diary of all your food. That way, you will not worry about if you are staying within your correct body budget for the day. The Apps can also help you keep track of how many calories you burn daily.

Side Note: All three *Slim Down Level Up Formulas* use a Low-Calorie Diet as a key player to help you lose weight. Regardless of which one you plan to follow, as you are losing weight be sure you are checking back with the Daily Body Budget Charts in Chapter 10, to reduce your daily intake accordingly. This step is needed because as you are losing, you will not require as many calories to sustain the weight you are. The reduction in calories can continue creating the daily calorie deficit needed, so you can keep losing more weight. For example, if you were taking in 1900 calories and 63 fat grams back when you were 25 pounds heavier, based on your new weight, you would make the adjustment and reduce your intake to 1600 calories and 53 fat grams. **What will make following a Low-Calorie Diet easier?** Using fitness apps, ordering food from meal kit delivery services, premeasured packaged foods from diet programs, and learning easier, simpler ways of cooking healthier, low-calorie meals at home.

WHAT ARE SOME EXAMPLES OF A LOW-CALORIE DIET?

Low-Calorie Foods: 3 oz Chicken Breast=138 calories, 3 oz Lean Ground Beef =182 calories, 3 oz Flank Steak=138 calories, 3 oz Salmon=177 calories, 1 cup Cucumbers=16 calories, 1 cup Spinach=7 calories, 1 cup Tomatoes=32 calories, 1 cup Watermelon=46 calories, 1 Apple= 95 calories, ½ cup Pinto Beans=123 calories, ½ cup Chickpeas=134 calories, ½ cup Lentils=115 calories, 1 cup Skim Milk=89 calories, 1 Egg=78 calories, ½ cup Non-Fat Cottage Cheese=80 calories, 1 cup Oats=150 calories, 1 oz Chia Seeds=137 calories, 1 oz Pistachios=159 calories, 1 oz Cashews=157 calories, 1 cup Quinoa=222 calories

EXAMPLES OF LOW-CALORIE MEALS

1200 Calorie Day Example:	1500 Calorie Day Example:
Breakfast:	**Breakfast:**
1 Cup of Berries	3 Cinnamon Vanilla Pancakes
1 Cup of Plain Yogurt	1 Apple
Lunch:	**Lunch:**
6-8 oz Turkey Sandwich on Wheat Bread	1 ½ Cup of Chicken Chili
1 Orange	12 Baby Carrots & 2 tbsp of Hummus
Dinner: 6 oz of Grilled Salmon	**Dinner:** Chicken Fajita Quesadilla
1 medium Sweet Potato	½ cup of Black or Red Beans
1 cup of Steamed Broccoli	1 cup of Steamed Green Beans

LOW CALORIE CONDIMENTS

*Sriracha – 5 calories *Hot Sauce – 5 calories *Mustard – 5 calories *Soy Sauce – 5 calories *Salsa – 10 calories *Sugar Free Ketchup – 10 calories *Pico de Gallo – 10 calories *Sugar Free BBQ sauce – 10 calories *Apple Cider Vinegar – 5 calories *Balsamic Vinegar – 15 calories

Take a look at the chart on the next page. Unlike the first chart, these are examples if you are *not* going to use the Intermittent Fasting Diet. But rather, your *Base Diet* would use the benefits of following a **Low-Calorie Diet.** Which can be combined with one of the *Remixx Diets* of your choosing.

Either one of the examples in the chart can provide you the power of combining different diets together, to help you lose more weight.

LOW-CALORIE BASE DIET EXAMPLES

BASE DIET	PLUS	REMIXX DIET
LOW-CALORIE		INTERMITTENT FASTING*
LOW-CALORIE		VEGAN
LOW-CALORIE		WEIGHT WATCHERS
LOW-CALORIE		KETO
LOW-CALORIE		MEDITERRANEAN
LOW-CALORIE		JENNY CRAIG
LOW-CALORIE		PALEO
LOW-CALORIE		SOUTH BEACH
LOW-CALORIE		NUTRISYSTEM
LOW-CALORIE		LOW-CARB

*You will see a variety of fasting schedule charts in Chapter 17.

You can refer to Chapter 10 and 11 for your Calories, Fat Grams and Net Carbs prior to starting the program.

Examples:

1. Low-Calorie with a Low-Carb Diet (Daily Body Budget is 1500 Calories, 50 Fat Grams and Moderate Low-Carb intake is 20-50 Net Carbs Max)

2. Low-Calorie with a Vegan Diet (Daily Body Budget is 1700 Calories, 56 Fat Grams, Liberal Low-Carb intake is, 50-100 Net Carbs Max)

Side Note: Structured diet programs like, South Beach, Weight Watchers, Nutrisystem and Jenny Craig, generally have a low-calorie diet included in their programs. However, if you are just purchasing their food, and supplementing it with other recipes etc. it is important to stick to your Daily Body Budget numbers to increase your weight loss success. The same thing applies to the Remixx Diets we will go over in the next chapter. Combining them with a Low-Calorie Diet will provide you the needed parameters for answering the *how* much and *what* you will eat while losing weight.

LOW-CARB DIET
WHAT IS THE DIET?

A Low-Carb Diet means you include fewer carbohydrates in your daily intake. For example, bread, rice, candy, pasta, ice cream. Your primary food source would come from fat. This diet includes small amounts of protein as well. The best part, of course, is with your body taking in fewer carbs, it will burn stored fat as fuel. A Low-Carb Diet can also be referred to as a Low-Carb, High-Fat Diet (LCHF).

For years, we have seen and heard stories of fat being detrimental to our overall health and how it can cause heart disease related problems. However, the trendy "low-fat diet" products promoted on our supermarket shelves can be a bigger problem for us. Many of those types of products make us believe we need to eat them over the others, as the better "weight loss" choice. But low-fat does not always mean it's weight loss friendly because often they are loaded with sugars and high carbs. For example, flavored yogurts and several types of granola bars disguise themselves as "low-fat" products. However, they can be equivalent to having a dessert with the amount of carbs and sugars they have.

A Low-Carb Diet is effective because it can lower your insulin levels and insulin resistance. It is a powerhouse player in the *Slim Down Level Up Formula #2* and is the reason behind why that combination works so well. Here is a recap of the chart from Chapter 11.

LOW-CARB CHART

1.	**Liberal Low-Carb** is taking in between 50-100 net carbs max daily
2.	**Moderate Low-Carb** is taking in between 20-50 net carbs max daily
3.	**Ketogenic Low-Carb (Keto)** is taking in at or below 20 net carbs max daily

CAN A LOW-CARB DIET HELP YOU LOSE WEIGHT?

Yes! Using a Low-Carb Diet can help you lose weight because it can increase your metabolism and decrease your hunger. Which is vital to losing weight long-term. By taking in the higher fat foods, you will feel full eating less. Creating a situation where you would be taking in fewer calories, allowing the calorie deficit to take place. The other benefits besides losing weight are lowering your blood pressure, reducing your belly fat, as well as lowering blood triglycerides. Which are the fat molecules that increases your risk of heart disease. Using a Low-Carb Diet can also increase your HDL, the good cholesterol. The diet primarily focuses on incorporating healthier foods like lean meats, fish, eggs, seeds, nuts, and healthy fats. By default, with you using this type of eating style, you can remove a lot of unnecessary processed food from your diet. This is not just beneficial to your weight loss goal, but also to improving your health.

"Research shows that women who are obese or have metabolic problems do better hormonally on lower carbs. Improved outcomes include better sleep, mental clarity and increased satiety." (35)

That can be seen, as great news because, being overweight or obese is a hormonal disorder of fat regulation. If by using a Low-Carb Diet, you experience better sleep patterns and mental clarity, they can decrease the stress hormone, cortisol, in your body. We talked about persistent high levels of cortisol over time, can cause you to gain weight, but it can also disrupt your sleep patterns, cause high blood pressure, as well as contribute to diabetes.

In that same study, the results were helpful in identifying how using a Low-Carb Diet can also provide feelings of satiety (fullness) and can decrease your appetite. Causing you to eat less. Which means, a decreased appetite equals successful weight loss.

IS A LOW-CARB DIET EASY TO FOLLOW?

A Low-Carb Diet can be a little challenging for carb lovers initially; however, with proper planning, it can make following the diet easier. Avoiding foods like chips, cookies, crackers, rice, bread, pasta, milk, bananas, ice cream, candy, beans, and lentils, can increase the effectiveness of the diet and produce better weight loss results. Having a Low-Carb daily intake makes you pay more attention to the number of processed food in your diet. The less you eat of those types of products, and reduce your overall carb intake, the sooner your body can make the change to burning fat as fuel instead of glucose. Making the diet easier to adjust to and adapt to the new way of eating. The diet can be easier to follow if you incorporate more foods like broccoli, zucchini, chicken, fish, olives, raspberries, and avocados. If you decide to add Intermittent Fasting with it, keep in mind, it can help your body get into ketosis a lot easier and faster.

There are additional benefits to using a Low-Carb Diet that can make it easier to lose weight. For example, there was a study conducted in 2016 on the benefits of using a low-carb diet in aiding in lowering insulin resistance. "People who ate three lower-carb meals (of less than 30 percent carbs each) reduced their insulin resistance by more than 30 percent compared with people who consumed higher-carb meals (60 percent carbs)." (36)

This is significant in losing weight because, as we learned in Chapter 3, controlling both insulin levels and insulin resistance are required. The results from the study provides another example to the benefits of using a Low-Carb and Low-Calorie Diet, together to help you reach your goals. This is the key to why *Slim Down Level Up Formula #2* works so efficiently.

WHAT ARE SOME EXAMPLES OF A LOW-CARB DIET?

Here Are Some Examples of Eating on a Low-Carb Diet

Ribeye Steak	Ground Beef	Lamb	Chicken Thighs & Wings
Bacon	Jerky Turkey	Veal	Bison Salmon
Sardines	Shellfish Shrimp	Lobster Catfish	Halibut
Cauliflower	Brussels Sprouts	Tomatoes Eggplant	Cucumbers
Kale Bell Peppers	Asparagus	Mushrooms Spinach	Cabbage

Here Are Examples of Low-Carb Diet Meals

Breakfast: Bacon and Scrambled Eggs with Spinach and Mushrooms
Lunch: Bunless Cheeseburger with Sliced Avocado
Dinner: Grilled Chicken Wings with a Cucumber Tomato Salad

Breakfast: Chocolate Coconut Smoothie with Heavy Cream and Protein Powder
Lunch: Chicken Fajita Soup and ½ cup of Raspberries
Dinner: Roasted Garlic Pork Chop with Steamed Vegetables

Following a Low-Carb Diet can be beneficial to your weight loss goals. There are a variety of tasty food options you will be able to choose from, that will be low-carb and low-calorie to help you stay within your daily body budget numbers.

CAN YOU EXERCISE WHILE USING ANY OF THE THREE DIETS?

Absolutely. Intermittent Fasting, Low-Calorie and Low-Carb Diets will determine what, when and how much you will eat. By adding physical activities, it can help you lose weight and improve your overall health. Low to moderate intensity is ideal for fat burning. As, mentioned earlier, things like brisk walking, bike riding and swimming, or even dancing are wonderful and can burn lots of calories. Light to moderate weightlifting is also a good idea to build muscle and increase your overall daily activity. Incorporating exercises into your routine will increase your metabolism and can also help to burn stored fat.

What is the Best Time to Work Out? Anytime you can fit it, into your schedule. For me, I had the most success working out in the mornings. I do not know if you are a morning person or not, but there are benefits to working out in the AM.

One, you can burn more fat on an empty stomach, and two, you can remove any excuses if for some reason unexpected things pop up as the day goes on. Three, it can help with decreasing your appetite and may push back breakfast until later in the morning (you can reap the benefits from an unintentional or intentional fast). Keep in mind, exercise also revs up your metabolism. I am recommending you work out in the mornings; however, if that is not possible with your schedule, workout whenever you can. The most important thing is, that you do add some form of physical activity to your daily routine.

In the first week of the *6-Week Program*, regardless of which *Slim Down Level Up Formula* you use, you will not add exercising to your weight loss routine. This is designed into the program for a reason. The first week of the program is all about your mental and physical preparedness, while you are making the *shift*. Instead of working out, you can use the time to shop, meal prep and make any additional necessary arrangements for cooking and/or you can sign up for meal plans.

During that same time, also work on increasing your daily activities, like parking the car farther away, taking the stairs instead of the elevator and talking on the phone while walking around instead of sitting. You can also work on preparing your exercise regimen by ordering, looking up or gathering all necessary workout items, shoes, clothes, leg or arm weights, YouTube videos, DVD's etc. or find out about the different fitness programs offered in your area.

When you do start incorporating exercise into your routine, refer to Chapter 19 for ideas and tips on getting started and on how to increase the duration and intensity as you are losing weight.

I recommend you lay out all your exercise items the night before each workout to have them ready to go first thing in the morning. This can help remove any excuses as to why you do not go. Plus, your workout items staring back at you, will be a reminder of what you had *planned* to do. Lastly, working out can force you to stay hydrated, by drinking more water to help cool you down during and after each workout.

On the next page is the final chart in this chapter and it includes examples of losing weight using a *Base Diet,* **Low-Carb** with a variety of *Remixx* and *Bonus Diets.* Take a look at the various ways you can combine the different eating styles.

Low-Carb Base with Remixx and Bonus Diets

BASE DIET   PLUS   REMIXX DIET   PLUS   BONUS DIET

BASE DIET	REMIXX DIET	BONUS DIET
LOW-CARB	**VEGAN**	Low Calorie Reduced to 1200 Calories and 40 Fat Grams Daily
LOW-CARB	**WEIGHT WATCHERS**	Enhanced Fasting Schedule Add Two 24-Hour or 36-Hour Fasting Days a Week
LOW-CARB	**MEDITERRANEAN**	4:3 Fasting Schedule 500-600 calories on fasting days Normal on other days
LOW-CARB	**JENNY CRAIG**	No Added Sugar 14-day Challenge
LOW-CARB	**SOUTH BEACH**	Meatless Days Added 3 Days a Week
LOW-CARB	**PALEO**	Liquid Dinner Meal Replacement 3 Days a Week
LOW-CARB	**NUTRISYSTEM**	5:2 Fasting Schedule 500-600 calories on fasting days Normal on other days
LOW-CARB	**LOW-CALORIE**	Liquid Dinner Meal Replacement 3 Days a Week

*You can refer to Chapter 10 and 11 for your Calories, Fat Grams and Net Carbs prior to starting the program.

SLIM DOWN LEVEL UP

Examples: Daily Body Budget is 1200-1400 Calories, 40-46 Fat Grams, Liberal: 50-100 Net Carbs

1. Low-Carb and Mediterranean Diet and a 5:2 Fasting Schedule

2. Low-Carb and Jenny Craig and a No Added Sugar Challenge

Before we talk about the four Remixx Diets, let us pause for a moment and point out a couple of things from the different examples in the charts. There was a total of three charts. They all used a different *Base Diet* and were combined with a variety of Remixx Diets. The first was Intermittent Fasting, the second Low-Calorie and the third Low-Carb. (The third chart also showed how to add in a Bonus Diet as well). The charts will give you so many options to choose from down the line. After following the *6-Week Program*, you can use any of them to continue dominating losing weight. Or you will have the option to move on to the next step of the program. You will be provided a number of options, to choose from to fit your diet preferences. All with examples guiding you along the way.

EXAMPLE TIME

Let us just say, for example purposes, now that you have seen the three *Slim Down Level Up Formulas,* and a few of the Base, Remixx and Bonus Diet examples, you are thinking about using *Formula #3* to lose weight. That would mean your *Base Diet* would be Keto, your *Remixx Diet* would be Low-Calorie and your *Bonus Diet,* would be Intermittent Fasting. What would the process look like to getting started?

It would involve 3 steps for you to select in the book from the different lists:

1. Which Intermittent Fasting Schedule you want to use to start with

2. Selecting the different types of Keto foods, shopping list, recipes, and snacks ideas

3. Locating your precalculated Daily Body Budget numbers on the charts provided (calories, fat grams and net carbs)

All designed to take the guesswork out for you, so you have an easier time deciding on which combination to use. Additional combinations will be available for you to either change up your fasting schedule routine, add in a different *Remixx Diet* or change the *Bonus Diet* to one of the other listed options.

The *Slim Down Level Up 6-Week Program* is about you. It is about learning new ways to take losing weight to another level. The battle of the bulge can be hard and learning how to apply the techniques to your day-to-day routine can make it easier.

In the coming chapters, we will discuss little tips I learned over the years that may be helpful to you on your journey. As well as additional key pieces to set you on a path to taking control of your health and transforming your body. But first I would like to share with you how, while on my weight loss journey, I discovered and created the power of the *Slim Down Level Up Formula #3*.

At the time, I combined Intermittent Fasting with Keto and a Low-Calorie Diet. I had previously already lost 64 pounds using other combination methods. But I had reached a plateau and decided to make the change. By combining Intermittent Fasting with Keto and reducing my caloric intake, I kicked my diet combination into full gear.

How? By, pushing my body into ketosis, and lowering my insulin levels and insulin resistance. **When I did, in a little over a month, my 64-pound weight loss went to 79 pounds.** What also contributed to my success was, I took it to the next level and incorporated alternating Meatless and Liquid Dinners 3 times a week. Needless, to say I was very, excited with the results.

*__Full Disclosure:__ I was also working out 4-5 days a week for 45-60 minutes during that time to help with losing the weight.

15

THE 4 REMIXX EATING STYLES

This chapter brings us to looking at the four key *Remixx Diet* options, Keto, Vegan, Mediterranean, and Weight Watchers. You can utilize them in conjunction with any of the previously mentioned *Base Diets*. Adding this step is where the power of combining different diets together will show you its magic. When that happens, you will begin to see the weight come off.

When looking at the diets in this chapter, again, not to sound like a broke down record but, you do not necessarily have to completely commit full on, per se, to one way of eating. What will be helpful is to keep an open mind when reading the different options for you to choose from. For example, when we look at the food from the Keto or Vegan Diet, you do not have to fully adopt their diet eating styles to try some of their food, to help you lose weight. Actually, some of the food and snack options may pleasantly surprise you, as they did me, with how good they tasted. **When making your food selections, remind yourself, meatless dinners can make you thinner and taking in lower carbs and having a liquid meal, can help seal your weight loss deal.**

As you read about some of the different diets, you may notice there are some similarities between the food options you can use in either of the other diets. A lot of the choices are interchangeable that is because the focus is on helping you make healthier food choices for weight loss and improved health. This is what will make the *Slim Down Level Up Formulas,* so much more enjoyable and maintainable for you.

After seeing all the diets, you will have a vast quantity of quality food choices at your disposal. (Recipes, prepackaged meal plans, support groups, cookbooks, tips and tools and meal kit delivery services). All of which will be ready to help assist you with reaching your goal weight.

KETOGENIC DIET

WHAT IS THE DIET?

The Ketogenic Diet (or Keto Diet, for short) is a low-carb, high-fat diet that offers many health benefits. Similar, to the Low-Carb Diet, however, this one involves drastically reducing your carbohydrate intake and replacing it with fat. This reduction in carbs puts your body into a metabolic state you now know so well, called Ketosis. When this happens, not only does your body become incredibly efficient at burning fat for energy, it also turns fat into ketones in the liver, which can supply energy for the brain.

A Keto Diet can help you lose much more weight than if you were to use a low-fat diet. This often happens without hunger. Because you cut back on most of the carbs that are easy to digest, which are, considered to be wasted calories. Like sugar, soda, pastries, and white bread.

There are four commonly used types of Keto Diets that can be used to lose weight.

4 DIFFERENT VERSIONS OF THE KETO DIET

- **Standard Keto Diet (SKD):** This is a low-carb, moderate-protein, and high-fat diet. The macronutrient breakdown is typically: 75% fat, 20% protein and only 5% carbs.

- **Cyclical Keto Diet (CKD):** This diet involves periods of higher-carb refeeds, such as 5 ketogenic days followed by 2 high-carb days.

- **Targeted Keto Diet (TKD):** This diet allows you to add carbs around workouts.

- **High-Protein Keto Diet:** This is similar, to a standard ketogenic diet but includes more protein. The macronutrient breakdown is typically: 60% fat, 35% protein and 5% carbs.

- There are several versions of the Keto Diet. The standard (SKD) version is the most recommended and researched out of all the options. (37)

CAN IT HELP YOU LOSE WEIGHT?

Yes, it can, specifically thanks to ketosis. But more importantly, let us take a look at what happens when your body goes into this stage. When you consistently eat fewer carbs, your body eventually runs out of its primary fuel, glucose, blood sugar. Which can typically take 3 to 4 days. After it runs out completely, your body will start to break down protein and fat for energy. This is when it enters the Ketosis stage. And the body turns into a constant fat burning, belly busting machine. How can you reach ketosis? By not eating too many carbs. What is too many carbs?

To follow a *Keto Diet* specifically and not just a Low-Carb Diet, it is a good idea to be at or below 20 net carbs. The fewer the carbs you eat daily, the more effective the diet can be in helping you reach ketosis. Which can lead to helping you lose weight.

Another benefit of following a Keto Diet is having a steady supply of energy (coming from stored fat) without repeated sugar peaks and valleys that can come from eating a high carb diet. By not having all the highs followed by the repeated lows, it can help you be more alert and focused throughout the day.

If you decide to use a Keto Diet as one of your diet combinations, at first it will be helpful to count your carbs. One of the easiest ways to do that is by using a fitness app. This would be a good idea to keep track of, until you are more comfortable with identifying what is good for you to eat. As well as to make sure you stay within the recommended numbers. In order, to calculate your macronutrient breakdown, you can refer to the Daily Body Budget Charts in Chapter 10 for your recommended intake.

Lastly, a Keto Diet can help you lose weight because, by cutting your carbs, it keeps your blood sugar and insulin levels low. It also helps with reducing cravings by lowering ghrelin, which is your hunger hormone. Another benefit is, "Ketogenic diets may help lower your risks of heart disease and can help people who have diseases, such as Metabolic Syndrome, Insulin Resistance and Type 2 Diabetes." (38)

IS A KETO DIET EASY TO FOLLOW?

You can use a Keto Diet for weight loss for a short period of time or cycle in and out as your weight loss needs change. Carbs are kept to a minimum, fat-rich foods are high on the list and your protein intake is moderate. If you are a carb lover, it can be a little difficult at first making the adjustments to reducing your overall daily intake. However, it is the simple carbs that you would primarily be cutting out. Like white bread, white rice, baked goods, soda, sugar, and honey. The good part is, nowadays, there are a variety of low-carb wraps, rice substitutes like cauliflower rice, low-carb pastas, and desserts that can make the transition a lot easier for you. The Keto Diet is not the typical daily intake of food most people are used to eating. Initially, it will take some time getting adjusted, as your body is preparing to make the shift to ketosis.

Here is an example of what you can expect when following a Keto Diet:

- The first 12-24 hours after reducing your carbs to between 20-50 grams, your body will start producing ketones

- The next 4-5 days, your body may shift into, what is referred as, the *Keto Flu*

- Some of the symptoms you may experience are dehydration, fatigue, and mind fog

- Staying hydrated during this time is so important

- Add high quality salts to your food and in your water to replace the electrolytes that will be lost initially due to the depletion of excess water

- It is recommended to drink water the equivalent to a minimum of half your body weight in ounces

- Drink a glass of water first thing in the morning, throughout the day and at least 16-20 ounces with every meal

By day 7, you will start seeing weight loss. Initially, it will be mostly water weight; that is why increasing your water intake will be essential in being successful and in helping to reduce the Keto flu symptoms. As you progress into the second and third week, you will not only see weight loss but also begin to feel better. You will experience more energy, less brain fog, and a decrease in hunger. That is because, at that point, your body is adjusting better to the diet.

By week four, you can expect additional weight loss, especially if you have been physically active and sticking closely to your daily body budget numbers and macronutrient breakdown. By week five and beyond, you should be experiencing less cravings for carbs, if any at all. You will also see more weight loss, hunger control increased and be more fat adapted to where your body is primarily using fat as fuel.

Key Point: Selecting the right food will begin to get a lot easier as you become accustomed to using the Keto Diet and are more familiar with the daily macronutrient breakdown. Here is a recap of using the (SKD) Standard Keto Diet.

Daily breakdown of how to spend your calories:

- Fat=75%

- Protein=20%

- Carbs=5%

Based on a 2,000 calories per day budget, your macronutrients on a Keto Diet will look like this:

1. Fat Intake at 75% =1500 calories

2. Protein Intake at 20% =400 calories

3. Carbohydrate Intake at 5% =100 calories/25 grams of carbs

To calculate carbs, use: 2,000 x .05 = 100 calories from carbs (4 calories per gram of carb) =25 grams of carb

WHAT ARE EXAMPLES OF A KETO DIET?

When Following a Keto Diet, Focus on Eating Meats Like:

*Rib-eye Steaks *Beef Brisket *Pork Shoulder
*Chicken Thighs (with the skin on)
*Grass-Fed Beef *Salmon *Bacon

Side Note: The Keto Diet is the powerhouse player in the *Slim Down Level Up Formula #3* and is the reason why that combination is so effective for weight loss. Even if you do not follow a Keto Diet, knowing which foods are low in carbs, can be helpful on the days when you are aiming to keep your carb intake low to lose more weight. In the next section to give you an idea of grocery shopping when following a Keto Diet, examples are provided.

KETO GROCERY STORE STAPLES
KETO PROTEIN OPTIONS

*Chicken *Bacon *Lamb *Turkey *Steak *Fish *Burgers
*Eggs *Pork *Shellfish *Sausages *Tofu

KETO DAIRY OPTIONS

*Cream Cheese *Sour Cream *Half and Half *Yogurt (full fat) *Butter Cream *Cheese *Cheddar *Parmesan *Swiss *Colby *Mozzarella *Blue cheese * Havarti

KETO VEGGIE OPTIONS

*Celery *Spinach *Radishes *Bell Peppers *Broccoli *Cauliflower
*Mushrooms *Cabbage *Eggplant *Arugula *Green Beans *Asparagus

KETO FRUIT OPTIONS

*Strawberries *Blackberries *Raspberries *Lemons *Limes *Avocado

*Tomatoes *Watermelon *Coconut *Apricot *Cantaloupe

KETO NUTS OPTIONS

*Macadamia *Brazil *Pecans *Walnuts *Hazelnuts *Flax Seeds

*Almonds *Pine Nuts *Peanuts *Chia Seeds *Sunflower Seeds *Pistachios

KETO FAT OPTIONS

*Full Fat *Dairy Oils *Avocado *Nuts *High Fat Meats *Lard

KETO PANTRY STAPLES

*Stevia *Almond Flour *Monkfruit *Erythritol *Coconut Flour *Protein Powder

KETO VEGETABLES

When it Comes to Vegetables You Can Also Focus on Eating:

Broccoli, Cucumbers, Spinach, Lettuce, Kale and Cauliflower. You can also add mineral rich foods like bone broth, celery, wild-caught, seafood, sea vegetables, pickles, olives, leafy, and cruciferous veggies, sauerkraut, and olives.

*Stay away from starchy vegetables like: Carrots, Turnips, Potatoes and Parsnips.

Avocado, olive, canola, flaxseed, and palm, oils, as well as mayonnaise can be used to flavor your salads while fattening them up at the same time. Since a Keto Diet is primarily high fat, instead of margarine, use clarified butter, or ghee, for cooking or as a spread. Use whole-fat milk, yogurt, cheese, and other whole dairy products.

However, be sure to measure the heavy creams and cheeses you are using because you could quickly go over your daily caloric intake budget with these items. Same goes for eating nuts, be sure to measure your portions. Another thing you can do while on a Keto

Diet is substitute stevia in place of using sugar and artificial sweeteners. This can help with keeping your carb intake low.

Examples of Eating on a Keto Diet

Breakfast: Poached Eggs, Salt & Pepper with Steamed Asparagus
Lunch: 2-3 Cups of Salad Veggies with Lemon Juice, Salt, Pepper, Garlic Powder & a Grilled Steak Strip
Dinner: Pork Lettuce Wraps, 1 cup of Baked Beans & ½ Tomato
Snack:1st: 1 Avocado- 2nd: Nuts or Seeds of Your Choice

Breakfast: 2 Scramble Eggs, ¼ Slice of Avocado, ½ Slice of Tomato & Ham
Lunch: Cabbage/Apple Slaw with a Grilled Salmon Fillet, Add Sliced Almonds
Dinner: Baked Chicken Thighs-skin on with Side Salad (can add walnuts)
Snack: 1st: 3 Celery Sticks & 2 tbsp Almond Butter 2nd: Kale Chips

The next eating style we will go over is the Vegan Diet and the ways it can help you lose weight. But before we do, take a look at the chart below and on the next page. It includes examples of using the **Low-Calorie Diet** as the *Base Diet* and a variety of *Remixx and Bonus Diets* together.

Low-Calorie Base with Remixx, and Bonus Diets

BASE DIET   PLUS   REMIXX DIET   PLUS   BONUS DIET

BASE DIET	REMIXX DIET	BONUS DIET
LOW-CALORIE	**VEGAN**	Liquid Dinner Meal Replacement 3 Days a Week
LOW-CALORIE	**KETO**	Low Calorie Reduced to 1200 Calories and 40 Fat Grams Daily
LOW-CALORIE	**WEIGHT WATCHERS**	Enhanced Fasting Schedule Add Two 24-Hour or 36-Hour Fasting Days a Week

LOW-CALORIE	MEDITERRANEAN	Low Carb/Reduce Intake: 50 Net Carbs Max
LOW-CALORIE	JENNY CRAIG	No Added Sugar 14-day Challenge
LOW-CALORIE	SOUTH BEACH	Meatless Days Added 3 Days a Week
LOW-CALORIE	PALEO	Liquid Dinner Meal Replacement 3 Days a Week
LOW-CALORIE	LOW-CARB	Meatless Dinner Added 3 Days a Week
LOW-CALORIE	NUTRISYSTEM	5:2 Fasting Schedule 500-600 calories on fasting days/Normal intake on other days*

*You can refer to Chapter 10 and 11 for your Calories, Fat Grams and Net Carbs prior to starting the program.

Examples: Daily Body Budget of 1600 Calories, 50-53 Fat Grams, Moderate: 20-50 Net Carbs

1. Low-Calorie with a Mediterranean Diet and Low-Carb

2. Low-Calorie with a Vegan Diet and 3 Liquid Dinners a week

Side Note: This chart highlights the power of using a Base, Remixx and Bonus Diet together, which will keep your body constantly guessing and allow you to continue losing weight. The slight change ups, like adding additional fasting enhancers, incorporating liquid meals and the no added sugar challenge will be the types of tools you can use to succeed.

VEGAN DIET
WHAT IS THE DIET?

Simply put, a Vegan Diet is centered around you, eating plant-based foods and does not include eating animal products of any sort. Eating as a Vegan or as a Vegetarian has come such a long way since, 20 years ago, when I first set out to incorporate this style of eating into my diet. Why did I go Vegan? To maximize my weight loss. When, I first started following a Vegan Diet, I slowly eliminated what I was eating in stages. In four stages to be exact.

The first step I took was to cut out eating all red meat. Second, I stopped eating chicken/poultry products. Third, seafood, and the final step was dairy. It made perfect sense to me back then because I realized, I could lose even more weight by learning to eat and make veggie products taste as good as meat products. The best part was they were a third of the calories, and fat grams compared to what I was eating prior.

Most people when they hear the words Vegan or Vegetarian, think of eating only plant-based foods. But did you know there are 6 different types of *vegetarian style diets?* Some include eating animal products, others do not. Either one can be used to help you lose weight. Deciding on which ones you would like to incorporate in your diet can be beneficial to your long-term success.

VEGAN/VEGETARIAN EATING OPTIONS EXPLAINED

- **Lacto-Vegetarian:** Excludes fish, seafood, poultry, meat, and eggs. However, dairy products like milk, cheese, yogurt, and butter, are included in the diet.

- **Ovo-Vegetarian**: Excludes fish, seafood, poultry, meat, and dairy products. Eggs are, included in this style of eating.

- **Lacto-Ovo Vegetarian**: Excludes fish, seafood, poultry, and meat. All dairy products and eggs are included in this diet.

- **Pescatarian**: Excludes seafood, poultry, meat, dairy, and eggs. However, fish is allowed.

- **Vegan**: Excludes fish, seafood, poultry, meat, eggs, and dairy products. Any food containing these products are also not included in the diet.

- **Flexitarian**: Primarily plant-based; however, it includes all food groups but limits the amount of consumption of animal products.

The key with using either of these diets is to make sure you are getting the proper nutrients when removing food groups. As I was eliminating each of the four stages, I made sure to introduce the proper nutrients back into my diet with new foods and supplements.

Here is a list of the nutrients I pay special attention to when eating primarily as a Vegan/Vegetarian:

*Protein *Omega-3 Fats *Calcium * Vitamin B12 *Iron * Vitamin C *Zinc * Iodine *Vitamin A

CAN A VEGAN DIET HELP YOU LOSE WEIGHT?

Yes, you can lose weight following a Vegan/Vegetarian Diet. Going Vegan or deciding to incorporate meatless meals into your weight loss routine, can deliver important health benefits also. Besides helping you lose weight, plant-based focused diets are associated with lowering cholesterol levels and reducing risk factors associated with type-2 diabetes. As well as plant-based foods, contain compounds with anti-cancer properties.

DO YOU HAVE TO BE A FULL VEGAN TO LOSE WEIGHT?

No, instead of diving into becoming a full Vegan, trying out the *Flexitarian Diet* is a more realistic eating style, if you do not completely want to give up eating meat. It can help you lose weight faster. As discussed throughout the book, the key to successful weight loss is lowering your insulin levels and insulin resistance. Eating a more plant-based diet can help you do just that and assist with you feeling fuller longer on low-calorie dense foods. Creating the desired calorie deficit for increased weight loss.

IS A VEGAN DIET EASY TO FOLLOW?

A Vegan Diet can be a lot easier to follow when you have a better understanding of the different foods and snack options available. If, and when you are ready to eat a mostly or entirely plant-based diet, it is a good idea to learn the basics of plant-based nutrition first. These types of diets can be easy to follow once you identify which nutrients are important. One of the great benefits of using a Vegan/Vegetarian/Flexitarian Diet is, by eating healthy fats and a variety of whole plant foods, you can decrease your chances of getting chronic diseases. Like heart disease, high blood pressure, diabetes, and high cholesterol.

Adopting plant-based diets will initially require you being a little creative in finding new ways to meet your daily nutrient needs. Nowadays, there are endless cookbooks, recipes, Pinterest ideas and YouTube videos, on how to prepare plant-based meals. Once you learn the basics of meal prepping and cooking the foods, following a healthy plant-based diet can become second nature.

Whether you are deciding to use a Vegan Diet or incorporate more plant-based meals into your diet regimen, be mindful to include a wide variety of vegetables, whole grains, beans, nuts, and seeds. Especially when you are losing or maintaining weight. Having Meatless Mondays and Try Tofu Thursdays can help you reach your weight loss goals and improve your long-term health. On the nights you decide to remove the meat from your meal, remember a few of my favorite weight loss words, **"My Meatless Dinner Makes Me Thinner!"**

One Key Tip: When cooking plant-based products like tofu or soy, heavy herbs and spices will be your best friend. You will want to look, into other seasonings besides the traditional salt, pepper, and garlic powder. Since you will be cooking natural plant-based products, keep in mind, they will not have the flavor that comes from animal fats. I will be honest, the products out of the package are, by all accounts, bland. That is until you spice them up with some of your favorite ingredients. By adding extra seasonings, you can enhance the flavors and take eating plant-based foods to another level for you. Especially when you add in sauteed vegetables, fresh garlic, and herbs to the dish.

WHAT IS AN EXAMPLE OF A VEGAN DIET?

By learning to cook and eat a Vegan/Vegetarian/Flexitarian Diet, you will be pleasantly surprised on how easy and tasty the meals can be. Weekly meal planning can help you be more successful on your weight loss journey. Knowing a variety of food and recipe options to turn to will help make your transition to a plant-based diet a lot easier. As well as helping you incorporate meatless meals your whole family can enjoy (refer to Chapter 13 when looking for Vegan/Vegetarian meal ideas and recipes).

For instance, I was able to convince my husband of the benefits of meatless meals, and how he would not feel deprived having dinner without meat. One night, I tried my luck and made him a portobello mushroom sandwich. I first sautéed the mushrooms in garlic and served it with a lightly seared and seasoned beef steak tomato. Added a piece of veggie cheese and lettuce and topped it off with vegan mayo on a toasted bun. He loved it and said, "Wow I'm actually full, and it was good." I almost fell over on our kitchen floor.

I share that story because I know convincing our loved ones to try new foods with us while we are losing weight, is not always an easy feat. It may take some time to get them to try new things with you, but do not give up. Especially when you know the diet changes can help benefit their health also.

To understand how the portobello mushroom sandwich breakthrough was significant in my household, and how being persistent can pay off, I have, to tell you a little bit about my husband. He spent a few months shy of 30 years serving in the United States Army. He retired as a Special Forces Brigadier General. He has been in more Countries than I can pronounce and has eaten things I do not even want to think about. He is a full-blown, warm-blooded, die-hard meat eating Solider. Loves it, and if I let him, he, and our son, would have a big juicy steak and any kind of pork product every day of the week! His health, as well as our son's health, is important to me. I knew continuing to watch them eat meat all the time was not good for them long-term. So, I started working on convincing them a few years back to have *Meatless Mondays and Try Tofu Thursdays* with me. Even though I knew it would be an up-hill battle, I kept trying my luck. After experimenting with several recipes and incorporating the seasonings and flavors they liked, it worked! Lord, was that "mission almost impossible."

If you decide to utilize a more plant-based diet into your weight loss plan, do not be discouraged if at first your family or friends do not want to try any of the foods with you. Over time, with practice and discovering new recipes and food options, you may eventually win them over and bring them on the plant-based side of eating healthier meals with you.

Side Note: When deciding on trying plant-based meals, you can initially leave it up to the professionals. Like eating out or ordering food from the meal kit delivery services. You can choose either option for the convenience and until you are more comfortable with the food. Also, look for coupons and specials when purchasing vegan items from the grocery store to help save money, as you are making the shift and introducing new items into your diet.

Here is an example of grocery shopping when following a Vegan Diet.

VEGAN GROCERY STORE STAPLES
VEGAN PROTEIN OPTIONS

*Veggie Chicken *Veggie Burger *Veggie Bacon
*Tofu *Soy *Veggie Sausages

VEGAN DAIRY OPTIONS

*Soy-Milk **Almond-Milk *Veggie Cheese *Veggie Ice Cream **Veggie Yogurt

VEGAN VEGGIE OPTIONS

*Celery *Spinach *Radishes *Bell Peppers *Broccoli *Cauliflower *Mushrooms

*Cabbage *Eggplant *Arugula *Green Beans *Asparagus

VEGAN LOW-CALORIE SNACK LIST

*1 Small Banana *1 Apple *2 Cups Diced Watermelon *1 Cup of Blueberries

*1/2 an Avocado *28 Grapes *20 Roasted Peanuts *4 Medium Carrots

*4 Slices of Veggie Meat *3 Small Clementine *1 Sweet Potato

*1/2 cup of Edamame *1/2 of Medium Cantaloupe

*1 1/4 Veggie Cheese *33 Cherry Tomatoes *14 Almonds

VEGAN FRUIT OPTIONS

*Strawberries *Blackberries *Raspberries *Lemons *Limes *Avocado

*Tomatoes *Watermelon *Coconut *Apricot *Cantaloupe

VEGAN NUTS OPTIONS

*Macadamia *Brazil *Pecans *Walnuts *Hazelnuts *Flax Seeds

*Almonds *Pine Nuts *Peanuts *Chia Seeds *Sunflower Seeds *Pistachios

Here Are a Few Examples of Some Plant-Based Foods

Guacamole	Grilled Veggies Mix	Vegan Quesadillas
Stuffed Peppers	Black Beans	Salad Mix
Baked Sweet Potatoes	Lentil Burger	Peanut Butter
Vegan Falafel	Roasted Potatoes	Red Lentils
Smoked Tofu	Salsa	Vegan Tacos
Cauliflower	Soy Burger	Snow Peas
Cashews	Hummus	Basmati Rice

Here Are a Couple of Days of Eating on a Vegan Diet

- **Breakfast:** Mango, Pineapple and Spinach Smoothie with Almond milk and a Banana-Flaxseed-Walnut Muffin

- **Lunch:** Baked Lemon Garlic Tofu Sandwich with a Tomato and Cucumber Salad

- **Dinner:** Vegan Chili with Cauliflower Rice and an Avocado

- **Breakfast:** Cinnamon Apple Pancakes, Veggie Bacon and Freshly Squeezed Orange Juice

- **Lunch:** Tofu Vegan Quiche with a side of Garlic Sautéed Mustard Greens

- **Dinner:** Vegan Spring Rolls and a side of Steamed Broccoli with Mushrooms

Before moving on to the Mediterranean Diet, let us take a look at the chart below and on the next page. It includes examples of using a *Base Diet* of **Intermittent Fasting** combined with a variety of *Remixx and Bonus Diets.* Either of the three-step combinations can be used to maximize your weight loss.

Intermittent Fasting Base, with Remixx, and Bonus Diets

BASE DIET PLUS REMIXX DIET PLUS BONUS DIET

INTERMITTENT FASTING	VEGAN	Enhanced Fasting Schedule Adding Two 24-Hour or 36-Hour Fasting Days a Week
INTERMITTENT FASTING	PALEO	Low Calorie Reduced to 1200 Calories and 40 Fat Grams Daily
INTERMITTENT FASTING	WEIGHT WATCHERS	Liquid Dinner Meal Replacement 3 Days a Week *Non-consecutive Days Ex. M W F

INTERMITTENT FASTING	LOW-CALORIE	Meatless Dinner Added 3 Days a Week*Non-consecutive Days Ex. M W F
INTERMITTENT FASTING	MEDITERRANEAN	Low Calorie Reduced to 1200 Calories and 40 Fat Grams Daily
INTERMITTENT FASTING	LOW-CARB	Enhanced Fasting Schedule Adding Two 24-Hour or 36-Hour Fasting Days a Week
INTERMITTENT FASTING	JENNY CRAIG	Low Carb Reduce Intake: to 50 Net Carbs max
INTERMITTENT FASTING	SOUTH BEACH	No Added Sugar 14-Day Challenge
INTERMITTENT FASTING	NUTRISYSTEM	Meatless Dinner Added 3 Days a Week *Non-consecutive Days Ex. M W F

*You will be able to select a Fasting Method and Schedule from the charts in Chapter 17.

Side Note: This chart highlights the power of a multi-layer strategy to fight against obesity. When you combine Intermittent Fasting with any of the Low-Calorie Diets and then take it to another level by adding in a Bonus Diet, you create the weapons needed to win against the battle of the bulge.

MEDITERRANEAN DIET
WHAT IS THE DIET?

The Mediterranean Diet is more of a plant-based, rather than meat based, eating style. It shares a few of the same principles of the Paleo and the Vegetarian/Flexitarian Diets. It has an emphasis on eliminating processed, refined grains, sugary foods and replacing them with more plant-based products. For example with, vegetables, fruits, eggs, whole grains, fish, and poultry. It also includes moderate portions of dairy products and limits the amount of red meat from your weekly diet regimen.

The diet is traditionally based on food consumed from countries bordering the Mediterranean Sea. Like Morocco, Italy, Spain, and Greece. You may find different definitions of the Mediterranean Diet, but overall, besides eating a majority, of fruits and vegetables, it consists of whole grains, beans, nuts, seeds, and olive oil.

One of the main components behind the Mediterranean Diet is the importance of slowing down and sharing meals with family and friends. It even allows for the enjoyment of a glass of red wine, in moderation.

The Mediterranean Diet is also high in omega-3 seafood. Like herring, lake trout, sardines, tuna, and salmon, and can help with reducing inflammation, decrease triglycerides as well as decrease the risk of heart disease and heart failure.

CAN YOU LOSE WEIGHT ON A MEDITERRANEAN DIET?

Yes, the Mediterranean Diet can be used to help you lose weight and improve your health. It can also help prevent heart attacks, strokes, type 2 diabetes, and premature deaths. Knowing these types of benefits, can be helpful when deciding if using this diet can work for you in reaching your weight loss goals. The Mediterranean Diet helps you lose weight by eliminating things like, added sugars found in white bread, soda, candy, and ice cream.

It also removes trans fats, like the ones found in margarine, refined oils, like canola oil and processed meats, like sausages, lunch meat and hot dogs. By reducing your red meat consumption and incorporating more fish, fruits, and vegetables in your diet, you will be able to see weight loss results. Eating more whole foods can make you feel fuller longer with fewer calories, creating the ever so desirable calorie deficit, needed for weight loss.

IS A MEDITERRANEAN DIET EASY TO FOLLOW?

The Mediterranean Diet is an eating pattern, so incorporating a Low-Calorie Diet with it can help you enjoy good foods and stay within your recommended daily intake. Stick to the Mediterranean Diet's eating philosophy and incorporate more fruits, vegetables, beans, nuts, whole grains, legumes, olive oil and herbs and spices. This can put you on the right track with consuming healthier foods. You can also eat fish and seafood two to three days a week, keep yogurt, poultry, eggs, and cheese in moderation. Lastly, red meat and sweets should be an occasional food option when following this diet. There are several cookbooks, recipes, Pinterest ideas and YouTube videos on how to cook and eat on a Mediterranean Diet. After seeing the eating examples in the next section, it may surprise you how many different delicious options are available to choose from, when eating on this type of diet.

WHAT ARE EXAMPLES OF A MEDITERRANEAN DIET?

You may find a variety of different options to follow when deciding to try a Mediterranean Diet, especially online. While doing some research, there was one I particularly liked, and it was similar, to how I had used the diet in the past. It came from the Mayo Clinic's website on the benefits and ways to follow a Mediterranean Diet. They provide good information on understanding the basics of the diet and give great tips on how to get started.

Eating on a Mediterranean Diet

- **Eat More Fruits and Vegetables:** Aim for 7 to 10 servings a day of fruit and vegetables.

- **OPT for Whole Grains:** Switch to whole-grain bread, cereal, and pasta.

- **Use Healthy Fats:** Try olive oil as a replacement for butter when cooking. Instead of putting butter or margarine on bread, try dipping it in flavored olive oil.

- **Eat More Seafood:** Eat fish twice a week. Fresh or water-packed tuna, salmon, trout, mackerel, and herring are healthy choices. Grilled fish is another good option, and requires little cleanup. (avoid deep-fried fish or make it a *sometimes* food. You can also cook it in an air fryer to reduce your fat and calorie intake).

- **Reduce Red Meat:** Substitute fish, poultry, or beans for meat. If you eat meat, make sure it is lean and keep portions small.

- **Enjoy Some Dairy:** Eat low-fat Greek or plain yogurt and small amounts of a variety of cheeses.

- **Spice It Up:** Herbs and spices boost flavor and lessen the need for salt.

Here is An Example of Eating a Mediterranean Diet

Breakfast: Veggie Omelet with Tomatoes and Spinach

Lunch: Whole-Grain, Grilled Salmon Sandwich with a Greek Yogurt

Dinner: Mediterranean Lasagna and a Side Salad

Dessert: Fresh Fruit

Mediterranean Diet Meals

*Lemon Shrimp Pasta *Cabbage Stuffed with Marinated Cod

*Chickpea and Eggplant Warm Salad *Lentil Soup with Kale

*Chicken Tagine with Apricots and Almonds *Grilled Fish in Saffron Sauce

*Eggplant Frittata *Calamari Salad *Fish Stew *Hummus & Veggie Sandwich

Healthy Salad Dressing Combos

*Lemon + Garlic + Olive Oil

*Balsamic Vinegar + Sea Salt + Olive Oil

*Apple Cider Vinegar + Mustard + Honey + Olive Oil

*Tahini + Maple Syrup + Lemon Water

*Red Wine Vinegar + Olive Oil + Garlic + Dried Herbs

Following a Mediterranean Diet can expose you to a world of new food options and improve your health, as well as help you lose weight. You can always refer to Chapter 13, for the list of over 2,000 recipes and additional food choices that can be incorporated, into your diet eating styles.

WEIGHT LOSS SUCCESS STORY TIME

In an article titled, "Combining Intermittent Fasting and Paleo Transformed My Body," one woman discovered the benefits of using a Paleo Diet along with Fasting to lose 35 pounds.

"Ultimately, after I developed an understanding of what foods fueled me best, I started following a Paleo Diet. I am also a huge believer in Intermittent Fasting and have been doing it for years. It was a game changer for me." (39)

Of course, I smiled when I read her story because once again, the power of combining different diets together showed its' magic of helping someone reach their weight loss goals. Like the Mediterranean Diet, a Paleo Diet shares similar principles in eliminating processed foods from your diet and incorporating more plant-based meals. This was key to her success.

Next up is the last Remixx Diet we will go over prior to getting to the best part of the book, laying out the *6-Week Program*.

(WW) WEIGHT WATCHERS PROGRAM
WHAT IS THE DIET?

Weight Watchers is a structured diet program you can utilize to lose weight. I have used it in the past and had much success with reaching my goal. It is definitely not, the same program my grandmother joined years ago. They are more recently referred to as WW, and are specifically designed to provide food, recipes, meal plans and support for those looking to lose weight. WW has come a long way since it first started in the early 1960's. Back then, members would join the program and would attend weekly in-person meetings for tips and support. The concept to start the program came from its founder, Jean Nidetch, who had been overweight most of her life. She wanted to have a support system in place to help her and other women while losing weight. Her concept quickly took off and gave members more than just a meal plan to follow. WW has been providing support and guidance to millions of people all over the world ever since.

The program emphasizes the importance of portion control, making healthier food choices and to focus more on slow, consistent, long-term weight loss. WW uses a science-based approach in helping its members lose weight. They created an accountability system similar, to tracking calories. However, instead of counting calories, they use a point system. Their system is what helps members keep track of what they are eating daily, to ensure they are creating the desired calorie deficit needed for weight loss. It also helps with teaching and encouraging members to make better eating choices, from their color-coded points system food lists (blue, green, purple). They offer three plans to choose from when getting started, and regardless of which plan you choose, there are a host of healthy, low calorie food options available.

The point system is a valuable tool to use when losing weight if, you need additional help with how to spend your calories more wisely throughout the day. For example, WW understands calories are not all equal. Therefore, 100 calories of cookies is not the same as 100 calories of broccoli.

The point system they designed has a lower point value for healthier food items. Those types of items are what members are encouraged to use their points towards while losing weight. A large percentage of the items tend to be more nutrient-rich, low-calorie dense, plant-based foods.

WEIGHT LOSS SUCCESS STORY TIME

There was an article titled, "WW and Intermittent Fasting How and Why I'm Doing it", by a woman who realized combining the two together made perfect sense in helping her to lose weight. Her discovery, by default, answered the three key questions to successful weight loss.

Wendy J.:

"There is no reason why these two can't be combined, since IF (Intermittent Fasting) is when you eat, and WW (Weight Watchers) is how much and what you eat. WW is a great way to track your food intake and pairing it with fasting could help the program work better for you. Especially if it helps cut down on the nighttime snacking!" (40)

Sound familiar? The *what,* the *when,* and the *how* much we eat will be essential in losing weight, no matter which *Slim Down Level Up Formula* you choose to use.

CAN IT HELP YOU LOSE WEIGHT?

Yes, using a WW Diet can help you lose weight. The key to utilizing their program is the flexibility to use your SmartPoints: Free Style, or Points Plus (calories) as you prefer. You can enjoy many of your favorite foods if you plan accordingly and be cognitive of your portion sizes. They also put an emphasis on spending the points wisely on healthier food choices to ensure weight loss can occur.

Unlike some other programs, WW sets realistic expectations with their members, that they can expect to lose half a pound to two pounds a week. They keep track of members' progress along the way and celebrate their wins with certificates and recognition. Besides the coaching support received from being a member, there are also large support groups on social media, some of which are even specific to each color-coded program.

When it comes to understanding WW's SmartPoints, they use several variables to calculate what your daily budget will be, including things like: your weight, height, age, and activity level. For instance, a younger, taller, and more active member would receive more SmartPoints points than an older, shorter member with a sedentary lifestyle. Here are two examples:

- A shorter woman who is less active may receive a daily budget of 24 SmartPoints.

- A tall, 28-year-old woman who exercises 3 or more days a week might get 29 SmartPoints. (41)

WW discourages people from trying to calculate their Smart-Points on their own. For exact calculations, refer to their program. After joining, they do have a feature on their app that helps with converting calories to points. Which can also be helpful in the grocery store and when eating out at restaurants. Bottom line, whether we are counting calories or counting points, losing weight is all about creating a calorie deficit and being accountable to what we are eating each day.

By incorporating more fruits, vegetables and making healthier meals, using a program like WW can assist with helping you reach your goal weight. Especially if you include it in with your *Slim Down Level Up Formula* of choice.

IS A WW DIET EASY TO FOLLOW?

With the latest technology, members do not have to attend in person meetings anymore, and can gain access to their digital program as soon as they join. They also provide a user-friendly app that can help with keeping track of your daily progress.

On their website, they provide a variety of plans to choose from which are tailored to your specific needs. After joining, a personal assessment is put together for you, based on your eating habits, food preferences, lifestyle, and activities. That is also when you are given one of the three plans to follow along with additional tips and tools.

Another great benefit of being a member is they offer food options for those who have dietary restrictions, and more recently, added additional Vegan options to choose from. If you need a little more support while losing weight, you can receive it by joining their program.

Besides the in person weekly meetings in helping to stay motivated, WW provides its members with a large support system. They have an online 24/7 chat support and community. They also offer magazines and newsletters for members.

Following a WW Diet has gotten more convenient over the years. As with some of the other diets, there are cookbooks, recipes, Pinterest ideas and easy to follow YouTube videos, showing weekly meal prep tips and how-to videos on shopping and cooking efficiently on a WW Diet.

You will also see on their website a variety of recipes, success stories and tips on losing weight enjoying real food. They also pride themselves in members feeling empowered to use their points eating out with family and friends.

When purchasing WW foods or using recipes from online or in cookbooks, most come with nutritional information. It will have the calories, fat grams, carbs, fiber, etc. breakdown. There are some websites that offer WW calculators to convert points to calories or vice versa.

To gain a little better understanding of how WW points calculates to calories here is an estimated example chart you can refer to:

- ***Free Style:** 1 WW Smart Point is equal to about 30 calories

- ***Points Plus:** 1 WW Points Plus is equal to about 35 calories

*Example: 23 SmartPoints equals approximately 690 calories. If you are limiting yourself to 1200 calories per day, that would equal 36-40 SmartPoints. (42)

Side Note: Based on my understanding and research of the points, WW SmartPoints are similar, to what your daily fat grams budget would be. Which would mean your caloric intake divided by 30, then minus 4 would equal your SmartPoints range. For example: 1200 calories divided by 30=40. Then minus 4=36. Putting your WW SmartPoints range at 36-40 points. The fat grams on the *Daily Body Budget Chart* in Chapter 10 for a 1200 calorie budget would be 36-40 fat grams. Same calculation. These numbers can be used as *estimates* to give you an idea about staying within a specific daily intake. However, if you do decide to use WW as one of your diet combinations, for more exact numbers and how to use their points system, you can refer to their program.

COST AND FOOD OPTIONS?

WW has a variety of plans to choose from if you decide to join. For the basic Digital Plan, they offer access to their app, which includes barcode scanning capabilities, a large database of restaurants and recipes. The app also includes expert techniques, live coaching, meditations, and audio workouts. The cost is about $3.00 a week. They have other plan options with more features on their website, Weightwatchers.com. Check for specials before joining. If you visit their website, they have a variety of tips and recipes you can view for free. You can purchase food and snacks from their website or from Walmart and Amazon. The app Pinterest has a variety of WW recipes, meal options and snack ideas as well.

WHAT ARE EXAMPLES OF WW FOOD?

Here is a list of some of the most tracked WW foods and their points.

Plain Almond Milk-1 Smart Point	3 oz Chicken Breast- 2 SmartPoints
¼ Avocado-2 SmartPoints	1 Medium Corn on the Cob- 4 SmartPoints
3 oz Cooked Ground Beef- 4 SmartPoints	1 Hard Boiled Egg- 2 SmartPoints
½ cup Black Beans-3 SmartPoints	3 oz Tilapia-1 SmartPoint
Broccoli-0 SmartPoints	Green Beans- 0 SmartPoints
Blackberries-0 SmartPoints	3 oz Cooked Shrimp-1 SmartPoint

Here are Examples of Eating on a WW Diet

Breakfast: Maple Brown Sugar Oatmeal with a Banana

Lunch: Shrimp Salad, Light Whole Grain Bread, and a Fruit Salad

Dinner: Baked Penne with Turkey Mushrooms with Pepper Ragu

Breakfast: Blueberry Lemon Basil Jam on an English Muffin and ½ cup of Mixed Fruit

Lunch: Grilled Chicken Fajita Wrap with ½ cup of Blueberries

Dinner: Spice Rubbed Flank Steak with 1 cup of Vegetables

CAN YOU EXERCISE WHILE USING ANY OF THE 4 DIETS?

As with the three previously mentioned diets in Chapter 14, to get the most out of using either a Keto, Vegan, Mediterranean, or Weight Watchers Diet, it can be beneficial when you are physically active more days than not. However, the same philosophy applies here, as it relates to not working out in the first week of the *6-Week Program*. The first week is all about you getting a handle on the food and making the new *shift* in your life.

Instead, of working out, 30-45 minutes, a few days a week, use the time to shop, meal prep and make necessary arrangements for cooking and/or signing up for whichever of the meal plans you decide to use. You can also search online at Pinterest or Google for new recipes and snack ideas that can help with satisfying your tastebuds and are low in calories.

During the first week, you can increase your daily activities so that you start burning additional calories and boost your metabolism.

When you do start incorporating exercise into your routine, remember to refer to Chapter 19 for ideas and tips on getting started. As stated earlier, there are lots of benefits to working out in the mornings. You can burn more fat on an empty stomach. If possible, try and incorporate a few morning exercises, each week to maximize your results.

Bonus Material? Besides, the key seven diets, that we just went over, in the back of the book, in the Bonus Material section, you will have access to the benefits, food and recipes from three additional structured diets, Jenny Craig, South Beach and Nutrisystem and the low-calorie, Paleo Diet. Either of the four can be an additional option you can use to lose weight.

Side Note: In 2018 Jenny Craig released its *Rapid* Results Program and it involved members adding a *mini 12:12 fast* to their eating routines. (43) Where they would eat during a 12-hour window, then fast/rejuvenate for the other 12 hours (The 12 hours would include the sleeping window also). The good news was, as you know, even a mini fast can help with weight loss. The concept behind Jenny Craig adding fasting to their Rapid Results Program, is based on the body's natural 24-hour cycle clock, called circadian rhythms. The new fasting addition helped their members lose weight more *rapidly*. Because it improved their insulin levels and insulin resistance. This is another example of why incorporating fasting into your weight loss strategy and using more than one diet can be beneficial and increase your overall weight loss success.

The last chart to look at, is an example of using the power of *four* diets together. I call it the **Ultimate 4 Punch Knockout Remixx Combination**. Do not let the name intimidate you. We are just adding one more layer we can use to fight the weight loss dragon. Over time while losing weight, I evolved to this level and reaped the benefits of being able to choose, how I wanted to continue reaching my goal. The way the program is designed, you can follow either combination created within the three formulas to reach your goal weight. However, in Phase 2 of the program, depending on which *Slim Down Level Up Formula* you choose, there will be alternative options of the program that use the 4-Punch technique, if you are an advanced dieter. No worries if you are not ready to jump out the gate at this level. If you are a beginner dieter, attaining this level will be for later in your journey. After you have gone through the *6-Week Program* and are more familiar and comfortable with combining the diet eating styles together. I wanted to share this technique because it will be available if you want to advance your weight loss to a higher level and need the additional *punch* to defeat the weight loss dragon.

THE ULTIMATE 4 PUNCH KNOCKOUT REMIXX COMBINATIONS

1, 2, 3, 4 Punch = Intermittent Fasting Base, a Remixx Diet, Bonus Diet, and a Level Up. Examples are provided to give you a snapshot of what it would look like to combine four of the options together. When you are ready, any one of the combinations can help you with your weight loss goals.

BASE DIET	PLUS	REMIXX DIET	PLUS	BONUS DIET	PLUS	LEVEL UP
INTER-MITTENT FASTING		**VEGAN**		No Added Sugar 14-Day Challenge		**LOW-CALORIE or LOW-CARB**
INTER-MITTENT FASTING		**KETO**		Liquid Meal Re-placement 3 Days a Week		**LOW-CALORIE**
INTER-MITTENT FASTING		**WEIGHT WATCHERS**		Meatless Dinner Added 3 Days a Week		**LOW-CALORIE or LOW-CARB**
INTER-MITTENT FASTING		**MEDITERRA-NEAN**		No Added Sugar 14-day Challenge		**LOW-CALORIE or LOW-CARB**
INTER-MITTENT FASTING		**JENNY CRAIG**		Liquid Meal Re-placement 3 Days a Week		**LOW-CALORIE or LOW-CARB**
INTER-MITTENT FASTING		**SOUTH BEACH**		No Added Sugar 14-day Challenge		**LOW-CALORIE or LOW-CARB**
INTER-MITTENT FASTING		**PALEO**		Meatless Dinner Added 3 Days a Week		**LOW-CALORIE or LOW-CARB**
INTER-MITTENT FASTING		**LOW-CARB**		Add 2 OMAD (24 Hour Fast)		**LOW-CALORIE**
INTER-MITTENT FASTING		**NUTRISYS-TEM**		Liquid Meal Re-placement 3 Days a Week		**LOW-CALORIE or LOW-CARB**

*Low-Calorie=1200 Calories and 40 Fat Grams * Moderate Low-Carbs=20-50 Net Carbs.

Examples: Both have a daily intake of 1800 Calories, 56-60 Fat Grams, 20-50 Net Carbs

1. Intermittent Fasting 18:6 Schedule and the WW Diet, with 3 Meatless Dinners and Low-Carb

2. Intermittent Fasting 16:8 Schedule and the South Beach Diet, 2 OMAD fast and Low-Calorie

288

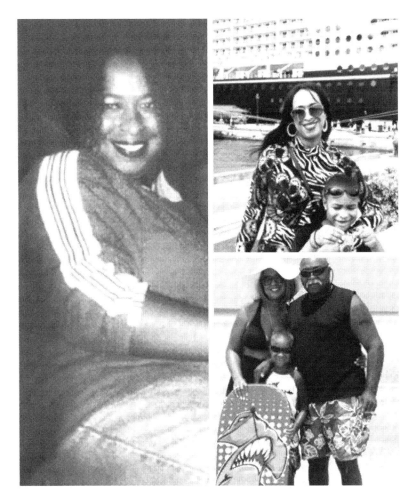

In the picture on the left, at that weight (265 pounds) if I would have stayed that size, it would have been hard for me to play with my son, for long without hurting. Especially, when he was little. Which would of made me feel bad, like I would have been letting him down. That was why I was so proud, for example, on his 7th birthday, in the pictures on the right, I could run around and keep up with him on the Disney Cruise with no problem. Especially since it was his only wish, and he had anxiously waited all year long to go. That trip reminded me of why I was so glad, years prior, I had stopped being in denial and mad at myself for gaining so much weight back and did something about it. Not just for myself but also for my family.

Enough about me. The excitement continues to build for you! In the next chapter, we will go over the actual *6-Week Program*. But first let us take a look at three different 6-Week examples of seeing the formulas in action.

All three examples utilize the *Slim Down Level Up Formula Chart* we went over in Chapter 8 and were created by using the three-step technique. The first of the examples is a slow and steady dieter who wants to start out not so aggressively by using a modified fasting schedule to lose weight. The second is a semi-aggressive dieter who is ready to lose weight at a medium fasting pace. Lastly, the third is an example of a dieter being more aggressive with their fasting schedule for weight loss. All three examples use the power of combining different diets together and can be referred to as various ways, in which you can reach your goal weight. They show you how to utilize up to *three* diet eating styles together at the same time.

SLIM DOWN LEVEL UP

6-WEEK PROGRAM EXAMPLES

Slow and Steady Sally

Example 1:   **Starting Weight:** 195 Pounds

PHASE 1-Week 1-2: Sally chooses Intermittent Fasting, with a 14:10 schedule as her *Base Diet* and uses the food and recipes from Weight Watchers as her *Remixx Diet*. Based on the Conservative Daily Body Budget Chart, she will take in no more than 1500-1600 calories a day and 50-53 Fat Grams (49-53 SmartPoints). She will add 30 minutes of exercise 2-3 days a week starting in week 2 of the program.

PHASE 2-Week 3-4: Sally continues to use Weight Watchers and makes an adjustment to her Intermittent Fasting schedule. She decreases her eating window to 15:9. She adds in a *Bonus Diet* of Low-Calorie to her combination and reduces her intake by 300 calories. Her new daily intake is 1200-1300 calories and 40-43 Fat Grams (40-43 SmartPoints). She increases her exercise to 3-4 days a week for 45 minutes.

PHASE 3 -Week 5-6: Sally stays on Weight Watchers and is now using a 16:8 Intermittent Fasting schedule and instead of a Low-Calorie *Bonus Diet,* she adds in 3 Meatless Dinners a Week and decides to do Meatless Mondays and Try Tofu Tuesdays and Thursdays. She continues using the same calories and fat grams (SmartPoints) from the previous week. She increases her exercise to 4-5 days a week for 45 minutes.

**BONUS WEEKS 7-8: Sally combines Weight Watchers with a Keto Diet and uses an Intermittent Fasting schedule of an 18:6 Monday-Friday and 16:8 on Saturday and Sunday. She exercises 5-6 days a week for 60 minutes.

Intermediate Ingrid

Example 2:   **Starting Weight:** 263 Pounds

PHASE 1-Week 1-2: Ingrid chooses Intermittent Fasting with a 16:8 schedule as her *Base Diet* and Keto as her *Remixx Diet*. Based on the Conservative Daily Body Budget Chart, her daily intake will not exceed 2,200 calories and 73 fat grams. Since she is following a Keto Diet, her max carb intake will be 20 net carbs. Her macronutrient breakdown would be 1,650 calories from fat (55 fat grams), 450 calories from protein (15 fat grams) and 100 calories from carbs (3 fat grams). Even on a Keto Diet, Ingrid understands the importance of not overeating fat. Having the daily budget helps her to create the calorie deficit needed so she can lose weight. She will exercise 3-4 days a week for 45 minutes, starting in week 2 of the program.

PHASE 2-Week 3-4: Ingrid keeps her same *Base Diet* and *Remixx Diet* but adds a *Bonus Diet* Low-Calorie to her combination and reduces her caloric intake by 400 calories. Her new max daily intake would be 1,800 calories and 60 fat grams. Her macronutrient breakdown would be 1,350 calories from fat (45 fat grams), 360 calories from protein (12 fat grams), and 90 calories from carbs (3 fat grams). She will exercise 4-5 days a week for 45 minutes.

PHASE 3-Week 5-6: Ingrid chooses to stay on the Keto Diet and increases her Intermittent Fasting to an 18:6 schedule, remains on the Low-Calorie Diet using the same macronutrient breakdown and adds 3 Meatless Dinners a Week. She exercises 3-4 days a week for 60 minutes.

**BONUS WEEKS 7-8: Ingrid continues using the Keto Diet but chooses to add a *Bonus Diet*: No Added Sugar and remains on the 18:6 Intermittent Fasting schedule but only for 5 days a week. She adds in 2 non-consecutive days of OMAD (24-hour fast), exercises 5-6 days a week for 60 minutes.

Advanced Alesha

Example 3:   **Starting Weight:** 237 Pounds

PHASE 1-Week 1-2: Alesha chooses Low-Calorie as her *Base Diet* and Intermittent Fasting as the *Remixx Diet* with a 16:8 schedule, and a *Bonus Diet* of 3 Liquid Dinner meals a Week. Based on the Aggressive Daily Body Budget Chart, her daily intake will be between 1400-1500 calories and 46-50 fat grams max. She will exercise 4-5 days a week for 45-60 minutes, starting in week 2 of the program.

PHASE 2-Week 3-4: Alesha keeps the Low-Calorie *Base Diet,* swaps her *Bonus Diet* with a Low-Carb Diet instead, and takes in between 40-50 Net Carbs max. She makes an adjustment the *Remixx Diet,* Intermittent Fasting schedule to an 18:6 Monday-Friday *Extra Diet* and 16:8 Saturday and Sunday. She exercises 5-6 days a week for 45-60 minutes *and* incorporates 15 minutes of strength training exercises 2-3 days a week.

PHASE 3-WEEK 5-6: Alesha remains using Low-Calorie as her *Base Diet* and keeps Low-Carb as the *Bonus Diet*. She uses the same *Remixx Diet* Intermittent Fasting schedule but adds OMAD (24 Hour Fast) once a week. She exercises 5-6 days a week for 60 minutes and incorporates 15-30 minutes of strength training exercises 3 days a week.

BONUS WEEKS 7-8: Alesha continues using a Low-Calorie *Base Diet*, adds 2 OMAD (24 Hour Fast) and instead of a Low-Carb *Bonus Diet*, she swaps it for 3 Meatless Dinners a Week (I recommend you do not plan meatless dinners on the same day as OMAD-24 Hour Fast days).

Side Note: Either one of the examples, could have started with a different *Base* and *Remixx Diet* based on your preferences. After following the *6-Week Program*, you will be able to make, adjustments as needed and swap out your *Base, Remixx* or *Bonus Diet* with one of the other options provided in the charts. To change up the combinations and keep your body guessing, so you can lose more weight.

PART SEVEN
THE 6-WEEK SLIM DOWN LEVEL UP PROGRAMS

16

THE 6-WEEK PROGRAMS

Yes! It's Transformation Time!

In, this section, a *6-Week Program* for all three *Slim Down Level Up Formulas* will be provided for you to follow. Here is a recap of the formulas. (IF=Intermittent Fasting)

<u>**Slim Down Level Up Formula #1**</u>: IF + Low-Calorie
<u>**Slim Down Level Up Formula #2**</u>: Low-Calorie + Low-Carb
<u>**Slim Down Level Up Formula #3**</u>: Keto + Low-Calorie + IF

Each of the three formulas has a **Deluxe** and **Advanced** option to choose from, depending on your level of comfort when first starting out. Between the three formulas, after starting with your initial *6-Week Program*, you will have access to an **additional 30 Weeks** of weight loss options you can use in reaching your goal. Each option has examples to guide you along the way.

6-Week Program: Deluxe and Advanced Options

*6-Week ***Deluxe*** Program: Intermittent Fasting + Low-Calorie Diets
*6-Week ***Advanced*** Program: Intermittent Fasting + Low-Calorie Diets
*6-Week ***Deluxe*** Program: Low-Calorie + Low-Carb Diets
*6-Week ***Advanced*** Program: Low-Calorie + Low-Carb Diets

*6-Week **Deluxe** Program: Keto + Low-Calorie + Intermittent Fasting Diets

*6-Week **Advanced** Program: Keto + Low-Calorie + Intermittent Fasting Diets

Before deciding on which of the formulas you would like to start with, you may want to briefly look over all the options. This will give you a better idea about some of the others you can use at, a later date on your journey. Or if you already know the formula you want to follow, you can go to that section and review the Deluxe and Advanced options. That way you will be able to see which one is best for you based on your comfort level and preference.

Using any of the *6-Week Programs* can get you to your goal weight and can be used to help you maintain your weight as well.

The 6-Week Programs

PHASE 1, 2, 3:

PHASE 1-Week 1-2: **REBOOT**
Reboot= To make a change in, order to establish a new beginning

PHASE 2-Week 3-4: **TRANSFORM**
Transform= To undergo a change in form, appearance

PHASE 3-Week 5-6: **DOMINATE**
Dominate= To rule over; control

Your new journey to a healthier and slimmer you, starts now. Everything you have read so far in the book is tied to this very moment. This is your time, and it will be a fresh start, to a new beginning, making this time different than any other time before, when you set out to lose weight.

In Phase 1, **Reboot** in Weeks 1-2 it will be all about you making the changes and adjusting to the *weight loss food shift*. Making those small changes daily will make a big difference in what, when and how much you will be eating. Positioning yourself to win.

Phase 2, **Transform**. Weeks 3-4 will be all about you seeing the changes in your body, and in how you feel. The transformation process, loving your curves, listening to your body, and taking it one day, one meal, and one pound at a time, will be your keys to success in this phase. In Phase 3, **Dominate**, by Weeks 5-6, you will feel more empowered to dominate losing weight, using the power of combining the different diets together. They can and will get you to the finish line.

Remember, when you start on your journey this time, the race is not to the swift, but rather to those that keep running. **You got this!**

Side Note: To get the most from combining any of the diets, and when using the three formulas, it is a good idea to refer to that *diet's eating style* section in the book for a recap on the tips, food, and recipe options. After reviewing the formulas, and prior to starting the program, we will go over a variety of Intermittent Fasting options and protocols you can follow. As, well as how to prepare for the Holidays/Special Events while losing weight and putting together your get moving plan, to maximize your weight loss.

Here is the chart you can refer to when deciding on your combinations.

SLIM DOWN LEVEL UP FORMULAS CHART

STEP 1: PICK A BASE DIET

> 1. Intermittent Fasting 2. Low-Calorie 3. Keto 4. Vegan
>
> 5. Mediterranean 6. Weight Watchers 7. Paleo 8. Jenny Craig
>
> 9. South Beach 10. Low-Carb 11. Nutrisystem

STEP 2: PICK A REMIXX DIET

> 1. Low-Calorie 2. Mediterranean 3. Weight Watchers 4. Paleo
>
> 5. Jenny Craig 6. Vegan 7. South Beach 8. Intermittent Fasting
>
> 9. Nutrisystem 10. Low-Carb 11. Keto

STEP 3: THE BONUS, EXTRA AND LEVEL UP OPTIONS

The **Bonus, Extra,** and *Level Up Diets*, can be selected as *Enhancers*. They can be combined and used in conjunction with the **Base** and the **Remixx Diets**:

1. **Meatless Dinner** (3 Days a Week)

2. **Low-Calorie** (Follow Body Budget Charts)

3. **Sugar Free** (2-Week Challenge with no Added Sugars)

4. **Liquid Dinner Meal Replacement** (3 Days a Week)

5. **Soup Dinner Meal Replacement** (3 Days a Week)

6. **Low-Carb** (Reduce daily intake to 40-50 Net Carbs max)

7. **Platinum Low-Carb** (20-30 Net Carbs max)

8. **Platinum Low-Calorie** (Reduced to 1200 calories and 40 fat grams)

9. **Fasting Extra** (Add 3 Days of an 18:6 Fast Schedule)

10. **Fasting Extra** (Add 5 Days of an 18:6 Fast Schedule)

11. **Fasting Extra** (Add 1- OMAD= 24-Hour Fast)

12. **Fasting Extra** (Add 1- 36 Hour Fast)

13. **Fasting Extra** (Add 2- OMAD= 24-Hour Fast)

14. **Fasting Extra** (Add 2- 36 Hour Fast)

15. **Fasting Extra** (Add a 5:2 Fast Schedule)

16. **Fasting Extra** (Add a 4:3 Fast Schedule)

SLIM DOWN LEVEL UP FORMULA #1

Intermittent Fasting + Low-Calorie Diets: Deluxe Option

This option is a *6-Week Deluxe**Program,* with 3 parts: Phase 1: **Reboot**, Phase 2: **Transform**, Phase 3: **Dominate**. Each phase last for two weeks and has a variety of different Bonus and Extra options included.

Bonus and Extra Options Chart

*Fasting Extra: Add (1) 36-Hour Fast	*Low-Carb (50 net carbs max)
*Liquid Dinner 3 Days a Week	*Fasting Extra: Add 1 OMAD (24-Hour Fast)
*No Added Sugar Challenge	*Fasting Extra: Add 1 Day of 18:6 Fast
*Meatless Dinner 3 Days a Week	*Fasting Extra: Add 3 Days of 18:6 Fast
*Platinum Low-Calorie = *(1200 calories, 40 fat grams)*	

You can choose to start with this **Deluxe Program or see the **Advanced Program** in the next section if you are an experienced faster. When referring to the weekly program, you will see some of the above listed Bonus and Extra options within the chart. These are recommended for optimum results each week. However, if you get to a certain week and the selected option is not one you prefer, select a different one from the chart and continue following the rest of the week's program.

STARTING OUT-PHASE 1:

NO SODAS, JUICES, SPORTS DRINKS, ALCOHOL, WHITE BREAD, WHITE RICE, PASTA, FRIED FOODS, OR WHOLE FAT DAIRY PRODUCTS

Important Note: If you are a first time *Faster*, or have not fasted in a while, start out using the 14:10 Schedule in the first two weeks of the program. Slowly decrease the eating window by 30 minutes every other day in the first 10-12 days to arrive at the 16:8 window by Week 3. If you are an *Advanced Faster,* you will start with a 16:8 Schedule for the first two weeks.

Low-Calorie*: You will see Low-Calorie listed in the weekly program as a *Remixx Diet.* You can choose any Low-Calorie Diet/ eating style you prefer. For help with making your decision, you can refer to Chapters 14-15 to see the seven previously mentioned diets.

Key Point: Keep in mind, while fasting, by using the decreased eating timeframe, you may not use your entire daily body budget. It is there as a guide to keep you from overeating. When starting out, if you are full on less food and your daily intake is not below 1200 calories or 40 fat grams, regularly, that is okay. It is showing your body is transitioning to the new eating schedule. As it continues adjusting to receiving less calories and as your fasting window increases, it will start relying more on your stored fat, as its primary fuel. Turning your body into a fat burning, belly busting machine.

Slim Down Level Up Formula #1 Deluxe Option Explained

PHASE 1: REBOOT

Week 1-2 Example: *You're ready for the weight loss food shift.*

Your Base Diet is Intermittent Fasting. You have not fasted before, so you will start out using the 14:10 Schedule, and you have decided to eat between the hours of 9 am-7 pm. Your Remixx Diet is Low-Calorie, and you will use a combination of food from the Weight Watchers Program and some low-calorie recipes you saw online. You also signed up for one of the meal delivery kit services for the days when you do not feel like cooking. Your Bonus Diet is Low-Carb, and you will keep your intake at 40-50 net carbs max daily. Your starting weight is 235 pounds. You check the Conservative Daily Body Budget Chart in Chapter 10 and see your intake is 1800-2000 calories and 60-66 fat grams max. You have downloaded apps to help you with daily tracking of your food and activities. In the first two weeks, you will decrease your, eating time by 30 minutes every other day, to make the transition easier, to arrive at the desired 16:8 Fasting Schedule, by the beginning of Week 3. (Decreasing Timeframe Example: 9:00-7:00 pm, 9:30-7:00pm, 10:00-7:00pm, 10:30-7:00pm, 11:00-7:00pm).

PHASE 2: TRANSFORM

Week 3-4 Example: *You're transforming your body and mind and continuing to believe in yourself again.*

You have a 16:8 Fasting Schedule, and you are continuing the Low-Calorie Diet. You are swapping your Bonus Diet to now having 3 Liquid Dinners a Week. By doing so, on those days, you are putting your heavier/larger meal in the middle of the day. You have an Extra Diet of 1 Day of an 18:6 Fast per week added to your combination. Reducing your eating window down by the additional two hours. You can choose any day of the week you prefer.

PHASE 3: DOMINATE

> **Week 5-6 Example:** *You're on the path to dominate losing weight.*
>
> You are continuing your 16:8 Intermittent Fasting Schedule and Low-Calorie Diet. You are swapping your Bonus Diet to now having 3 Meatless Dinners a Week. And adjusting your Extra Diet to 3 days a week of an 18:6 Fasting Schedule. You have decided to make them non-consecutive days. Example: Monday, Wednesday, Friday, Sunday 16:8 Schedule and Tuesday, Thursday, Saturday an 18:6 Schedule.

*Alternative: If you are not ready to add the fasting Extra Diet 18:6 Schedule in Week 5-6, continue using the 16:8 Schedule. Also, continue following the other steps and stick to your daily body budget numbers. For increased weight loss and maintenance, you can add in 3 Days of an 18:6 fasting schedule once a month. You can also add, 1 to 2 OMAD (24-Hour) or 2 36-Hour Fast once or twice a month. (You can check fasting schedules in Chapter 17).

SLIM DOWN LEVEL UP FORMULA #1

Intermittent Fasting + Low-Calorie Diets: Deluxe Option

6-WEEK DELUXE PROGRAM

Phase	Timeframe	Base Diet	Remixx	Bonus	Extra
Phase 1: **Reboot**	Week 1-2	Intermittent Fasting 14:10 Schedule	Low-Calorie*	Low-Carb**	N/A
Phase 2: **Transform**	Week 3-4	Intermittent Fasting 16:8 Schedule	Low-Calorie*	Liquid Dinner 3 Days a Week	Add 1 Day of 18:6 Fast per Week
Phase 3: **Dominate**	Week 5-6	Intermittent Fasting 16:8 Schedule	Low-Calorie*	Meatless Dinner 3 Days a Week	Add 3 Days of 18:6 Fast per Week

*Low-Calorie-Check with the Daily Body Budget Charts in Chapter 10 for calories and fat grams allowance.

**Low-Carb-Choose Either:

Liberal Low-Carbs: 50-100 Net Carbs Max
Moderate Low-Carbs: 20-50 Net Carbs Max
Ketogenic Low-Carbs: 20 Net Carbs or Less Max

Formula to Calculate Net Carbs:

Total Carbohydrates – Dietary Fiber = Net Carbs

*After completing the 6-week session, you can circle back starting at Week 1 using a 16:8 fasting schedule. The second time around, you can choose a different Bonus, Remixx, Extra or Level Up combination based on your preferences. You can refer to the chart on page 298 for more eating style options when making your selections.

SLIM DOWN LEVEL UP FORMULA #1

Intermittent Fasting + Low-Calorie Diets: Advanced Option

This option is a *6-Week Advanced** Program,* with 3 parts: Phase 1: **Reboot**, Phase 2: **Transform**, Phase 3: **Dominate**. Each phase last for two weeks and has a variety of different Bonus, Extra and Level Up options included.

Bonus, Extra and Level Up Options Chart

*Fasting Extra: Add (1) 36-Hour Fast	*Low-Carb (50 net carbs max)
*Liquid Dinner 3 Days a Week	*Fasting Extra: Add 1 OMAD (24-Hour Fast)
*No Added Sugar Challenge	*Fasting Extra: Add 3 Days of 18:6 Fast
*Meatless Dinner 3 Days a Week	*Fasting Extra: Add 5 Days of 18:6 Fast
*Platinum Low-Calorie**	*Ketogenic Low-Carb*** (20 Net Carbs Max)

You can choose the **Deluxe Program to begin or use this **Advanced Program** if you are an experienced faster. When referring to the weekly program, you will see some of the above Bonus, Extra and Level Up options listed within the chart. These are recommended for optimum results each week. However, if you get to a certain week and the selected option is not one you prefer, select a different one from the chart and continue following the rest of the week's program.

STARTING OUT-PHASE 1:

NO SODAS, JUICES, SPORTS DRINKS, ALCOHOL, WHITE BREAD, WHITE RICE, PASTA, OR WHOLE FAT DAIRY PRODUCTS

Important Note: If you are an experienced faster but need a few days to jumpstart your body and would like to follow the *Advanced Program,* use the first 5-7 days to get your body adjusted to eating in the reduced timeframe. Slowly decrease your, eating window by 30 minutes to an hour, every other day in the first few days, to arrive at the 16:8 window by the end of Week 1.

Low-Calorie*: You will see Low-Calorie listed in the weekly program as a Remixx Diet. You can choose any Low-Calorie Diet or eating style you prefer. For help with making your decision, you can refer to Chapters 14-15 to see the seven previously mentioned diets.

Key Point: Keep in mind, by fasting and using the decreased eating timeframe, you may not use your entire daily body budget. It is there as a guide to keep you from overeating. When starting out, if you are full on less food and your daily intake is not below 1200 calories or 40 fat grams, regularly, that is okay. It is showing your body is transitioning to the new eating schedule. As it continues adjusting to receiving less calories and as your fasting window increases, it will start relying more on your stored fat as its primary fuel. Allowing your body to reap the benefits of being in ketosis.

Slim Down Level Up Formula #1 Advanced Option Explained

PHASE 1: REBOOT

Week 1-2 Example: *You're ready for the weight loss food shift.*

You are starting out using a 16:8 Fasting Schedule with a Low-Calorie Diet. Your Bonus Diet is Low-Carb. Since you are advanced, you decide to start with the Moderate Low-Carb range and stay between 20-50 net carbs max. Your starting weight is 185-pounds, and you check the Conservative Body Budget Chart in Chapter 10 for your starting numbers. Your budget is 1400-1500 calories and 46-50 fat grams. In Week 2, everything remains the same except your new Extra Diet is OMAD (24-Hour Fast) is added to your fasting schedule (any day you choose).

PHASE 2: TRANSFORM

Week 3-4 Example: *You're transforming your body and mind and continuing to believe in yourself again.*

You continue the same Fasting Schedule and Low-Calorie Diet. You swap your Bonus Diet to the No Added Sugar Challenge and swap your Extra Diet to add 3 Days of an 18:6 Fasting Schedule. You are adding a Level Up Diet and will have 3 Liquid Dinners a Week. (You can do 3 alternating days for the 18:6 schedule). Example: Monday, Wednesday, Friday 18:6 schedule, Tuesday, Thursday, Saturday, Sunday 16:8 schedule.

PHASE 3: DOMINATE

Week 5-6 Example: *You're on the path to dominate losing weight.*

You keep the same Fasting Schedule and are continuing your Low-Calorie Diet. You swap your Bonus Diet to 3 Meatless Dinners a Week. And your Extra Diet will swap to 5 Days a Week of an 18:6 Fasting Schedule. You will change your Level Up Diet to now being Platinum Low-Calorie (1200 calories, 40 fat grams max). For your new fasting schedule: you could do 18:6 M-F and 16:8 on SAT-SUN.

**Alternative: If you are not ready to add the fasting Extra Diet 18:6 Schedule in Week 5-6, continue using the 16:8 Schedule. Also, continue following the other steps and stick to your daily body budget numbers.

For increased weight loss and maintenance, you can add in 3 Days of an 18:6 fasting schedule once a month. You can also add, 1 to 2 OMAD (24-Hour) or 2 36-Hour Fast once or twice a month. (You can check fasting schedules in Chapter 17).

*After completing the 6-week session, you can circle back starting at Week 1. The second time around, you can choose a different Bonus, Remixx, Extra or Level Up combination based on your preferences. You can refer to the chart on page 298 for more eating style options when making your selections.

SLIM DOWN LEVEL UP FORMULA #1

Intermittent Fasting + Low-Calorie Diets: Advanced Option

6-WEEK ADVANCED PROGRAM

Phase	Time frame	Base Diet	Re-mixx	Bonus	Extra	Level Up
Phase 1: **Reboot**	Week 1-2	Intermittent Fasting 16:8 Schedule	Low-Calorie*	Low-Carb**	Add 1 OMAD Fast (24-Hour) in Week 2	N/A
Phase 2: **Transform**	Week 3-4	Intermittent Fasting 16:8 Schedule	Low-Calorie*	No Added Sugar Challenge	Add 3 Days of 18:6 Fast per Week	Add Liquid Dinner 3 Days a Week
Phase 3: **Dominate**	Week 5-6	Intermittent Fasting 16:8 Schedule	Low-Calorie*	Meat-less Dinner 3 Days a Week	Add 5 Days of 18:6 Fast per Week	Platinum Low-Calorie

*__Low-Calorie-__Check with the Daily Body Budget Charts in Chapter 10 for calories and fat grams allowance.

Platinum Low-Calorie=1200 calories and 40 Fat Grams (Used in Week 5-6)

***__Low-Carbs__-Choose Either:

Liberal Low-Carbs: 50-100 Net Carbs Max
Moderate Low-Carbs: 20-50 Net Carbs Max
Ketogenic Low-Carbs: 20 Net Carbs or Less Max

Formula to Calculate Net Carbs:

Total Carbohydrates – Dietary Fiber = Net Carbs

SLIM DOWN LEVEL UP FORMULA #2

Low-Calorie + Low-Carb Diets: Deluxe Option

This option is a *6-Week Deluxe**Program,* with 3 parts: Phase 1: **Reboot**, Phase 2: **Transform**, Phase 3: **Dominate**. Each phase last for two weeks and has a variety of different Bonus and Extra options included.

Bonus and Extra Options Chart

*Liquid Dinner 3 Days a Week	*Liberal Low-Carbs (50-100 Net Carbs Max)
*Meatless Dinner 3 Days a Week	*Moderate Low-Carbs (20-50 Net Carbs Max)
*No Added Sugar Challenge	*Ketogenic Low-Carbs*** (20 Net Carbs Max)
*Platinum Low-Calorie = *(1200 calories, 40 fat grams)*	

You can choose this **Deluxe Program for a semi-aggressive start or see the **Advanced Program** in the next section if you are a more aggressive dieter. When referring to the weekly program, you will see some of the above Bonus and Extra options listed within the chart. These are recommended for optimum results each week. However, if you get to a certain week and the selected option is not one you prefer, select a different one from the chart and continue following the rest of the week's program.

STARTING OUT-PHASE 1:

NO SODAS, JUICES, SPORTS DRINKS, ALCOHOL, WHITE BREAD, WHITE RICE, PASTA, FRIED FOODS, OR WHOLE FAT DAIRY PRODUCTS

Low-Calorie*: You will see Low-Calorie listed in the weekly program as a Remixx Diet. You can choose any Low-Calorie Diet or eating style you prefer. For help with making your decision, you can refer to Chapters 14-15 to see the seven previously mentioned diets.

Key Point: When starting out and reducing your daily overall intake, if you are full on less food and it is not below 1200 calories or 40 fat grams, regularly, that is okay. It is showing your body is transitioning to the new eating habits. As it continues adjusting to receiving less calories, and you reduce your net carb intake to ketogenic levels (20 or less), it will start relying more on your stored fat, as its primary fuel. Turning your body into a fat burning, belly busting machine.

Slim Down Level Up Formula #2 Deluxe Option Explained

PHASE 1: REBOOT

Week 1-2 Example: *You're ready for the weight loss food shift.*

You weigh 195 pounds. You have Low-Calorie as your Base Diet and have chosen to follow several low-calorie recipes you saw online and use some of the food from the Jenny Craig Program. You also signed up for one of the meal delivery kit services for on the days when you do not feel like cooking. You have a Remixx Diet of Low-Carb and will keep your intake between 20-50 net carbs max daily. You checked the Aggressive Daily Body Budget Chart in Chapter 10 and saw your intake is 1300-1400 calories and 43-46 fat grams max. You have downloaded apps to help you with daily tracking of your food and activities. You do not have a Bonus or Extra Diet in Phase 1 they will be added in Phase 2.

PHASE 2: TRANSFORM

Week 3-4 Example: *You're transforming your body and mind and continuing to believe in yourself again.*

You continue following your Low-Calorie and Low-Carb Diet and the numbers from the Aggressive Body Budget Chart. You now will add in a Bonus Diet of 3 Liquid Dinners a Week and an Extra Diet of the No Added Sugar Challenge for 14 days. On the days you have liquid dinners, you can put your heavier meal in the middle of the day. This will increase your weight loss.

PHASE 3: DOMINATE

Week 5-6 Example: *You're on the path to dominate losing weight.*

You are keeping your same Base Diet and Remixx Diet of Low-Calorie and Low-Carb, but you are adding in a new Bonus Diet of having 3 Meatless Dinners a Week and an Extra Diet of going Platinum Low-Calorie (1200 calories, 40 fat grams max). Going meatless three days a week will also help with your lower caloric intake because you can spend your budget on more low-calorie dense plant-based foods. Making it easier to stay within your daily body budget. (Remember: Meatless Dinners Will Help You Get Thinner).

SLIM DOWN LEVEL UP FORMULA #2

Low-Calorie + Low-Carb Diets: Deluxe Option

6-WEEK DELUXE PROGRAM

Phase	Time-frame	Base Diet	Remixx	Bonus	Extra
Phase 1: Reboot	Week 1-2	Low-Calorie*	Low-Carb**	N/A	N/A
Phase 2: Transform	Week 3-4	Low-Calorie*	Low-Carb**	Liquid Dinner 3 Days a Week	No Added Sugar Challenge
Phase 3: Dominate	Week 5-6	Low-Calorie*	Low-Carb**	Meatless Dinner 3 Days a Week	Platinum Low-Calorie

*__Low-Calorie__ = Check with the Daily Body Budget Charts in Chapter 10 for calories and fat grams allowance.

Platinum Low-Calorie = 1200 calories and 40 Fat Grams (Used in Week 5-6) *Meatless Dinners: Refer to pages 204-210 for Keto-Vegan-Low-Carb recipes*

***__Low-Carb__-Choose Either:

Liberal Low-Carbs: 50-100 Net Carbs Max
Moderate Low-Carbs: 20-50 Net Carbs Max
Ketogenic Low-Carbs: 20 Net Carbs or Less Max

Formula to Calculate Net Carbs:

Total Carbohydrates – Dietary Fiber = Net Carbs

*After completing the 6-week session, you can circle back starting at Week 1. The second time around, you can choose a different Remixx, Bonus or Extra option to change up your combination based on your preferences. You can refer to the chart on page 298 for more eating style options.

Alternative: If you are not ready to add the Extra in Week 5-6, continue following the rest of the steps in those weeks and you can choose to add another option from the chart to your combination. For increased weight loss, you can add in a 5:2 or 4:3 fasting schedule once a month to your routine. (You can refer to the Intermittent Fasting Schedule Examples in Chapter 17).

SLIM DOWN LEVEL UP FORMULA #2

Low-Calorie + Low-Carb Diets: Advanced Option

This option is a *6-Week Advanced**Program,* with 3 parts: Phase 1: **Reboot**, Phase 2: **Transform**, Phase 3: **Dominate**. Each phase last for two weeks and has a variety of different Bonus, Extra and Level Up options included.

Bonus, Extra and Level Up Options Chart

*Liquid Dinner 3 Days a Week	*Liberal Low-Carb (50-100 Net Carbs Max)
*Meatless Dinner 3 Days a Week	*Moderate Low-Carb (20-50 Net Carbs Max)
*No Added Sugar Challenge	*Ketogenic Low-Carb*** (20 Net Carbs Max)
*Add a 5:2 Fasting Schedule	*Platinum Low-Calorie = *(1200 calories, 40 fat grams)*

You can choose to start with the **Deluxe Program for a semi-aggressive start or use this **Advanced Program** if you are a more aggressive dieter. When referring to the weekly program, you will see some of the above Bonus, Extra and Level Up options listed within the chart. These are recommended for optimum results each week. However, if you get to a certain week and the selected option is not one you prefer, select a different one from the chart and continue following the rest of the week's program.

STARTING OUT-PHASE 1:

NO SODAS, JUICES, SPORTS DRINKS, ALCOHOL, WHITE BREAD, WHITE RICE, PASTA, FRIED FOODS, OR WHOLE FAT DAIRY PRODUCTS

Low-Calorie*: You will see Low-Calorie listed in the weekly program as a Remixx Diet. You can choose any Low-Calorie Diet/ eating style you prefer. For help with making your decision, you can refer to Chapters 14-15 to see the seven previously mentioned diets.

Key Point: When starting out and reducing your daily overall intake, if you are full on less food and it is not below 1200 calories or 40 fat grams, regularly, that is okay. It is showing your body is transitioning to the new eating habits. As it continues adjusting to receiving less calories, and you reduce your net carb intake to ketogenic levels, (20 or less), it will start relying more on your stored fat as its primary fuel. Turning your body into a fat burning, belly busting machine.

Slim Down Level Up Formula #2 Advanced Option Explained

PHASE 1: REBOOT

Week 1-2 Example: *You're ready for the weight loss food shift.*

You have a Base Diet of Low-Calorie and a Remixx Diet of Low-Carb. You have decided to order your food from one of the meal kit delivery services and stick to the premeasured meals weekly. You will cook occasionally following some of the recipes you found on pages 204-210 in the book. You weigh 260 pounds and have checked with the Aggressive Body Budget Chart in Chapter 10 and will take in 1400-1500 calories and 46-50 fat grams max daily. And you have decided to use the moderate carbs and will keep them between 20-50 net carbs. You have a Bonus Diet of having Meatless Dinners 3 Days a Week. You have no Extra or Level Up Diets in Phase 1; they will be added in Phase 2.

PHASE 2: TRANSFORM

Week 3-4 Example: *You're transforming your body and mind and continuing to believe in yourself again.*

You are sticking with the same Base Diet, Low-Calorie and Remixx Diet of Low-Carb. You will swap your Bonus Diet to the No Added Sugar 14 Day Challenge. You are adding an Extra Diet of having 3 Liquid Dinners a Week and a Level Up Diet of Ketogenic Low-Carbs (20 net carbs max). You continue to follow the Aggressive Daily Body Budget Chart for your calories and fat grams intake.

PHASE 3: DOMINATE

> **Week 5-6 Example:** *You're on the path to dominate losing weight.*
>
> You are keeping the same Low-Calorie and Low-Carb Diets, and now you will swap your Bonus Diet to 3 Meatless Dinners a Week and change your Extra Diet to Platinum Low-Calories (1200 calories, 40 fat grams). Then you will swap your Level Up Diet to adding in a 5:2 Fasting Schedule. Where you will follow the Platinum Low-Calories five days a week, and for two non-consecutive days, you will fast. On the two fasting days, you will only take in 500-600 calories. To help you not overeat and stay within the lower calories, you order premeasured plant-based meals to use on the two fasting days.

*Alternative: If you are not ready to add the Level Up fasting schedule in Week 5-6, continue following the rest of the steps in those weeks and you can choose to add another option from the chart to your combination. Or, for increased weight loss, you can add in the 5:2 or 4:3 fasting schedule once a month. (See Fasting Schedule Examples in Chapter 17).

SLIM DOWN LEVEL UP FORMULA #2

Low-Calorie + Low-Carb Diets: Advanced Option

6-WEEK ADVANCED PROGRAM

Phase	Time-frame	Base Diet	Re-mixx	Bonus	Extra	Level Up
Phase 1: **Reboot**	Week 1-2	Low-Calorie*	Low-Carb	Meat-less Dinner 3 Days a Week	N/A	N/A
Phase 2: **Trans-form**	Week 3-4	Low-Calorie*	Low-Carb	No Added Sugar Chal-lenge	Add Liquid Dinner 3 Days a Week	Keto-genic Low-Carbs
Phase 3: **Dominate**	Week 5-6	Low-Calorie*	Low-Carb	Meat-less Dinner 3 Days a Week	**Plat-inum Low-Cal-orie	Add 5:2 Fasting Sched-ule

*__Low-Calorie__ = Check with the Daily Body Budget Charts in Chapter 10 for calories and fat grams allowance.

**__Platinum Low-Calorie = 1200 calories and 40 Fat Grams__ (Used in Week 5-6) *Meatless Dinners: Refer to pages 204-210 for Keto-Vegan-Low-Carb recipes*

***__Low-Carb__-Choose Either:

Liberal Low-Carbs: 50-100 Net Carbs Max

Moderate Low-Carbs: 20-50 Net Carbs Max

Ketogenic Low-Carbs: 20 Net Carbs or Less Max

Formula to Calculate Net Carbs:

Total Carbohydrates – Dietary Fiber = Net Carbs

*After completing the 6-week session, you can circle back starting at Week 1. The second time around, you can choose a different Remixx, Bonus, Extra or Level Up combination based on your preferences. You can refer to the chart on page 298 for more eating style options when making your selections.

**Again, if you are not ready to add the Level Up fasting schedule in Week 5-6, continue following the rest of the steps in those weeks and you can choose to add another option from the chart to your combination.

SLIM DOWN LEVEL UP FORMULA #3

Keto + Low-Calorie + Intermittent Fasting Diets: Deluxe Option

This option is a *6-Week Deluxe** Program,* with 3 parts: Phase 1: **Reboot**, Phase 2: **Transform**, Phase 3: **Dominate**. Each phase last for two weeks and has a variety of different Bonus, Extra and Level Up options included.

Bonus, Extra and Level Up Options Chart

*Fasting Extra: Add (1) 36-Hour Fast	*Low-Carb (50 net carbs max)
*Liquid Dinner 3 Days a Week	*Fasting Extra: Add 1 OMAD (24-Hour Fast)
*No Added Sugar Challenge	*Fasting Extra: Add 3 Days of 18:6 Fast
*Meatless Dinner 3 Days a Week	*Fasting Extra: Add 5 Days of 18:6 Fast
*Platinum Low-Calorie	*Ketogenic Low-Carb*** (20 net carbs max)

You can choose this **Deluxe Program to begin or use the **Advanced Program** in the next section if you are an experienced faster and experienced with using a Keto Diet. When referring to the weekly program, you will see some of the above Bonus, Extra and Level Up options listed within the chart. These are recommended for optimum results each week. However, if you get to a certain week and the selected option is not one you prefer, select a different one from the chart and continue following the rest of the week's program.

STARTING OUT- PHASE 1:

NO SODAS, JUICES, SPORTS DRINKS, ALCOHOL, WHITE BREAD, WHITE RICE, PASTA, FRIED FOODS

Important Note: If you are a first time *Faster*, or have not fasted in a while, you will start out using the 14:10 Schedule in the first two weeks of the program. Slowly decrease the eating window by 30 minutes every other day in the first 10-12 days, to arrive at the

16:8 window by Week 3. If you are an *Advanced Faster,* you can start with a 16:8 Schedule for the first two weeks.

Low-Calorie*: You will see Low-Calorie listed in the weekly program as a Remixx Diet. You can choose any Low-Calorie Diet/ eating style you prefer. For help with making your decision, you can refer to Chapters 14-15 to see the seven previously mentioned diets.

Key Point: Keep in mind, by fasting and using the decreased timeframe, you may not use your entire daily body budget. It is there as a guide to keep you from overeating. When starting out, if you are full on less food and your daily intake is not below 1200 calories or 40 fat grams, regularly, that is okay. It is showing your body is transitioning to the new eating schedule. As it continues adjusting to receiving less calories and as your fasting window increases, combined with the low-carb intake, it will start relying more on your stored fat as its primary fuel. Turning your body into a fat burning, belly busting machine.

Slim Down Level Up Formula #3 Deluxe Option Explained

PHASE 1: REBOOT

Week 1-2 Example: *You're ready for the weight loss food shift.*

You weigh 220-pounds, you will follow the numbers in the Conservative Daily Body Budget Chart in Chapter 10 and take in 1600-1800 calories and 53-60 fat grams max. Your Base Diet, is Keto and you will take in 20 net carbs max daily. Your Remixx Diet is Low-Calorie, and you will follow some recipes you found on Pinterest and order some food from the meal kit delivery services. Your Bonus Diet is Intermittent Fasting. You have not fasted before, so you will start out using the 14:10 Schedule, and you have decided to eat between the hours of 8:30 am-6:30 pm. You have downloaded apps to help you with daily tracking of your food and activities. In the first two weeks, you will decrease your, eating time by 30 minutes every other day, to make the transition easier to arrive at the desired 16:8 Fasting Schedule, by the beginning of Week 3. (Decreasing Timeframe Example: 9:00-7:00 pm, 9:30-7:00pm, 10:00-7:00pm, 10:30-7:00pm, 11:00-7:00pm). You do not have an Extra or Level Up Diet in Phase 1, they will be added in Phase 2.

PHASE 2: TRANSFORM

Week 3-4 Example: *You're transforming your body and mind and continuing to believe in yourself again.*

You are continuing to follow the Base Diet, Keto, the Remixx Diet, Low-Calorie and now have a Bonus Diet of a 16:8 Fasting Schedule. You are adding an Extra Diet of having OMAD 24-Hour Fast added to your routine on any day of your choosing, in Week 4. Lastly, you, are adding the Level Up Diet of having 3 Liquid Dinners a Week. By doing so, on those days, you are putting your heavier/larger meal in the middle of the day (remember the saying, "My Liquid Dinner Makes Me Thinner").

PHASE 3: DOMINATE

Week 5-6 Example: *You're on the path to dominate losing weight.*

You are continuing to follow your Base Diet, Keto, and Remixx Diet, Low-Calorie. Your Bonus Diet is now changing to having 3 Meatless Dinners a Week. There is a change to your Intermittent Fasting schedule, you will now have 4 days using the16:8 Schedule. And 3 days at 18:6 Schedule, reducing your, eating window by 2 additional hours on those days. They can be consecutive or non-consecutive, depending on your schedule. Example: Monday 16:8, Tuesday 18:6, Wednesday 18:6, Thursday 16:8, Friday 16:8, Saturday 18:6, Sunday 16:8.

---

*Alternative: If you are not ready to add the Extra 18:6 fasting schedule in Week 5-6, continue using the 16:8 schedule. For increased weight loss and maintenance, you can add in 3 Days of an 18:6 schedule once a month or 1 to 2 OMAD (24-Hour) or 2 36-Hour Fast twice a month.

SLIM DOWN LEVEL UP FORMULA #3

Keto + Low-Calorie + Intermittent Fasting Diets: Deluxe Option

6-WEEK DELUXE PROGRAM

Phase	Time-frame	Base Diet	Remixx	Bonus	Extra	Level Up
Phase 1: Reboot	Week 1-2	KETO	Low-Calorie*	Intermittent Fasting 14:10 Schedule	N/A	N/A
Phase 2: Transform	Week 3-4	KETO	Low-Calorie*	Intermittent Fasting 16:8 Schedule	Add 1-OMAD Fast (24-Hour) in Week 4	Add Liquid Dinner 3 Days a Week
Phase 3: Dominate	Week 5-6	KETO	Low-Calorie*	Meatless Dinner 3 Days a Week	Add 3 Days of 18:6 Fast	Platinum Low-Calorie

*Low-Calorie=Check with the Daily Body Budget Charts in Chapter 10 for calories and fat grams allowance.

Platinum Low-Calorie=1200 calories and 40 Fat Grams (Used in Week 5-6) *Meatless Dinners: Refer to pages 204-210 for Keto-Vegan-Low-Calorie recipes*

Ketogenic Low-Carb: 20 Net Carbs or Less Max

Formula to Calculate Net Carbs:

Total Carbohydrates – Dietary Fiber = Net Carbs

*After completing the 6-week session, you can circle back starting at Week 1. The second time around, you can choose a different Bonus, Remixx, Extra or Level Up combination based on your preferences. You can refer to the chart on page 298 for more eating style options when making your selections.

SLIM DOWN LEVEL UP FORMULA #3

Keto + Low-Calorie + Intermittent Fasting Diets: Advanced Option

This option is a *6-Week Advanced** Program,* with 3 parts: Phase 1: **Reboot**, Phase 2: **Transform**, Phase 3: **Dominate**. Each phase last for two weeks and has a variety of different Bonus, Extra and Level Up options included.

Bonus, Extra and Level Up Options Chart

*Fasting Extra: Add (1) 36-Hour Fast	*Low-Carb (50 net carbs max)
*Liquid Dinner 3 Days a Week	*Fasting Extra: Add 1 OMAD (24-Hour Fast)
*No Added Sugar Challenge	*Fasting Extra: Add 3-Days of 18:6 Fast
*Meatless Dinner 3 Days a Week	*Fasting Extra: Add 5 Days of 18:6 Fast
*Platinum Low-Calorie	*Ketogenic Low-Carb*** (20 net carbs max)

You can choose the **Deluxe Program to begin or use this **Advanced Program** if you are an experienced faster and experienced with using a Keto Diet. When referring to the weekly program, you will see some of the above Bonus, Extra and Level Up options listed within the chart. These are recommended for optimum results each week. However, if you get to a certain week and the selected option is not one you prefer, select a different one from the chart and continue following the rest of the week's program.

STARTING OUT-PHASE 1:

NO SODAS, JUICES, SPORTS DRINKS, ALCOHOL, WHITE BREAD, WHITE RICE, PASTA, FRIED FOODS

Important Note: If you are an experienced faster but need a few days to jumpstart your body and would like to use the *Advanced*

Program, use the first 5-7 days to get your body adjusted to eating in the reduced timeframe. Slowly decrease your, eating window by 30 minutes to an hour every other day in the first few days, to arrive at the 16:8 window by the end of Week 1.

Low-Calorie*: You will see Low-Calorie listed in the weekly program as a *Remixx Diet*. You can choose any Low-Calorie Diet/eating style you prefer. For help with making your decision, you can refer to Chapters 14-15 to see the seven previously mentioned diets.

Key Point: Keep in mind, by fasting and using the decreased eating timeframe, you may not use your entire daily body budget. It is there as a guide to keep you from overeating. When starting out, if you are full on less food and your daily intake is not below 1200 calories or 40 fat grams, regularly, that is okay. It is showing your body is transitioning to the new eating schedule. As it continues adjusting to receiving less calories and as your fasting window increases, as well as the reduced carb intake, it will start relying more on your stored fat as its primary fuel. Allowing your body to reap the benefits of being in ketosis.

Slim Down Level Up Formula #3 Advanced Option Explained

PHASE 1: REBOOT

Week 1-2 Example: *You're ready for the weight loss food shift.*

You weigh 250-pounds, you will follow the numbers in the Aggressive Daily Body Budget Chart in Chapter 10 and take in 1400-1500 calories and 46-50 fat grams max. You have a Base Diet of Keto and will take in 20 net carbs max daily. Your Remixx Diet is Low-Calorie, and you will follow some recipes you found on pages 204-210 in the book and order some food from the South Beach Diet. Your Bonus Diet is Intermittent Fasting. You will start out using a 16:8 Schedule and you have an Extra Diet of adding OMAD (24-hour fast) in Week 2. It can be on any day you choose. You do not have a Level Up Diet in Phase 1; it will be added in Phase 2.

PHASE 2: TRANSFORM

Week 3-4 Example: *You're transforming your body and mind and continuing to believe in yourself again.*

Your Base Diet is still Keto, your Remixx Diet is Low-Calorie, and your Bonus Diet is still the 16:8 Fasting Schedule. You are swapping your Extra Diet to now adding in 3 days of an 18:6 Fast to your routine. Reducing your, eating window down by two hours on those days. You will add a Level Up Diet of 3 Liquid Dinners a Week (remember to say, "My Liquid Dinner Makes Me Thinner").

PHASE 3: DOMINATE

Week 5-6 Example: *You're on the path to dominate losing weight.*

Your Base Diet is still Keto, your Remixx Diet is Low-Calorie, and your Bonus Diet is still the 16:8 Fasting Schedule. You are swapping your Extra Diet to having 3 Meatless Dinners a Week. And your Level Up Diet is now adding in 5 days of an 18:6 Fast to your routine. For example, Monday 16:8, Tuesday 18:6, Wednesday 18:6, Thursday 18:6, Friday 16:8, Saturday 18:6, Sunday 18:6.

Alternative: If you are not ready to add the Level Up 18:6 fasting schedule in Week 5-6, continue using the 16:8 schedule. For increased weight loss and maintenance, you can add in 3-5 Days of an 18:6 schedule once a month or 1 to 2 OMAD (24-Hour) or 2 36-Hour Fast twice a month.

SLIM DOWN LEVEL UP FORMULA #3

Keto + Low-Calorie + Intermittent Fasting Diets: Advanced Option

6-WEEK ADVANCED PROGRAM

Phase	Time-frame	Base Diet	Remixx	Bonus	Extra	Level Up
Phase 1: Reboot	Week 1-2	KETO	Low-Calorie*	Intermittent Fasting 16:8 Schedule	Add 1-OMAD Fast (24-Hour) in Week 2	N/A
Phase 2: Transform	Week 3-4	KETO	Low-Calorie*	Intermittent Fasting 16:8 Schedule	Add 3 Days of 18:6 Fast per Week	Add Liquid Dinner 3 Days
Phase 3: Dominate	Week 5-6	KETO	Low-Calorie*	Intermittent Fasting 16:8 Schedule	Meatless Dinner 3 Days a Week	Add 5 Days of 18:6 Fast

*Low-Calorie=Check with the Daily Body Budget Charts in Chapter 10 for calories and fat grams allowance.

Platinum Low-Calorie=1200 calories and 40 Fat Grams (Can be used in Week 5-6 to lower your daily intake as an added, Bonus) *Meatless Dinners: Refer to pages 204-210 for Keto-Vegan-Low-Calorie recipes*

Ketogenic Low-Carb: 20 Net Carbs or Less Max

Formula to Calculate Net Carbs:

Total Carbohydrates − Dietary Fiber = Net Carbs

*After completing the 6-week session, you can circle back starting at Week 1. The second time around, you can choose a different Bonus, Remixx, Extra or Level Up combination based on your preferences. You can refer to the chart on page 298 for more eating style options when making your selections.

***Yes, weight loss is near! The formulas have been laid out and examples have been shown to paint a better picture, of how your weight loss journey will look once you get started. In the next chapter we will go over Intermittent Fasting protocols, timeframes, and schedules.

17

FASTING CHARTS EXAMPLES AND TIMEFRAMES

As discussed in Chapter 14, there are so many amazing benefits from fasting, and it can be an added, bonus to you losing weight. If you decide to use one of the *Slim Down Level Up Formulas* that includes Intermittent Fasting, (#1 or #3) you can refer to the charts in this chapter. There are multiple options to choose from and a variety of fasting schedules. In case you are a night owl or work third shift, there are fasting examples provided if you need a later timeframe to accommodate your schedule. There are also examples provided if you prefer to have an earlier fasting window, to cut your eating off prior to 5 pm. The fasting charts include, **14:10, 16:8, 18:6, 20:4, 5:2, 4:3 and Spontaneous Meal Skipping.** Which, the latter, can be a great option to use if you want the flexibility of randomly skipping meals and are starting with formula #2. Here is some information on getting started with using Intermittent Fasting.

TIPS ON HOW TO START FASTING

The first key step to using Intermittent Fasting as one of your weight loss tools is, to decide on which fasting schedule will work best for your lifestyle. If you normally eat later in the evenings, shift your fasting window until later in the day. Same thing on the flip side; if you are an early riser and early to bed kind of person, you can plan accordingly. The most important thing to remember is fasting is something you can do for life. Take it easy on yourself, when first starting out, and if you are within 15-20 minutes of breaking fast and feel the need to eat or drink something, do so. You can always reset yourself back the next day. Keep in mind, when fasting, even for shorter periods of time, you can still allow your body to benefit from all the health perks that come with limiting your, eating window. Like helping you to lose weight, autophagy (the removal of those old and damaged cells), lowering your insulin levels and insulin resistance. As well as its ability to fight stubborn belly fat.

DRINK LOTS OF WATER WHEN FASTING

One of the most common side effects when first starting out fasting is the feeling of fatigue. This can be due to the reduction in fluids you would normally receive from the additional foods you eat. Staying hydrated by drinking plenty of water can help with increasing energy lost from not receiving the additional calories. Water is the number one choice to go with. However, you can also have coffee, tea, or non-caloric beverages like sparkling or tonic water. There is a chart in the next section, following the fasting schedules, with what are approved drinks while fasting and what constitutes a clean fast, dirty fast and what breaks a fast. (A clean fast is strict on what you are and are not allowed to have inside the fasting timeframe. While a dirty fast has a little more wiggle room. But still allows you to reap the benefits of incorporating the smaller eating window into your weight loss routine).

DON'T BREAK FAST BY FEASTING

How you break-fast is significant as it relates to your weight loss success. For best results when breaking your fast, try to choose lighter food options to start with. Like bone broth, a handful of nuts or a small salad and slowly introduce the heavier foods as the day goes on. This will help to eliminate bloating, stomach pain and will be a lot easier on the digestive tract. You may be tempted to overeat when breaking a fast with a feasting type of meal. That can hinder your weight loss goals. Gradually spreading out the calories over a few hours is ideal. Like sliced avocado, scrambled eggs with spinach, Greek Yogurt, or a salad with tuna. Then, your second meal could be something like, grilled chicken, baked salmon with rice, or a turkey sandwich wrap. I love spicy food; however, I avoid it first thing when breaking fast, to eliminate having an upset stomach. You may want to do the same. For breakfast/brunch ideas and recipes, you can refer to Chapter 13, page 204 for a list of food options that may be helpful when deciding what to eat.

STOP FASTING IF YOU ARE FEELING SICK

Other common side effects when first starting out fasting can be dizziness, lightheadedness, and headaches. This can be due to being dehydrated and needing more fluids or from the reduction in sodium that is usually received from eating. You can add pink salt or unsweetened electrolytes to your water to help with reducing these feelings. Also, to minimize the side effects, slowly ease out of bed in the mornings, as, well as allow yourself time to go from a seated position to standing throughout the day. If you are feeling sick while fasting, stop immediately and get fluids or food in your system. Monitoring your blood pressure while fasting is also suggested to see how your body is responding.

CONSIDER TAKING SUPPLEMENTS

While dieting and fasting, it is important to make sure you are getting adequate amounts of nutrients. Incorporating supplements into your daily routine may be beneficial for you, to ensure you are receiving the necessary vitamins and minerals daily. Especially if you have a chronic health condition or type 2 diabetes. Also, it is okay to take your medications with water while fasting. However, if your medications need to be taken with food, you may have to adjust your eating window to accommodate those needs.

These are the supplements I make sure to take while fasting: a multi-vitamin, B12, iron, calcium, vitamin C, and vitamin D. Always consult your physician about the safest supplements for your needs.

Fasting Tip: When starting Intermittent Fasting, just remember you do not have to jump in the deep end of the pool to get in. Starting out using a modified schedule like a 12:12 or 14:10 and work yourself up to the desired 16:8 Schedule, will allow your body time to adapt to the eating changes.

Besides taking supplements, when using Intermittent Fasting, it is important to receive adequate amounts of electrolytes, magnesium, calcium, and sodium through food intake. Here is a list of a few items you can incorporate in your diet that can provide these nutrients.

*Olives *Pickles *Pickle Juice *Salty Foods *Leafy Green Vegetables (Kale, Collard Greens, Spinach) *Avocado *Sweet Potato *Squash *Bananas *Dried Apricots *Yogurt *Cheese *Nuts *Beans *Lentils *Milk *Coconut Water *Soy Milk *Tomato Juice

Side Note: When I first started out using Intermittent Fasting, in the early days, I would feel weak and a little tired. I increased my fluid intake by drinking tea and water. Then inside my eating window, I drank pickle juice and ate olives to help with increasing my electrolytes lost from not eating. I also increased my fat intake and reduced my carbs. By increasing my electrolytes and making the changes to what I was eating during my 8-hour window, it helped eliminate the early signs of fasting I was experiencing.

Bonus Meal Plan: As you view through the different fasting charts, you will see a total of 8-weeks of meal plans provided within the examples. You can use them as a guide when first starting the program. You will be able to choose from low-calorie and low-carb as, well as a few vegan options. And in the coming chapters you will be provided a 2-Week Grocery Shopping List and a 4-Week 1500 Calorie Meal Plan to use as well. In total, you will have **12-Weeks of a Sample Meal Plan** on ways to spend your Daily Body Budget (portion sizes will vary depending on how much you are making, which brand of food you are using and how much of your daily budget you will have, to spend).

INTERMITTENT FASTING 16:8 SCHEDULE WITH AN EARLY DINNER 7:30AM-3:30PM

16:8 EARLY SCHEDULE	BREAKFAST 7:30AM	LUNCH – 12PM	DINNER – 3:30PM	EVENING 3:30PM-BEDTIME
MONDAY	Greek Yogurt with Mixed Berries	**Soup and Sandwich**	Ginger Chicken Lettuce Wraps	**FAST**
TUESDAY	Smoothie	**Grilled Chicken Salad**	Portobello Mushroom Wraps	**FAST**
WEDNESDAY	Overnight Oats	**Steak & Grilled Vegetables**	Curry Eggplant & Cauliflower Rice	**FAST**
THURSDAY	Omelet & Fruit	**2 Turkey Wraps**	Spaghetti Squash Bowl	**FAST**
FRIDAY	Pancakes	**Chili & Rice**	Grilled Salmon, Rice &Vegetables	**FAST**
SATURDAY	Breakfast Burrito	**Pork Chop & Salad**	Chicken Caesar Salad	**FAST**
SUNDAY	Eggs and Bacon	**Asian Grilled Shrimp & Veggies**	Veggie Burger & Sweet Potato Fries	**FAST**

*One-Week Sample Meal Plan

INTERMITTENT FASTING 16:8 SCHEDULE WITH A LATE DINNER 11:30AM-7:30PM

16:8 LATE SCHEDULE	BREAKFAST 7:30AM	BRUNCH 11:30 AM	AFTERNOON-4PM	DINNER – 7:30PM
MONDAY	FAST	Quesadilla	Soup and Sandwich	Curry Eggplant & Cauliflower Rice
TUESDAY	FAST	Oatmeal & Strawberries	Chicken Salad	Chicken Caesar Salad
WEDNESDAY	FAST	Smoothie	Pork Chop & Salad	Soup & Sandwich
THURSDAY	FAST	Omelet & Fruit	Smoothie	Asian Grilled Shrimp & Veggies
FRIDAY	FAST	Pancakes	Grilled Salmon, Rice &Vegetables	2 Turkey Wraps
SATURDAY	FAST	Breakfast Burrito	Steak & Grilled Vegetables	Smoothie
SUNDAY	FAST	Eggs and Bacon	Ginger Chicken Lettuce Wraps	Chili & Rice

*One-Week Sample Meal Plan

INTERMITTENT FASTING 16:8 SCHEDULE WITH 2 MEALS A DAY- EARLY DINNER 7:30AM-3:30PM

16:8 EARLY SCHED-ULE 2 MEALS	BREAK-FAST 7:30AM	LUNCH – 12PM	DINNER – 3:30PM	EVENING 3:30PM-BEDTIME
MONDAY	Quesadilla	**SNACK***	Grilled Salmon & Veggies	**FAST**
TUESDAY	Breakfast Burrito	**SNACK***	Soup and Sandwich	**FAST**
WEDNES-DAY	Overnight Oats	**SNACK***	Curry Egg-plant & Cauli-flower Rice	**FAST**
THURS-DAY	Omelet & Fruit	**SNACK***	Asian Grilled Shrimp & Veggies	**FAST**
FRIDAY	Eggs and Bacon	**SNACK***	2 Turkey Wraps & Salad	**FAST**
SATUR-DAY	Breakfast Burrito	**SNACK***	Chicken Caesar Salad	**FAST**
SUNDAY	Pancakes	**SNACK***	Pepper Steak & Rice	**FAST**

*Snack is optional-One-Week Sample Meal Plan

INTERMITTENT FASTING 16:8 SCHEDULE WITH 2 MEALS A DAY- LATE DINNER 11:30AM-7:30PM

16:8 LATE SCHEDULE 2 MEALS	BREAKFAST 11:30AM	LUNCH – 4PM	DINNER – 7:30PM	EVENING 7:30PM-BED-TIME
MONDAY	Sandwich & Soup	SNACK*	Turkey Wrap & Soup	FAST
TUESDAY	Breakfast Burrito	SNACK*	Chicken Caesar Salad	FAST
WEDNES-DAY	Quesadilla	SNACK*	Curry Eggplant & Cauliflower Rice	FAST
THURS-DAY	Omelet & Fruit	SNACK*	Veggie Burger & Sweet Potato Fries	FAST
FRIDAY	Pancakes & Sausage	SNACK*	Pork Chop & a Salad	FAST
SATUR-DAY	Cobb Salad	SNACK*	Asian Grilled Shrimp & Veggies	FAST
SUNDAY	Eggs and Bacon	SNACK*	Pepper Steak & Rice	FAST

*Snack is optional-One-Week Sample Meal Plan

INTERMITTENT FASTING 18:6 SCHEDULE WITH AN EARLY DINNER 9:30AM-3:30PM

18:6 EARLY-SCHEDULE	BREAK-FAST 9:30AM	LUNCH-12PM	DIN-NER-3:30 PM	EVENING 3:30PM-BEDTIME
MONDAY	Pancakes	SNACK*	Zucchini Crush Pizza	FAST
TUESDAY	Breakfast Burrito	SNACK*	Turkey Mole Tacos	FAST
WEDNES-DAY	Overnight Oats	SNACK*	Moo Shu Mushrooms Wraps	FAST
THURS-DAY	Omelet	SNACK*	Chicken-Steak Fajitas	FAST
FRIDAY	Eggs and Bacon	SNACK*	Pork Chop & Asparagus	FAST
SATUR-DAY	Breakfast Burrito	SNACK*	Grilled Tilapia with Veggies	FAST
SUNDAY	Quesadilla	SNACK*	Greek Stuffed Banana Peppers	FAST

*Snack is optional-One-Week Sample Meal Plan

INTERMITTENT FASTING 18:6 SCHEDULE WITH A LATE DINNER 1:00PM-7:00PM

18:6 LATE-SCHEDULE	BREAK-FAST 7AM	LUNCH-1PM	DINNER-7:00PM	EVENING 7:00PM-BED-TIME
MONDAY	FAST	Soup and Sandwich	Turkey Stroganoff	FAST
TUESDAY	FAST	Salmon & Veggies	Chicken Noodle Soup & Sandwich	FAST
WEDNESDAY	FAST	Chicken Caesar Salad	Baked Cheddar Eggs & Potatoes	FAST
THURSDAY	FAST	Curry Eggplant & Cauliflower Rice	Moroccan Chicken with Rice	FAST
FRIDAY	FAST	Steak & Grilled Vegetables	Vegetarian Bean Tacos, w/ Rice	FAST
SATURDAY	FAST	2 Turkey Wraps & Salad	Tilapia, w/ Veggies	FAST
SUNDAY	FAST	Asian Grilled Shrimp & Veggies	Chicken Caesar Salad	FAST

* One Week Sample Meal Plan

INTERMITTENT FASTING 4:3 SCHEDULE (ALTERNATING DAY FASTING)

4:3 ALTER- NATE DAYS SCHED- ULE	BREAKFAST	LUNCH	DINNER - 6PM
MONDAY	FAST	FAST	**500-600 Calories Max**
TUESDAY	Breakfast Burrito	Chicken Caesar Salad	Pepper Steak & Rice
WEDNES-DAY	FAST	FAST	**500-600 Calories Max**
THURS-DAY	Smoothie	Asian Grilled Shrimp & Veggies	Turkey Wrap & Soup
FRIDAY	FAST	FAST	**500-600 Calories Max**
SATUR-DAY	Eggs and Bacon	Veggie Burger & Sweet Potato Fries	Grilled Salmon, Rice &Vegetables
SUNDAY	Granola +Berry Coconut Parfaits	Steak & Grilled Vegetables	Vegan Taco Salad Bowl

* One Week Sample Meal Plan

INTERMITTENT FASTING WARRIOR 20:4 SCHEDULE

20:4 WARRIOR SCHEDULE	BREAK-FAST	LUNCH	EAT 5-9 PM	EVENING 9PM-BED-TIME
MONDAY	FAST	**FAST**	Pinto Beans Tostadas w/ Rice	**FAST**
TUESDAY	FAST	**FAST**	Mediterra-nean Turkey Skillet	**FAST**
WEDNES-DAY	FAST	**FAST**	Curry Rice Noodles w/ Chicken	**FAST**
THURS-DAY	FAST	**FAST**	Grilled Salm-on & Potato Salad	**FAST**
FRIDAY	FAST	**FAST**	Greek Stuffed Pep-pers	**FAST**
SATUR-DAY	FAST	**FAST**	Soup & Sandwich	**FAST**
SUNDAY	FAST	**FAST**	Mango Chut-ney Chicken & Veggies	**FAST**

* One Week Sample Meal Plan

INTERMITTENT FASTING SCHEDULE ENHANCERS*

20:4 SCHED-ULE WAR-RIOR	0MAD 24-HOUR Fast SCHED-ULE	36 HOUR-SCHEDULE (A Day & A Half Fast)	5:2 SCHED-ULE Non-Con-secutive Days	4:3 SCHED-ULE Alternat-ing Days
11AM-3PM	EAT AT 3PM	Monday Eat 6pm-Wednes-day Eat 6am	Fast: M/TH	Fast: M/W/F
12PM-4PM	EAT AT 4PM	Monday Eat 7pm-Wednes-day Eat 7am	Fast: T/SAT	Fast: T/TH/SAT
1PM-5PM	EAT AT 5PM	Monday Eat 8pm-Wednes-day Eat 8am	Fast: W/FRI	Fast: W/F/SUN
2PM-6PM	EAT AT 6PM	Monday Eat 9pm-Wednes-day Eat 9am	Fast: TH/SAT	Fast: TH/SAT/M
3PM-7PM	EAT AT 7PM	Monday Eat 10pm-Wednes-day Eat 10am	Fast: FRI/SUN	Fast: F/SUN/T
4PM-8PM	EAT AT 8PM	Monday Eat 11pm-Wednes-day Eat 11am	Fast: M/W	Fast: SAT/M/W
5PM-9PM	EAT AT 9PM	Monday Eat 12pm-Wednes-day Eat 12am	Fast: TH/SAT	Fast: SUN/T/TH
6PM-10PM	EAT AT 10PM	Monday Eat 1am-Wednes-day Eat 1pm	Fast: T/TH	Fast: M/W/SAT

*These can be used by themselves or added to any fasting schedule to enhance your weight loss

INTERMITTENT FASTING OPTIONS

12:12 SCHED-ULE	14:10 SCHED-ULE	15:9 SCHED-ULE	16:8 SCHED-ULE	18:6 SCHED-ULE
6AM-6PM	7AM-5PM	9AM-6PM	9AM-5PM	9AM-3PM
7AM-7PM	8AM-6PM	10AM-7PM	10AM-6PM	10AM-4PM
8AM-8PM	9AM-7PM	11AM-8PM	11AM-7PM	11AM-5PM
9AM-9PM	10AM-8PM	12PM-9PM	12PM-8PM	12PM-6PM
10AM-10PM	11AM-9PM	1PM-10PM	1PM-9PM	1PM-7PM
11AM-11PM	12PM-10PM	2PM-11PM	2PM-10PM	2PM-8PM
12PM-12AM	1PM-11PM	3PM-12AM	3PM-11PM	3PM-9PM
1AM-1PM	2PM-12AM	4PM-1AM	4PM-12AM	4PM-10PM

14:10 FASTING METHOD EXAMPLE

	DAY 1	DAY 2	DAY 3	DAY 4	DAY 5	DAY 6	DAY 7
MID-NIGHT 7AM	Fast	Fast	Fast	Fast	Fast	Fast	Fast
9 AM	FIRST MEAL	FIRST MEAL	FIRST MEAL	FIRST MEAL	FIRST MEAL	FIRST MEAL	FIRST MEAL
4 PM	Last Meal BY 7PM	Last Meal BY 7PM	Last Meal BY 7PM	Last Meal BY 7PM	Last Meal BY 7PM	Last Meal BY 7PM	Last Meal BY 7PM
7PM MID-NIGHT	Fast	Fast	Fast	Fast	Fast	Fast	Fast

16/8 FASTING METHOD EXAMPLE

	DAY 1	DAY 2	DAY 3	DAY 4	DAY 5	DAY 6	DAY 7
MID-NIGHT 7AM	Fast	Fast	Fast	Fast	Fast	Fast	Fast
11 AM	FIRST MEAL	FIRST MEAL	FIRST MEAL	FIRST MEAL	FIRST MEAL	FIRST MEAL	FIRST MEAL
4 PM	Last Meal BY 7PM	Last Meal BY 7PM	Last Meal BY 7PM	Last Meal BY 7PM	Last Meal BY 7PM	Last Meal BY 7PM	Last Meal BY 7PM
7PM MID-NIGHT	Fast	Fast	Fast	Fast	Fast	Fast	Fast

24-HOUR FAST-OMAD- EAT STOP EAT EXAMPLE

DAY 1	DAY 2	DAY 3	DAY 4	DAY 5	DAY 6	DAY 7
Eat Daily Intake*	Fast Day Only One Meal	Eat Daily Intake*	Eat Daily Intake*	Fast Day Only One Meal	Eat Daily Intake*	Eat Daily Intake*

*Follow Daily Body Budget Charts in Chapter 10 on Non-Fasting Days

36-HOUR FAST EXAMPLE

36-Hours	DAY 1	DAY 2	DAY 3	DAY 4	DAY 5	DAY 6	DAY 7
AM	Break-fast	Fast	Break/Fast*	Fast	Break/Fast*	Fast	Break-fast
After-noon	Lunch	Fast	Lunch	Fast	Lunch	Fast	Lunch
PM	Dinner	Fast	Dinner	Fast	Dinner	Fast	Din-ner

Break-Fast 36 hours from your last meal a day and a half prior

5:2 FASTING SCHEDULE EXAMPLE

DAY 1	DAY 2	DAY 3	DAY 4	DAY 5	DAY 6	DAY 7
Eat Daily Intake*	Fast Day 500-600 Calories	Eat Daily Intake*	Eat Daily Intake*	Fast Day 500-600 Calories	Eat Daily Intake*	Eat Daily Intake*

4:3 ALTERNATE DAY FASTING EXAMPLE

DAY 1	DAY 2	DAY 3	DAY 4	DAY 5	DAY 6	DAY 7
Eat Daily Intake*	Fast Day 500-600 Calories	Eat Daily Intake*	Fast Day 500-600 Calories	Eat Daily Intake*	Fast Day 500-600 Calories	Eat Daily Intake*

SPONTANEOUS MEAL SKIPPING EXAMPLE

DAY 1	DAY 2	DAY 3	DAY 4	DAY 5	DAY 6	DAY 7
Breakfast	Skip Meal	Breakfast	Break-fast	Break-fast	Break-fast	Break-fast
Lunch	Lunch	Lunch	Lunch	Lunch	Skip Meal	Lunch
Dinner	Dinner	Dinner	Skip Meal	Dinner	Dinner	Skip Meal

*Follow Daily Body Budget Charts in Chapter 10 for either fasting schedule

WHAT SHOULD YOU DRINK WHILE FASTING?

CLEAN FASTING	DIRTY FASTING	BREAKS-FAST	TIPS
Drink Plenty of Water, Sparkling Water, Carbonated Water, (all non-flavored) Black Coffee, Black, Green and Herbal Tea	Apple Cider Vinegar, Herbal Teas, Essential Oils, Noncaloric Sweeteners* Splash of Fresh Lemon, Lime or Cucumber Cream, Almond Milk (no added sugar-100ml max=39 calories)	Any Food, Bone Broth** Flavored Coffee or Tea, Soda, (regular or diet) Caloric Sweeteners, (sugar, honey) Coconut Oil, MCT Oil, Butter, BCAAs/ Pre-Workout Drinks	Stay hydrated during your fasting time by sipping on your beverages and keep busy to avoid breaking fast too soon, Use meditation, prayer, or workout prior to breaking fast to help, Sparkling, mineral water can help with quieting your stomach and cramping

CLEAN FASTING	DIRTY FASTING	BREAKS-FAST	TIPS
You can add to your drinks: Cinnamon, Nutmeg, Mint, Chia Seeds, Pink Salt or Unsweetened Electrolytes, You can take Vitamins and Medications (if can be taken w/out food)	*Stevia, Monk Fruit, Aspartame, Erythritol (check the labels some brands have glucose and sugar alcohols- avoid the ones that do)	**This along with milk and cream are heavily debated whether it breaks-fast or not-I have used them occasionally and was still able to fast successfully and lose weight	If you are within 15-20 minutes of breaking fast and need to eat or drink something, go ahead-do not become super strict on yourself, listen to your body, if you feel dizzy, or nauseous, eat or drink something, and just reset your fast the next day
Drinks can be cold or hot based on your preference	Gum or Mints but keep to a minimum (sugar-free)	**If you choose to drink any keep calories under 40	Avoid Alcohol, Juices, Sports Drinks, Flavored Waters, Flavored Teas, Sugar

Side Note: Drinking water not only keeps you hydrated but can also boost your metabolism up to 30%, helping you to feel full and eat less calories. Especially when you drink some prior to and during a meal. It also aids in flushing your body of toxins, which can give you clearer skin. As well as helping the body rid excrement (waste), so you are not constipated.

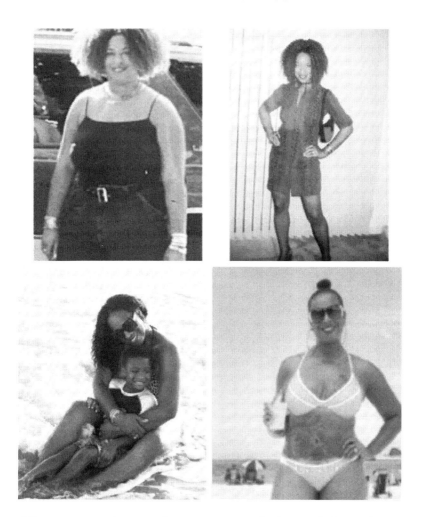

The top two pictures show moments during and then after on my weight loss journey. I have been asked why do, I not have a lot of loose skin all over my body. Especially because I lost so much weight. I do not know which of the Slim Down Level Up Formulas you plan to follow, but I can tell you, fasting helps with aiding in reducing not just belly fat but also the amount of loose skin when losing large amounts of weight. I do have some loose skin. What helped reduce the amount was my age, how long I was carrying the excess weight, and that I incorporated cardio and weightlifting as well as Intermittent Fasting into my routine.

Full Disclosure: In the two pictures at the bottom, after giving birth to my son, and getting all 115 pounds of pregnancy weight off that I had gained, the stomach bib, or I refer to it as my kangaroo pouch in my belly area was not going anywhere. I tried for years. No matter how hard I exercised or changed my diet, it was still there. I did not have the visceral fat, but the extra skin was causing me to have repeated rashes in my skinfolds. So, to feel better and as a reward to myself, I had a tummy tuck. If you want to reduce the amount of skin you may have, adding fasting to your weight loss regimen would be beneficial to you. I am not saying you will not have any loose skin, because you might, but it can help with reducing the amount and help to tighten up the skin all over your body.

18
PREPARING FOR THE HOLIDAYS/ SPECIAL EVENTS

Now that we have talked about the Formulas, making the Weight Loss Food Shift, the 6-Week Programs and Fasting Schedules, let us talk about, what to do, and how to prepare, to be successful for the Holidays and Special Events.

Do you have any special holiday food beliefs? Like the kind that could interfere with you reaching your goal weight? Is losing weight hard when special events come up? It was for me.

While losing weight and adjusting to the *shift,* I needed to address and make a couple more specific changes to my eating behaviors, if I was going to be successful. The time had come, I needed to say goodbye to the two long-standing beliefs that, year after year, was doing nothing except sabotaging my weight loss goals.

For example, besides eating and enjoying different events throughout the year, I used to have a specific seasonal all-you-can-eat food ritual. Every winter, from the week of Thanksgiving all the way through to the New Year, I was allowed to eat whatever I wanted to. **I accepted the yearly fact, it was inevitable, I was going to gain weight. I called it The Winter Spread** (please tell me you know what I am talking about).

I would try to be good, but with holiday cakes, cookies, and tons of food everywhere, like honey baked ham, deep fried turkey, and cheesy corn with bacon, I would wreck my diet. My plan of action would be to worry about fixing it on the backend. You know, the beginning of the year after all my traveling and special events were done.

It was never a good strategy and was not helpful to my weight loss goals. Instead of maintaining whatever weight I had already lost (or in most cases, gained back), I kept increasing the number on my scale. Those choices always made my battle even harder come January with the added weight, I would also have to lose.

So, the first belief to go was, to do away with the mindset of, *I only have a weight problem because the Holidays and Special Events keep throwing me off my diet.* The second was I had to let go of the travel pass I gave myself. It was the pass that convinced me, *calories on vacation really did not count* (seriously, I used to tell myself that). With that belief, I was able to use my all-you-can-eat and drink pass, whenever I wanted.

Those two, main beliefs were what I used to justify my eating and being obese. I believed it was not technically my fault. There were just *too* many holidays, special events and trips that happened. But were there really that many?

Let us take a look at how many of those, all-you-can-eat/drink days there really were, that *caused* me to have a weight problem. The major U.S. Federal Holidays are New Year's Day, the Birthday of Dr. Martin Luther King Jr., Washington's Birthday, Memorial Day, Independence Day, Labor Day, Columbus Day, Veterans Day, Thanksgiving Day, and Christmas Day. All together account for 10 days.

You probably already guessed those were not all the days I was celebrating and excessively eating. So, let us add to that number a couple of birthday parties for each of the twelve months to accommodate for family, friends, and co-workers on their special days. Adding an additional 24 more days to the calculation. Which would bring the number to 34 days so far.

I will also add 6 additional days for the invites to events over the Christmas Holidays, and for the family get-togethers throughout the year. As well as an additional 10 days for other events I would attend. Like fundraisers, Galas, cookouts, happy-hour events, and dinner party invites.

Let us add it all up: 50 days of celebrating and eating more than my share of food and drinks. Enjoying time with family, friends, and indulging in good food.

Does fifty days sound like a lot? In the bigger picture, it is less than 14% of the 365 days in a year. In truth, if I would have made better eating choices on the bulk of the other 315 days, the 50 days I went overboard would have been able to balance itself out.

However, that wasn't what was happening in my world of food choices. In reality, I knew it was in reverse. My eating poorly, was closer to the 315 days mark. All while trying to convince myself by eating healthy 50 days out of the year, it would somehow make up for the bulk of my excessive eating.

The ratio I created could not keep up with the larger percentage of days, I was eating an unhealthy diet. What I could have done, was taken those 50 days of celebrating, and looked at them as my weight loss treat days and enjoyed myself. Then, had I made better choices with my food intake the bulk of the other 315 days, I would have lost or maintained weight. While still being able to have almost one treat day a week throughout the year. Would you like to have the flexibility while losing weight, to be able to use treat days as needed for planned or even last-minute events?

Every year, we know the holidays are going to happen and special events will come up. The best way to be successful is to realize they are just that, *occasions*. They do not happen all the time. They are events we can plan for and enjoy ourselves, guilt free and stress free. Especially during the holidays.

Life is going to happen, and you should enjoy it, even while dieting or in maintenance mode. Being prepared on the days when you go to events, will be key. As, well as, doing away with thinking you messed up, or have fallen off the horse when you indulge at special occasions or events throughout the year. You can go to any event, enjoy the food and feel empowered to have a good time. How?

By being cognizant of your lifestyle habits on the other days, you will be able to create a more balanced nutritional food philosophy and develop a healthier environment, to continue losing and maintaining weight. In essence, you will Dominate Losing Weight!

In the next section, you will see three protocols I used and continue to use when preparing for the holidays, special events, last-minute invites, or weekend getaways. You can follow the steps, accordingly, based on which stage you are in when preparing for each occasion.

Taking the necessary preparations prior to attending an event always made me feel more in control of my eating. It also gave me the ability to enjoy my time with family and friends and not stress about whether, or not I was over my daily body budget numbers. Knowing what to do the day after the event was also key because it reset my body back on track without skipping a beat.

Two of the Protocols are for either 3 days or 7 days preparation for whether you are:

1. Still in the losing weight mode of the program

or,

2. In the weight maintenance mode

Lastly, the, third Protocol provides a few scenarios, to give examples regarding how to prepare for certain occasions.

9 Habits to Develop for Successful Dieting

1. Plan and Meal Prep

2. Take it One Day and One Pound at a Time

3. Prioritize Eating Protein with Each Meal

4. Drink Plenty of Water (aim for a gallon a day)

5. Incorporate "fun" Foods into Your Diet

6. Get Back on Track the Very Next Meal After a Treat Day/Meal

7. Be Kind to Your Mind and Believe in Yourself

8. Aim for Progress Not Perfection

9. Reboot, Transform, Dominate, Lose the Weight

PREPARING FOR THE HOLIDAYS/SPECIAL EVENTS PROTOCOLS

WHILE STILL LOSING WEIGHT

7-Day Pre-Set for the Holidays and Special Events Protocol.

Set yourself up for success for the coming event by Pre-Setting your body ahead of time.

Follow the steps below if you are still in the losing weight stage:

1. 7 Days prior to the event, reduce your daily body budget to 1400 calories, 42-46 fat grams, 20-40 net carbs max (If you are already at or near these numbers based on your current weight, then reduce your intake to a, 1200 calories, 40 fat grams and 20-40 net carbs budget).

2. If you are not already using Intermittent Fasting, then incorporate using the 5:2 Fasting Schedule in those 7 days. If you are already following a fasting schedule, then add in two-OMAD Fast within those 7 days. (You can refer to the Fasting Charts in Chapter 17).

3. For 7 days, no sodas, juices, fried foods, or junk food.

4. Incorporate 3 Meatless Dinners or 3 Liquid Dinners within the 7 days.

5. Increase your activity/exercise to 3-5 days, if you are not already doing so.

6. The day of the event – if it is an evening event – eat a small/medium breakfast (300-350 calories) and have a liquid lunch, if it is a mid-day event – have a liquid breakfast

and a small snack before the event to curve hunger and to not overeat.

7. At the event, use the One Plate/One Trip Rule* and allow yourself one dessert.

8. Enjoy the festivities, the company: no stress on what you are eating.

9. The day after the event or later that evening, use one of your MRE Kits to eat a well-balanced meal and set your body back on track.

10. Remind yourself, your new changes are for life and having fun and enjoying *sometimes* food is allowed.

*One Trip/One Plate Rule is either one trip up to the self-serve buffet or one plate-meal when ordering/dining out.

Important Side Note: In my experience, fasting and liquid meals do not blend well, if you plan on drinking adult-beverages, on the day of the event. You will want to plan accordingly and make sure you have adequate food intake prior to consuming alcohol or wine. This applies to all three protocols.

PREPARING FOR THE HOLIDAYS/SPECIAL EVENTS PROTOCOLS

IN WEIGHT MAINTENANCE MODE

3 Day Pre-Set for the Holidays and Special Events Protocol.

Prepare yourself for the upcoming event by Pre-Setting your body a few days before.

Follow the steps below if you are in the maintenance stage of your weight loss:

1. 3 Days prior to the event, have 1 Liquid Dinner or 1 Meatless Dinner.

2. Keep your daily body budget intake at or under 1300 calories, 40-43 fat grams and 20-50 net carbs (If you are already at or near this number based on your current weight, then

use the 1200 calories, 40 fat grams and 20-40 net carbs budget).

3. Whether you are using Intermittent Fasting or not, you can add (1) OMAD Fast within the 3 days.

4. Increase your activity/exercise daily that week if you are not already doing so.

5. The day of the event, if it is an evening event, eat a light/medium breakfast (300-350 calories) and have a liquid lunch.

6. If it is a mid-day event, have a liquid breakfast and a small snack before the event to curb hunger and to not overeat.

7. At the event, use the One Plate/One Trip Rule* and allow yourself to have one dessert.

8. Enjoy the event, the company, and the festivities; no stress on what the exact calories, etc. you will be eating.

9. The day after the event, use your MRE Kits to eat a well-balanced meal and get right back on track.

10. Remind yourself, your new changes are for life which includes having sometimes food and having fun.

Side Note: If you are in maintenance mode and will be going on vacation for a few days or have multiple events to attend over a span of a few days, you can follow the 7 Day Protocol to prepare your body for the additional events.

PREPARING FOR SAME DAY/NEXT DAY/WEEKEND EVENTS PROTOCOLS

WHILE STILL LOSING WEIGHT OR IN WEIGHT MAINTENANCE MODE

1. Prior to the event, keep your daily body budget intake at or under 1200 calories, 40-43 fat grams and 20 net carbs.

2. Add OMAD Fast prior to the event, if possible or add Spontaneous Meal Skipping the day after the event.

3. Just as with the previous protocol, the day of the event: If it is a mid-day event, have a liquid breakfast and a small lunch/snack before the event to curb hunger and to help you with not overeating. You can even carry a snack with you to the event if need be. If it is an evening event, eat a light/medium breakfast (300-350 calories) and have a liquid lunch.

4. At the event, you would also use the One Plate/One Trip Rule* and allow yourself to have one dessert.

5. Enjoy the event and the festivities and absolutely, no stress on what you will be eating.

6. The day after the event, use your MRE Kits and get right back on track. Remind yourself, your new changes are for life and having fun with family and friends is more than okay.

SCENARIOS

Follow the steps accordingly depending on what time of day it is, when you are asked to attend the event or depending on how many days prior to the event you are asked to attend.

1. While at work, your co-workers or friends invite you out to have dinner and drinks after work (Happy Hour, etc.).

2. Your job is having a potluck at work in 2 days.

3. Family/Friend invites you to dinner or to meet them for lunch tomorrow.

4. Attending a Holiday Party or Cookout.

5. Going to Birthday or Anniversary Parties.

6. Weekend Getaway - you can follow the steps accordingly based on how you plan your "vacation meals". Be sure to enjoy them as well (be cognitive of not overeating and if you do, just reset yourself back once you return home and remember steps #8-10 on the previous page).

NO FAMILY/FRIENDS SUPPORT?

What do you do when your family or friends, do not support you and doubt your success with your new lifestyle changes? Or how do you handle it if they judge your new eating habits and your decision to better your health? You can do what I did. Turn their doubts into your determination and continue making the changes for yourself!

For example, while losing weight, I had family and friends try to get me to give up and go back to my old unhealthy ways. I had people doubting my decisions and talked bad about my eating choices. As though choosing to reduce red meat from my diet and having some meatless meals was a bad thing. I even had "so-called" friends betting against me behind my back to see how long I would keep the weight off. I realized when you take a stance and decide to make healthier eating choices for yourself, it can make others feel bad or awkward about their eating habits and their lifestyles remaining the same. As though your healthier food options make theirs bad. It is the total opposite. **This journey is about you.** Your new choices are not about their current choices. You have decided to make changes for your own reasons, and having their support would be nice, but remind yourself, it is not needed. You can and you will dominate and defeat the weight loss dragon this time. With or without them.

When you are making the *weight loss food shift*, family or friends will sometimes go out of their way to tempt and test your discipline. By offering you food all the time, encouraging you to eat like them. To see if you will backslide. For me, it was so bad that I decided to stop going around some of them for a while. That was until I got stronger in my new food convictions and way of eating.

I know it can be challenging when we decide to make a lifestyle change, but just focus on you and how you are feeling. Block out the noise. At the end of the day, it is your body not theirs. Do this for you.

The sad part is, when you set out to transform your body, not everyone will be happy for you and your new lifestyle change. But just remember why you started in the first place. Try and connect with other like-minded people, support groups and clubs where you can get encouragement and additional tools on being success-ful long-term. Keep believing in your choices, because your future self is so proud of you and is happy about your decision to fight for your health.

Weight Loss Tip: While losing weight, until I was strong enough and could handle the temptations, I did not watch regular TV at night. It was a recipe for disaster when I did because the food commercials were too tempting for me. This is what would happen when I did watch TV at night. I would see a juicy cheeseburger or fried chicken commercial and find myself quickly heading downstairs out the front door on a mission. I would drive to my favorite fast-food restaurant and order my signature *#4 with extra cheese and a coke*. Or find myself standing up in my kitchen cooking something greasy to eat. Being successful on your journey will involve removing as much temptation as possible while you are making the *shift*. That may even require you asking loved ones or friends not to cook or eat in front of you at night. Especially when you are fasting or cutting your, eating time off early.

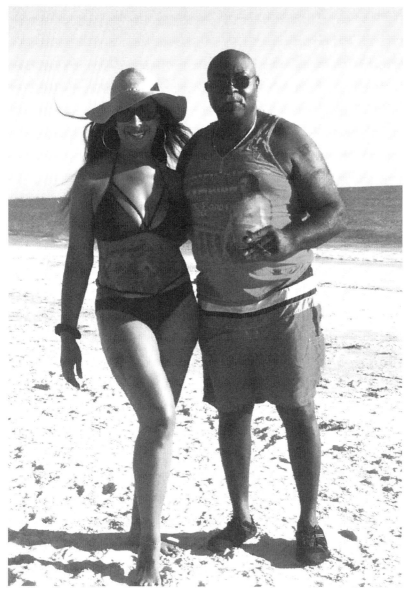

This is a picture of my husband and I on vacation. I was so proud because it was after we both were slimmer and wanted to go to the beach for another getaway. And guess what? We rode on one jet ski together! Winning! Confession: When we got back from our jet ski ride that day, and while we laid on the beach, I ate some chicken wings and had a couple of cocktails. But, unlike the initial jet ski incident, it was not because I was mad, but rather I wanted to enjoy them. I planned for the trip and prepped my body a week prior by following the special events protocol. I had a wonderful time on our trip, I did not completely lose my mind with eating, but I ate a little more than I normally would. So, what I did was just reset my body back when we returned with my MRE's and did not stress about it. Simple, right? **No stress, because stress will never be your friend, planning will be.** Planning for your events is how you can be successful and feel more in control, while on your weight loss journey and in the maintenance stage.

PART EIGHT
YOUR GET
MOVING PLAN

19

WALK, DANCE, HIIT, EXERCISE

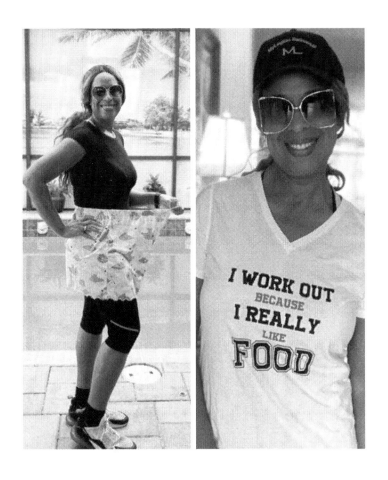

You may have noticed I spent a lot of time in the book on the food part of the program. Going over the different diets and meal kit food options. Cooking at home, eating out and preparing your Weight Loss MRE's. That is because we cannot out-work a poor diet.

As much as I wish it were possible, and as my T-shirt jokingly alludes to, we cannot beat or out-exercise unhealthy eating habits. (Trust me, I tried it doesn't work).

We could talk exercise all day long: which routines are best and how long to do each one. But if the food intake is still out of control, the exercise will not help undo the weight already gained and the excess amount of food continuing to be eaten.

With your eating under control and by incorporating physical activities you enjoy, into your lifestyle, it can be beneficial to your weight loss success and improve your health. Exercising 4-5 days a week is an ideal goal to aim for, especially, while losing weight. In, the next section, there are a variety of walking, running, dancing, jumping, and HIIT (high intensity interval training) examples you can incorporate in *your get moving plan*. First, here are five key steps to take when it comes to losing weight and exercising.

1. FOLLOW AN EXERCISE & EATING PROGRAM

This is highly recommended when first starting out and can lead to you being more successful. Having a set exercise program to follow or scheduled routine to assist your exercise activities, can take the guesswork out of the equation for you. Also, following an eating plan with set parameters regarding the amount of food intake can be helpful. Like using the *6-Week Program* and sticking to the numbers in the Daily Body Budget Charts. As well as, using prepackaged foods from structured diets or meal delivery kits, can be helpful with providing convenience when planning meals. Remember, this time around on your journey is all about convenience and working smarter, not harder, to lose weight.

2. **WALK BEFORE YOU RUN**

You can walk yourself slimmer by realizing the benefits to a brisk walk daily. Walking is an excellent form of exercise and can be the catalyst to jumpstarting your workout routine. Walking at a pace that increases your heart rate and over time adding to the distance and intensity of the walk, can be beneficial in losing more weight. The key is, as you are losing, to add weight back onto your body with leg or arm weights or even a weight vest (they can cost anywhere between $15-$25). This will cause you to work a little harder during your walk and help burn more calories and fat.

3. **INVEST IN A FITNESS TRACKER**

If you can, get a fitness tracker. This is a great way to set a goal and know if you are reaching your desired steps for the day. Fitness Trackers can also keep a record of your heart rate, activities, and speed to see how you are improving while on your weight loss journey (they can cost anywhere between $25-$50). You can also use your phone. That is, if you keep it on you all day and download free tracking apps, to see your daily steps and progress (you can refer to Chapter 13 again for the list of 5 free tracking/fitness Apps).

4. **MODIFIED WORKOUTS CAN BURN CALORIES**

It is okay if you decide to join an exercise class or use a video that is a little more advanced than your current abilities. Because you can go at your own speed and modify the moves to accommodate your current fitness level. It is about moving and getting your heart rate up. As you continue working out and getting stronger, you will be able to add the additional moves or exercises to your routine. The same thing applies to doing modified pushups, jumping jacks, sit ups or squats. When exercising, the key is to listen to your body, and if you need a break while working out, take one. Listening to your body may also mean you need a day off to rest from being active while losing weight.

5. ADD RESISTANCE TRAINING TO YOUR FITNESS ROUTINE

Lifting weights is a great way to build lean muscle and lose weight. Doing multiple reps with light weights can help increase your muscle tone and burn fat. Starting out using 5 or 10-pound dumb bells or a kettle bell is adequate, enough and can do the job. As a bonus workout, you can incorporate doing some of the exercises during the commercials while watching your favorite shows.

SOME KEY BENEFITS TO BEING MORE ACTIVE

*Lifts Mood *Improves Learning Abilities *Builds Self-Esteem *Keeps the Brain Fit

*Keeps the Body Fit & Able *Boosts Mental Health *Boosts Immune System

*Reduces Stress *Creates a Happy Mood *Has Anti-Aging Effects

*Improves Skin Tone and Color *Improves Sleeping Patterns *Helps Prevent Strokes

*Improves Joint Function *Improves Muscle Strength *Alleviates Anxiety

*Sharpens Memory *Helps to Control Addictions *Boosts Productivity

*Boosts Creative Thinking *Improves Body Image *Gives Confidence

*More Focused in Life *Improves Eating Habits *Increases Longevity

*Strengthens Bones *Improves Posture *Lowers Risk of Diabetes

*Prevents Colds *Reduces Knee Pain *Improves Cholesterol Levels

*Lower Risk of (certain) Cancers *Lowers High Blood Pressure

*Fights Dementia *Eases Back Pain *Increase Sports Performance

*Decreases Osteoporosis Risk *Reduces Feelings of Depression

*Reduces Muscle Loss *Increases Energy and Endurance

*Lessens Fatigue *Increases Pain Resistance

*Improves Balance and Coordination *Improves Oxygen Supply to Cells

*Strengthens the Heart *Improves Concentration *Helps with Self-Control

*Makes Life More Exciting *Improves Quality of Life (44)

HIIT EXERCISES

Years ago, I used to be one of those crazed workout people you may have seen in the gym. Doing an hour or more of cardio, hopping between two to three different machines. After my first cardio session, I would go and do 30-45 minutes of weight training and then finish off the last 15 minutes, of my **two-hour workout**, doing additional cardio exercises. Preferably on my favorite cardio machine, the elliptical. Those two-hour workout sessions were able to happen before three significant things took place in my life. 1. Marriage, 2. Children, and 3. Discovering HIIT exercises. The last thing I have nowadays is two hours to commit to a workout between being an entrepreneur, a wife, and a mother.

High-Intensity Interval Training is a great alternative to maximizing your workout time and results. Do not let the name scare you off. It is intense, but for only short bursts of time. Like 30 seconds to a minute of kicked up, sped up, heart pounding activities. For example, instead of doing a 60-minute cardio exercise, like walking or bike riding at a comfortable pace, you could do a 20-30 minute, HIIT rotation. By adding in one-minute power walking, jogging, or sprinting every four-minutes, you could change up the intensity of your workouts. Allowing you to burn up just as much, if not more, calories in the 20-30 minutes, than you would in the 60-minute session timeframe. This is how you can lose weight without spending hours working out. Making your exercises about working smarter not harder. Saving you time and, also increasing your body's oxygen intake by exerting yourself in small bursts.

If you have not done so already, you can find several different HIIT exercises online, some with videos and step-by-step instructions. You can specifically search for them based on which activities you like to do. For instance, HIIT dancing exercises, walking, weightlifting, and targeting specific areas of the body. Like stronger arms, legs or to slim your thighs. YouTube is a good resource to use because you will be able to find videos showing some of the exact moves you can use, in case you are not familiar with them. You can also find HIIT workout ideas on Pinterest.

As previously mentioned, investing in some free weights, if you do not have any already, would be a good idea also. Strength training is a faster way to lose weight and build muscle. You can burn more calories and help to reduce stubborn fat by lifting weights compared to doing cardio alone. They do not have to be heavy weights. I have 5-pound, 10-pound and 15-pound dumbbells. As well as an 8-pound kettle bell that I do several of my weight training exercises with. I also have a fitness mat I use when exercising on the floor. Online, you can find a set of dumbbells at Walmart, Target, or Amazon for about $45.00 or less. Usually, the sets come with 3-pound, 5-pound and 8-pound weights. As well as a stand to hold them when not in use.

If you do not have free weights or prefer not to use them, you can still do some HIIT exercises and take advantage of the interval training. There are a variety of options to choose from that do not involve using weights. Like Jumping Squats, Pushups, Jumping Jacks, Sit Ups, Planks, and using a wall to do chest presses, to name a few. Below is a chart to show the importance of six key factors and how they rank, in your weight loss success. As you will be able to see, going back to my first point in this chapter, we cannot out-work a poor diet. Exercise, adding resistance training, managing stress levels, better sleep, and adequate protein intake, all play major roles in how you will lose weight. However, the daily calorie deficit leads the pack as the powerhouse player behind your overall success.

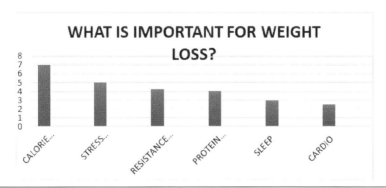

#1 Calorie Deficit #2 Stress Management #3 Resistance Training #4 Protein Intake #5 Sleep #6 Cardio

THE WALK YOURSELF SLIM SCHEDULE

Following this schedule for 3-5 days a week is ideal for weight loss. Starting in week 2, every 4 minutes on your walk, go ahead and power walk for 1 minute at a fast pace, then walk for 4 more minutes and repeat, until "walk for" time is complete. (45) MIN=Minute.

INTERMEDIATE 12-WEEK WALKING/POWER WALKING SCHEDULE

WEEK	WARM-UP	WALK FOR	COOL DOWN	TOTAL TIME
1	5MIN	15MIN	5MIN	25MIN
2	5MIN	20MIN	5MIN	30MIN
3	5MIN	20MIN	5MIN	30MIN
4	5MIN	25MIN	5MIN	35MIN
5	5MIN	25MIN	5MIN	35MIN
6	5MIN	30MIN	5MIN	40MIN
7	5MIN	30MIN	5MIN	40MIN
8	5MIN	35MIN	5MIN	45MIN
9	5MIN	40MIN	5MIN	50MIN
10	5MIN	40MIN	5MIN	50MIN
11	5MIN	45MIN	5MIN	55MIN
12	5MIN	45MIN	5MIN	55MIN

For example, in a 30-minute walk, that would be five one-minute power walking intervals during your workout, not including warmup or cooldown.

Weight Loss Tip: As mentioned earlier, while losing weight, you can intensify your workout routine and build muscle by adding weight back to your body. This can be helpful because the heavier you are, the more calories you burn. You can use ankle weights, arm weights or a body weight vest. If you have problems with your knees or ankles, I recommend you try the body vest option instead. That way, the weight is more distributed throughout the upper part of your body. Adding this technique to your walking exercise routine can help you maximize your weight loss.

While moving through the walking schedule, at any time, if you want to challenge yourself, you can start power walking for longer periods of time. As well as trying a light jog. I used to challenge myself on my walk/runs and power walk or jog between every seventh mailbox. My neighbors probably thought I was crazy, but the weight came off doing that technique.

You can use the walking time interval schedule, from the previous page, for almost any other cardio exercise you choose. Like dancing, swimming, or even bike riding. While losing weight, for example, I used this type of schedule as my *dance trainer* in my living room. I used my stopwatch to set the timers to remind me when to speed up my dancing and when to cool it back down. Prior to starting, I would put on some of my favorite music and would use the warmup time to move around and stretch. Then once the walk time started, I got to dancing like no one was watching. Every four-minutes, I did the one-minute intensified dancing moves to speed up my heartrate. Before bringing it back down during the next four-minute session.

Another example, you can use the flexibility of the schedule to speed up a bike ride, kickboxing or water aerobics for one minute. Then you could go at the normal pace for four minutes before starting again. Your options are endless as to how you can use the schedule.

Are You Burning the Most Calories? A good rule of thumb to know if you are in the desired state of aerobic exercise, to burn more calories is, you should not be in your normal breath. You should definitely not be to where you are going to pass out either. However, if you see your neighbor or are talking on your cellphone, while exercising, and are speaking normally with no change in your breathing, I have something to tell you. You are not working out Sis, you are what is, considered to be *moving*. There is a difference. You have already committed to using the time to be more active, so let us see how to make sure, you are taking advantage of your workout. Your workout gauge of burning calories is where you can say three words without needing a breath. Not out of breath, not normal breath, but being able to talk and say a few words before pausing to inhale is ideal.

For example, you see your neighbor out on your 30-minute walk/power walk. She calls out to you and asks, "How are you doing?" While being able to continue walking or pausing to answer her question, you should be able to say things like this in between taking a breath. "Hi, I'm fine. (breath) 30 minutes today (breath) is my goal (breath). You take care (breath)." By doing the three words to a breath strategy while exercising, whether it be walking, dancing, swimming, or kickboxing, you will know if you are getting the most from your workout. (You can also use a fitness tracker).

In the next section, you will see a series of charts that can be used to help you lose weight.

The first chart is using the HIIT format of interval training. It is an advanced 30-Day, Power Walk/Run Schedule. You can choose to start with this schedule or use the intermediate schedule previously listed and work yourself up to this one after completing the first 4-6 weeks.

The second chart, you can also use as a HIIT style format interval training. You can choose to follow that 30-Day schedule using either skipping, jumping in place, Jump Squats or Jumping Jacks as your cardio. You may also use a combination of them as well. As I said with the Intermediate Chart, you can use the time sequence with any exercise you choose. The key is to follow the intervals and create a situation to where you are aerobic and then kicking it up to intense levels for the specific times.

POWER WALKING/RUNNING 30 DAY ADVANCED PLAN

DAY 1:	DAY 2:	DAY 3:	DAY 4:	DAY 5:
4 MIN WALK	4 MIN WALK	2 MIN WALK	15 MIN WALK	1 MIN WALK
1 MIN RUN	1 MIN RUN	2 MIN RUN		10 SEC SPRINT
3 SETS	4 SETS	2 SETS		5 SETS

DAY 6:	DAY 7:	DAY 8:	DAY 9:	DAY 10:
2 MIN WALK	3 MIN WALK	15 MIN WALK	2 MIN WALK	2 MIN WALK
2 MIN RUN	2 MIN RUN		2 MIN RUN	10 SEC SPRINT
3 SETS	3 SETS		4 SETS	5 SETS
DAY 11:	DAY 12:	DAY 13:	DAY 14:	DAY 15:
5 MIN WALK	15 MIN WALK	2 MIN WALK	2 MIN WALK	2 MIN WALK
2 MIN RUN		3 MIN RUN	2 MIN RUN	20 SEC SPRINT
3 SETS		3 SETS	4 SETS	5 SETS
DAY 16:	DAY 17:	DAY 18:	DAY 19:	DAY 20:
15 MIN WALK	3 MIN WALK	2 MIN WALK	3 MIN WALK	15 MIN WALK
	3 MIN RUN	3 MIN RUN	3 MIN RUN	
	4 SETS	4 SETS	5 SETS	
DAY 21:	DAY 22:	DAY 23:	DAY 24:	DAY 25:
1 MIN WALK	1 MIN WALK	1 MIN WALK	15 MIN WALK	2 MIN WALK
1 MIN RUN	2 MIN RUN	3 MIN RUN		25 SEC SPRINT
5 SETS	3 SETS	3 SETS		5 SETS
DAY 26:	DAY 27:	DAY 28:	DAY 29:	DAY 30:
1 MIN WALK	2 MIN WALK	15 MIN WALK	2 MIN WALK	2 MIN WALK
4 MIN RUN	4 MIN RUN		5 MIN RUN	5 MIN RUN
3 SETS	4 SETS		3 SETS	4 SETS

*MIN=Minute **For the intervals you can do power walking, jogging, running or a combination of them all (46)**

JUMP START YOUR WEIGHT LOSS

DAY 1:	DAY 2:	DAY 3:	DAY 4:	DAY 5:
1 MIN JACKS* 1 MIN REST 3 SETS TOTAL	4 MIN TOTAL 4 SETS	2 MIN JACKS* NON-STOP	1 MIN JACKS* 1 MIN REST 3 SETS IN TOTAL	200 JACKS* ONE WORKOUT
DAY 6:	**DAY 7:**	**DAY 8:**	**DAY 9:**	**DAY 10:**
1 MIN JACKS* 1 MIN REST 3 SETS IN TOTAL	4 MIN TOTAL 4 SETS	2 MIN JACKS* NON-STOP	1 MIN JACKS* 1 MIN REST 3 SETS IN TOTAL	400 JACKS* ONE WORKOUT
DAY 11:	**DAY 12:**	**DAY 13:**	**DAY 14:**	**DAY 15:**
1 MIN JACKS* 1 MIN REST 4 SETS TOTAL	6 MIN TOTAL 6 SETS	3 MIN JACKS* NON-STOP	1 MIN JACKS* 1 MIN REST 4 SETS IN TOTAL	450 JACKS* ONE WORKOUT
DAY 16:	**DAY 17:**	**DAY 18:**	**DAY 19:**	**DAY 20:**
1 MIN JACKS* 1 MIN REST 4 SETS TOTAL	6 MIN TOTAL 6 SETS	3 MIN JACKS* NON-STOP	1 MIN JACKS* 1 MIN REST 4 SETS IN TOTAL	500 JACKS* ONE WORKOUT

DAY 21:	DAY 22:	DAY 23:	DAY 24:	DAY 25:
1 MIN JACKS*	8 MIN TOTAL	4 MIN JACKS*	1 MIN JACKS*	600 JACKS*
1 MIN REST	8 SETS	NON-STOP	1 MIN REST	ONE WORKOUT
4 SETS TOTAL			4 SETS IN TOTAL	
DAY 26:	DAY 27:	DAY 28:	DAY 29:	DAY 30:
1 MIN JACKS*	10 MIN TOTAL	4 MIN JACKS*	1 MIN JACKS*	700 JACKS*
1 MIN REST	10 SETS	NON-STOP	1 MIN REST	ONE WORKOUT
5 SETS TOTAL			5 SETS IN TOTAL	

*For the intervals you can do jumping jacks, jump rope, jump squats, skipping, or a combination of them all. MIN=Minute. (47)

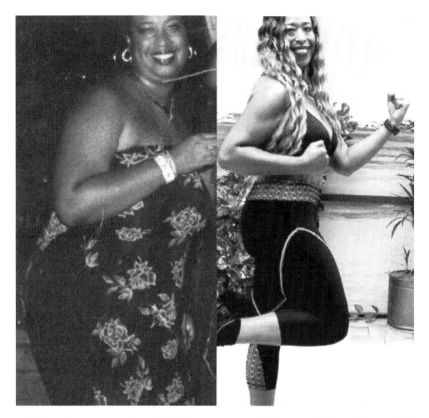

The picture on the left shows me smiling, weighing in at 250 pounds, and at that time I was about 4 months into my weight loss journey. I still had a long way to go, but I was 53 pounds down, and I knew I was on the right track. **You would be amazed with what can happen when you start believing in yourself again.** Don't give up, I believe in you. Now it is your turn to start believing in yourself again. You are unstoppable, resilient, powerful. You are woman and you were made for this!

PART NINE
SLIM DOWN
LEVEL UP QUICK
START GUIDE

20

SLIM DOWN LEVEL UP QUICKSTART GUIDE

B reathe. You made it. The time has come - the moment you have been waiting for.

You have read, and digested, hundreds of pages. Heard testimonies, research, examples and probably by now have gained a new perspective on dieting and losing weight. Hopefully, with the tools provided, you feel more prepared to stand in the ring and dominate losing weight. If so, that means you are ready to start my *6-Week Slim Down Level Up Program.*

To make things go as smoothly as possible, I am going to give you a checklist to get you started and guide you along the way. After, reviewing the checklist, there is a form you can use to fill in some of the information needed, to get you started. Regardless of which of the *Slim Down Level Up Formulas* you start with and whether it is the **Deluxe** or **Advanced** Program, there is a form for each of the six options you can use.

In this chapter, you will find a **2-Week Grocery Shopping List** and a **4-Week 1500 Calorie Meal Plan** provided with various breakfast, lunch, dinner, and snack options you can use as a guide to getting started. Remember you can also refer to Chapter 17 for the other 8-weeks of meal plan examples within the fasting charts.

KEY STEPS TO GETTING STARTED

WHICH FORMULA ARE YOU FOLLOWING?

Based on your food and dieting preferences, and if you have not decided yet, refer to Chapter 16 in making your decision on which of the *Slim Down Level Up Formulas,* you will start with first. If you are starting with a formula that includes fasting, you can refer to Chapter 17 and review the charts again to see which schedule timeframe will work best for you. Modified fasting timeframe examples were provided, and if you are starting with the Deluxe version with the 14:10 Schedule, remember to work on decreasing your fasting timeframe by thirty minutes, every other day until you arrive at the desired 16:8 Schedule.

WHO IS COOKING YOUR FOOD?

Decide on whether you are going to order food from meal delivery kit services, sign up for structured diet programs, cook at home or a combination. Make your grocery shopping list and write down how many days and meals you plan to cook. Have a two-week meal plan in place for how you will eat and who is cooking the food, prior to you starting the program. Also have three backup meals planned for the days when unexpected things come up. Like soups, prepackaged meals and healthier quick meal options available to use. Download calorie and fitness tracker apps if you have not done so already. They can be very helpful for you on your journey. You can refer to Chapter 13 again for the list of free apps and their features. And most importantly, put your MRE Kits together.

Look for meatless meal options to use ahead of time, that way when you get to the part of the program when you will have meatless dinners you will be prepared. Also, look for liquid dinner meal options. Like Smoothies, Slim Fast Shakes, V-8 Juice, etc. and decide whether you are making them or buying them already made.

You can refer to page 204 to see the list of recipes, meatless meal options, smoothies and more. Order any necessary kitchen instruments needed to get started that will make the shift easier and more convenient. Like a Crockpot, Instant-Pot, Air Fryer or Blender.

TRACKING YOUR PROGRESS

Take your, before pictures in a variety of poses, front, back and side views. Write down your measurements and starting weight. After your initial weigh in, do not weigh yourself daily. Only once a week on Wednesdays. You can refer to Chapter 5 again, to see the tips on weighing yourself successfully. Take your weight loss goal and break it up into five stages. For example, if your goal is to lose 90 pounds, that would be five stages with 18 pounds being the goal weight in each stage. After completing each stage and before moving on to the next, be sure you are celebrating your accomplishments and taking time to appreciate how far you have come. By breaking the weight up in stages, it does not make the mountain seem impossible to climb. In a matter of time, with using the formulas, you will look up and be at stage five of your goal. Just remember to celebrate all the wins, big and small, and the NSV's, non-scale victories also.

Be sure to make your weight loss vision board with motivating words, pictures and any images that will inspire you along the way.

YOUR GET MOVING PLAN AND SUPPLIES

Decide on what your get moving plan will be and sign up for any gym memberships and fitness programs. Order or download your workout videos. Gather your fitness gear, shoes, clothes, water bottles, free weights, arm, or leg weights, fitness tracker watch, and any other gear you will need to get started. Decide on what days and times you will exercise and write it down so that you are ready to go in week two of the program. As you are losing weight and your body is getting used to the exercises, you may need to make, adjustments in your routine and increase the time and intensity of your workouts. Remember, when all else fails and you are not sure what to do, you can always go for a nice brisk walk, and as a bonus, add on your arm, or leg weights or your body weight vest to increase the intensity of the walk. Be sure to set up your support team and ask them to check in with you weekly. You can also join weight loss support groups on social media. As well as create a weight loss accountability page on Instagram or Facebook, to track and show your progress. Take it one day at a time and remember, slow and steady wins the race.

WEIGHT LOSS READY CHECKLIST

1. Which Slim Down Level Up Formula are you going to use?

2. If choosing Intermittent Fasting, which schedule, and time-frame will you start with?

3. What is your start date?

4. Take the amount of weight you want to lose and break it into 5 stages

5. Download calorie/fitness tracker apps

6. Using meal kit delivery services and/or ordering food from structured diet plans?

7. Decide on and have a two-week meal plan to start, so you can have an easier time sticking to your daily budget

8. Order or locate any kitchen instruments needed for an easier shift with cooking your meals

9. Build your support team and decide who, how often and on what day they will check in with you (Check in can be once a week on the same day)

10. What is your get moving plan? Exercise? How long and what days and times?

11. Get workout supplies ready for week 2 of the program

12. Have 3 back up meal plan options for busy unexpected days (liquid meal replacements, frozen meals, or soups)

13. Weigh and measure yourself and take pictures (to track the transformation)

14. Make your weight loss vision board

15. Look up 2-3 meatless, low-carb and low-calorie meal options

16. Find non-processed dessert options (see reference list in Chapter 13)

17. Prepare your MRE Kits (for work, school, the homes of family/friends, or for the car, purse, etc.)

18. Look for salty, crunchy, and sweet cravings-healthy options

19. Join local or social media support groups

20. Fill out your starting *6-Week Program* Form (Deluxe or Advanced)

WEIGHT LOSS PLATEAUS PROTOCOLS

Weight loss is not a straight line. After selecting which *Slim Down Level Up Formula* you will start with and confirming your daily body budget numbers, you will begin to lose weight. However, while on your journey, you may experience plateaus along the way to reaching your goal. This is normal, and there are ways to overcome this when they happen.

The first thing to do when you reach a plateau is:

1. Check to see what your daily food intake has been over the last couple of weeks and that you have been sticking to your numbers. You can always confirm with the Daily Body Budget Charts listed in Chapter 10.

2. Be sure you are reducing your daily body budget intake as you are *losing weight*. Stick to the numbers and lower your calories and fat grams based on your new weight. Also make any necessary adjustments to your net carbs intake. For example, if you were more on the liberal side of the chart, try reducing it to the moderate range (20-50 Net Carbs max).

3. Take note of your sugar intake and what you are eating when breaking fast.

4. Check to see if you have been dealing with more stress, which can increase your cortisol levels and cause your metabolism to decrease. You can use relaxation techniques, prayer, and meditation to help.

5. Observe if your sleep patterns have changed and if are you getting enough rest or not. Inadequate sleep can cause a decrease in your metabolism as well.

6. If you are taking any new medications, they can also affect your metabolism and hormones and cause you to plateau.

7. It could be your time of the month, or if you are going through Pre-Menopause or Menopause, these can also have, an effect on your metabolism.

*You can also check with your doctor to see if anything else may be going on that needs attention. As we age, our metabolism and hormones change. Often, our lifestyle and diet will need to accommodate those shifts, in order, for us to continue to lose weight.

If after evaluating all those things, and you still need to make an adjustment, you can try one or more of the **8 Options** listed, to break through your plateau. Remember, on your journey, to be kind to your mind and celebrate all scale and non-scale victories as well. Keep taking it one day and one pound at a time. In a matter of time, you will look up and be at your goal weight.

8 OPTIONS TO OVERCOME WEIGHT LOSS PLATEAUS

OPTION 1:

Add a 5:2 Fasting Schedule with a 16:8 or 18:6 Schedule, keep your calories between 500-600 on the 2 non-consecutive fasting days and the other 5 days follow your Daily Body Budget numbers

OPTION 2:

Add a 4:3 Fasting Schedule to a 16:8 or 18:6 Schedule, keep your calories between 500-600 calories on the 3 fasting days and the other 4 days follow your Daily Body Budget numbers

OPTION 3:

Reduce your carb intake to 20-30 net carbs max

OPTION 4:

Reduce your daily intake to 1200-1300 calories, 40-45 fat grams, and 20-50 net carbs

OPTION 5:

Add 2 OMAD with an 18:6 Fasting Schedule

OPTION 6:

Add (2) 36-Hour Fast with an 18:6 Schedule

OPTION 7:

Add Ketogenic Low-Carb (20 net carbs max) with 3 days of Liquid Dinners

OPTION 8:

Add Ketogenic Low-Carbs (20 net carbs max) with 3 Meatless Dinners

Side Note: Regardless of which option you use, always refer to the Daily Body Budget Charts in Chapter 10, to make sure you are sticking as closely to your numbers as possible, to continue losing weight.

*Lastly, you can also use the:

7 DAY OR 14 DAY WEIGHT LOSS CHALLENGE

*No Burgers *No Chips *No Ice Cream *No Fast Food

*No Chocolate

*No White Bread *No Soda *No Cake or Donuts *No Cookies or Candy

REFERENCE CHARTS FOR TRACKING SHEETS ON GETTING STARTED

STEP 1: PICK A BASE DIET

1. Intermittent Fasting 2. Low-Calorie 3. Keto 4. Vegan

5. Mediterranean 6. Weight Watchers 7. Paleo 8. Jenny Craig

9. South Beach 10. Low-Carb 11. Nutrisystem

STEP 2: PICK A REMIXX DIET

1. Low-Calorie 2. Mediterranean 3. Weight Watchers 4. Paleo

5. Jenny Craig 6. Vegan 7. South Beach 8. Intermittent Fasting

9. Nutrisystem 10. Low-Carb 11. Keto

STEP 3: THE BONUS, EXTRA AND LEVEL UP OPTIONS

*The **Bonus, Extra and Level Up Diets,** can be selected as En-hancers.* They can be combined into and used in conjunction with the **Base** and the **Remixx Diets**:

1. **Meatless Dinner** (3 Days a Week)

2. **Low-Calorie** (Follow Body Budget Charts)

3. **Sugar Free** (2-Week No Added Sugar Challenge)

4. **Liquid Dinner Meal Replacement** (3 Days a week)

5. **Soup Dinner Meal Replacement** (3 Days a week)

6. **Low-Carb** (Reduce carb intake to 40-50 net carbs max)

7. **Platinum Low-Carb** (20-30 net carbs max)

8. **Platinum Low-Calorie** (Reduce to 1200 calories and 40 fat grams)

9. **Fasting Extra** (Add 3 Days of an 18:6 Fast Schedule)

10. **Fasting Extra** (Add 5 Days of an 18:6 Fast Schedule)

11. **Fasting Extra** (Add 1-OMAD 24-Hour Fast)

12. **Fasting Extra** (Add 1-36-Hour Fast)

13. **Fasting Extra** (Add 2-OMAD 24-Hour Fast)

14. **Fasting Extra** (Add 2-36-Hour Fast)

15. **Fasting Extra** (Add a 5:2 Fast Schedule)

16. **Fasting Extra** (Add a 4:3 Fast Schedule)

Slim Down Level Formula #1

Getting Started: 6-Week Deluxe Form

Phase	Time-frame	Base Diet	Remixx	Bonus	Extra
Phase 1: Reboot	Week 1-2	Intermittent Fasting 14:10 Schedule	Low-Calorie*	Low-Carb**	N/A
Phase 2: Transform	Week 3-4	Intermittent Fasting 16:8 Schedule	Low-Calorie*	Liquid Dinner 3 Days a Week	Add 1 Day of 18:6 Fast per Week
Phase 3: Dominate	Week 5-6	Intermittent Fasting 16:8 Schedule	Low-Calorie*	Meatless Dinner 3 Days a Week	Add 3 Days of 18:6 Fast per Week

Intermittent Fasting Schedule Hours: Phase 1_____
Phase 2_____ **Phase 3**_____

Remixx-Low-Calorie Diet:_____

Daily Body Budget Numbers

Calories:_____

Fat Grams:_____

Net Carbs:_____

Meal Delivery Kit/Food Service Sign Ups:_____

Start Date:_____

Slim Down Level Formula #1

Getting Started: 6-Week Advanced Form

Phase	Time-frame	Base Diet	Remixx	Bonus	Extra	Level Up
Phase 1: Reboot	Week 1-2	Inter-mittent Fasting 16:8 Sched-ule	Low-Calorie*	Low-Carbs**	Add 1-OMAD Fast (24-Hour) in Week 2	N/A
Phase 2: Trans-form	Week 3-4	Inter-mittent Fasting 16:8 Sched-ule	Low-Calorie*	No Added Sugar Chal-lenge	Add 3 Days of 18:6 Fast	Add Liquid Dinner 3 Days a Week
Phase 3: Domi-nate	Week 5-6	Inter-mittent Fasting 18:6 Sched-ule	Low-Calorie*	Meat-less Dinner 3 Days a Week	Add 5 Days of 18:6 Fast	Platinum Low-Cal-orie

Intermittent Fasting Schedule Hours: Phase 1＿＿＿＿＿＿＿＿
Phase 2＿＿＿＿＿＿＿Phase 3＿＿＿＿＿＿＿

Remixx-Low-Calorie Diet:＿＿＿＿＿＿＿＿＿＿＿＿＿＿＿

Daily Body Budget Numbers

Calories:＿＿＿＿＿＿＿＿＿＿＿＿＿＿＿＿＿＿＿＿＿＿

Fat Grams:＿＿＿＿＿＿＿＿＿＿＿＿＿＿＿＿＿＿＿＿＿

Net Carbs:＿＿＿＿＿＿＿＿＿＿＿＿＿＿＿＿＿＿＿＿＿

Meal Delivery Kit/Food Service Sign Ups:＿＿＿＿＿＿＿＿

Start Date:＿＿＿＿＿＿＿＿＿＿＿＿＿＿＿＿＿＿＿＿＿

Slim Down Level Up Formula #2

Getting Started: 6-Week Deluxe Form

Phase	Time-frame	Base Diet	Remixx	Bonus	Extra
Phase 1: **Reboot**	Week 1-2	Low-Calorie*	Low-Carb**	N/A	N/A
Phase 2: **Trans-form**	Week 3-4	Low-Calorie*	Low-Carb**	Liquid Dinner 3 Days a Week	No Added Sugar Challenge
Phase 3: **Domi-nate**	Week 5-6	Low-Calorie*	Low-Carb**	Meatless Dinner 3 Days a Week	Platinum Low-Calorie

Optional Intermittent Fasting Schedule Hours: Phase 1_____ Phase 2_____Phase3_____

Remixx-Low-Calorie Diet:_____

Daily Body Budget Numbers

Calories:_____

Fat Grams:_____

Net Carbs:_____

Meal Delivery Kit/Food Service Sign Ups:_____

Start Date:_____

Slim Down Level Up Formula #2

Getting Started: 6-Week Advanced Form

Phase	Time-frame	Base Diet	Re-mixx	Bonus	Extra	Level Up
Phase 1: Reboot	Week 1-2	Low-Calorie*	Low-Carb**	Meatless Dinner 3 Days a Week	N/A	N/A
Phase 2: Trans-form	Week 3-4	Low-Calorie*	Low-Carb**	No Add-ed Sugar Challenge	Add Liquid Dinner 3 Days a Week	Keto-genic Low-Carbs
Phase 3: Domi-nate	Week 5-6	Low-Calorie*	Low-Carb**	Meatless Dinner 3 Days a Week	Platinum Low-Cal-orie	Add 5:2 Fasting Sched-ule

Optional Intermittent Fasting Schedule Hours: Phase 1_____Phase2_____Phase3_____

Remixx-Low-Calorie Diet:_____

Daily Body Budget Numbers

Calories:_____

Fat Grams:_____

Net Carbs:_____

Meal Delivery Kit/Food Service Sign Ups:_____

Start Date:_____

SLIM DOWN LEVEL UP

Slim Down Level Up Formula #3

Getting Started: 6-Week Deluxe Form

Phase	Time-frame	Base Diet	Remixx	Bonus	Extra	Level Up
Phase 1: **Reboot**	Week 1-2	KETO	Low-Calorie*	Inter-mittent Fasting 14:10 Sched-ule	N/A	N/A
Phase 2: **Trans-form**	Week 3-4	KETO	Low-Calorie*	Inter-mittent Fasting 16:8 Sched-ule	Add 1-OMAD Fast (24-Hour) in Week 4	Add Liquid Dinner 3 Days
Phase 3: **Domi-nate**	Week 5-6	KETO	Low-Calorie*	Meat-less Dinner 3 Days a Week	Add 3 Days of 18:6 Fast	Platinum Low-Calorie

Intermittent Fasting Schedule Hours: Phase 1_____

Phase 2_____Phase 3_____

Remixx-Low-Calorie Diet:_____

Daily Body Budget Numbers

Calories:_____

Fat Grams:_____

Net Carbs:_____

Meal Delivery Kit/Food Service Sign Ups:_____

Start Date:_____

Slim Down Level Up Formula #3

Getting Started: 6-Week Advanced Form

Phase	Time-frame	Base Diet	Remixx	Bonus	Extra	Level Up
Phase 1: **Reboot**	Week 1-2	KETO	Low-Calorie*	Inter-mittent Fasting 16:8 Schedule	Add 1-OMAD Fast (24-Hour) in Week 2	N/A
Phase 2: **Trans-form**	Week 3-4	KETO	Low-Calorie*	Inter-mittent Fasting 16:8 Schedule	Add 3 Days of 18:6 Fast	Add Liquid Dinner 3 Days
Phase 3: **Domi-nate**	Week 5-6	KETO	Low-Calorie*	Inter-mittent Fasting 18:6 Schedule	Meatless Dinner 3 Days a Week	Add 5 Days of 18:6 Fast

Intermittent Fasting Schedule Hours: Phase 1_____
Phase 2_____ Phase 3_____

Remixx-Low-Calorie Diet:_____

Daily Body Budget Numbers

Calories:_____

Fat Grams:_____

Net Carbs:_____

Meal Delivery Kit/Food Service Sign Ups:_____

Start Date:_____

4-WEEK JUMPSTART 1500 CALORIE MEAL PLAN

MONDAY:

Breakfast: 2 Eggs and Steamed Spinach

Lunch: Garlic and Ginger Tofu with Broccoli

Dinner: Steak, Pasta and Vegetables

Snack: Raspberries and Almonds

TUESDAY:

Breakfast: Mango/Green Smoothie

Lunch: Grilled Chicken and Sliced Avocado

Dinner: Salmon and Cauliflower Rice and Steamed Vegetables

Snack: Grapes/Air Popped Popcorn

WEDNESDAY:

Breakfast: Vegetable Omelet

Lunch: Tacos

Dinner: Chicken Lettuce Wraps

Snack: Granola Bar/Sliced Apples

THURSDAY:

Breakfast: Breakfast Burrito

Lunch: Smoothie

Dinner: Steak and Sweet Potato

Snack: Tomato and Basil with Salad Dressing

FRIDAY:

Breakfast: Strawberry Protein Smoothie

Lunch: Half a Sandwich and Cup of Soup

Dinner: Honey Sriracha Meatballs with Cauliflower Rice

Snack: Baked Asparagus Fries and Chipotle Dip

SATURDAY:

Breakfast: Scrambled Eggs & Bacon

Lunch: Avocado Tomato, Turkey Wrap

Dinner: Caprese Grilled Cheese Sandwich

Snack: Trail Mix and Honeydew

SUNDAY:

Breakfast: Sausage and Zucchini Frittata

Lunch: Smoothie

Dinner: Chicken Blueberries Arugula Salad

Snack: Hummus and Carrots

MONDAY:

Breakfast: Banana Oatmeal Pancakes

Lunch: Cheeseburger and Oven Baked Zucchini Chips

Dinner: Smoothie

Snack: Pretzels and Cheese Wheel

TUESDAY:

Breakfast: Blueberry Smoothie

Lunch: Roasted Chicken Breast with Pasta and Vegetables

Dinner: Bowl of Soup

Snack: 1 Orange and Handful of Nuts

WEDNESDAY:

Breakfast: Greek Yogurt and Cereal Parfait

Lunch: Smoothie

Dinner: Vegetable and Tofu Stir-Fry

Snack: Mini Banana Pudding

THURSDAY:

Breakfast: Smoked Salmon Crepes

Lunch: Spinach Salad with Hard Boiled Eggs and Avocado

Dinner: Half of a Sandwich and a Cup of Soup

Snack: Fresh Fruit

FRIDAY:

Breakfast: Overnight Oats

Lunch: Spinach Avocado Quesadilla

Dinner: Tuna Pasta Salad

Snack: Celery Stalks with Peanut Butter

SATURDAY:

Breakfast: Smoothie

Lunch: Baked Ziti

Dinner: Shrimp with Steamed Vegetables

Snack: LARABAR

SUNDAY:

Breakfast: Waffles with Fruit

Lunch: Bacon Lettuce Tomato Wrap

Dinner: Chicken with Rice and Beans

Snack: Cucumber Slices with Guacamole Dip

MONDAY:

Breakfast: Oatmeal and a Banana

Lunch: Grilled Chicken Salad

Dinner: Smoothie

Snack: Apple Slices with Peanut Butter

TUESDAY:

Breakfast: Granola Cereal with Soy Milk

Lunch: Turkey Sandwich

Dinner: Veggie Stir Fry with Tofu and Cauliflower Rice

Snack: Mixed Fruit

WEDNESDAY:

Breakfast: Eggs and Bacon

Lunch: Smoothie and Granola Bar

Dinner: Steak Peppercorn with Carrots and Green Beans

Snack: Mini Pretzels and String of Cheese

THURSDAY:

Breakfast: Cinnamon Pancakes

Lunch: Sicilian-Style Chicken Parm with Broccoli

Dinner: Sausage Baked Penne with Zucchini Spinach

Snack: Greek Yogurt with Mixed Berries

FRIDAY:

Breakfast: Peach/Pineapple Smoothie

Lunch: Soup and a Sandwich Wrap

Dinner: White Bean Turkey Chili with Cilantro-Lime Rice

Snack: Sherbet Ice Cream

SATURDAY:

Breakfast: Sliced Tomato, Spinach and Cheese McMuffin

Lunch: Grilled Salmon with Asparagus

Dinner: One-Pot Chicken and Spanish Rice

Snack: Protein Bar and Banana

SUNDAY:

Breakfast: Eggs and Turkey Sausage

Lunch: Smoothie

Dinner: Gingered Steak Stir-Fry with Steamed Vegetables

Snack: Hummus with Celery

MONDAY:

Breakfast: Turkey Bacon and Scrambled Eggs

Lunch: Tuna Salad on wheat or low-carb bread

Dinner: Grilled Beef with Vegetable Stir-Fry

Snack: Carrots with Mozzarella Cheese

TUESDAY:

Breakfast: Oatmeal with a Banana

Lunch: Grilled Chicken Salad

Dinner: Cauliflower Rice and Sauteed Shrimp with Broccoli

Snack: Apple Slices with Peanut Butter

WEDNESDAY:

Breakfast: Strawberry, Berries, Banana Smoothie

Lunch: Chicken Sausage low-carb Pita with Grilled Mushrooms

Dinner: Lemon Butter Grilled Tilapia, Zucchini and Brown Rice

Snack: Mixed Fruit

THURSDAY:

Breakfast: Pancakes and Turkey Bacon

Lunch: Roast Beef with Provolone Sandwich

Dinner: Steak with Cauliflower Rice and Black Beans

Snack: Celery with Peanut Butter

FRIDAY:

Breakfast: Peach Banana Smoothie

Lunch: Bacon, Lettuce, Tomato Wrap

Dinner: Honey Dijon Mustard Grilled Chicken Breast, Brown-Rice and Vegetable Medley

Snack: An Orange with Dried Cranberries

SATURDAY:

Breakfast: Greek Yogurt with Berries and Granola

Lunch: Soup with a piece of Grilled Salmon

Dinner: Turkey Stuffed Bell Peppers and Pasta

Snack: Sliced Avocado and Tomatoes

SUNDAY:

Breakfast: Sausage and Hard-Boiled Eggs

Lunch: Pork Tenderloin with Grilled Vegetables and Brown Rice

Dinner: Sesame Tofu Wrap

Snack: Banana

*Portion sizes will vary based on the brand of the foods you choose to use and your daily body budget. You can adjust portion sizes and swap out menu items to accommodate your daily intake allowance.

2 WEEK GROCERY SHOPPING IDEAS

Week 1:

* Produce (Fresh)

Avocados, Bananas, Bell Peppers, Banana Peppers, Berries, Broccoli, Cauliflower, Tomatoes, Fresh Cilantro, Kale, Lime, Mushrooms, White or Yellow Onions, Potatoes, Spinach, Sweet Potatoes

* Produce (Frozen or Canned)

Corn, Broccoli, Squash, Green Beans, Vegetable Medley, Strawberries, Blueberries, Pears

* Grains

Bread (whole grain), Brown Rice, Oats, Pasta (whole grain, or low-carb) Pitas (whole grain, or low-carb), Tortillas (whole grain, or low-carb)

* Meat & Protein

Bacon (Pork or Turkey), Lean Beef, Red Beans, Breakfast Sausage, Chicken Breast, Chicken Sausage, Eggs, Shrimp (frozen and ready to eat), Soy Meatballs, Tuna, (packaged in water)

* Dairy

Cheddar Shredded Cheese, Reduce Fat-Cream Cheese, Plain-Greek Yogurt, Mozzarella Cheese, Parmesan Cheese, Swiss Cheese, or American Cheese, Veggie Cheese

* Pantry Items

Almonds, Baking Powder, Low-Sodium Vegetable Broth, Butter, Chili (in a can), Dijon Mustard, Granola, Herbs (Dried Thyme, Sage, or Rosemary), Honey, Marinara Sauce, Olive Oil (Extra Virgin), Salsa, Taco Seasoning, Vanilla Extract

Week 2:

* Produce (Fresh)

Basil, Bananas, Strawberries, Berries, Lemons, Cilantro, Kale, Mixed Greens, Apples, Red Onions, Celery, Oranges, Mushrooms, Parsley, Salad (in a bag), Rosemary

* Produce (Frozen or Canned)

Cauliflower, Spinach, Carrots, Zucchini, Green Beans, Vegetable Medley, Strawberries, Blueberries, Peaches,

* Grains

Bread (whole grain), Brown Rice, Crackers (whole grain), Frozen Waffles (whole grain) Ravioli, Frozen Pasta (whole grain), Rolls (whole grain) Tortillas (corn, 6 inches), Tortillas (whole grain, 8 inches), Cauliflower Rice

* Meat & Protein

Black Beans, Chicken Breast (cooked), Eggs, Pork Tenderloin, Deli-Style Roast Beef, Salmon, (fresh or canned), Sausage, Chicken, (ready to eat), Steak, Tilapia, Deli-Style Turkey, Tofu, Turkey Bacon, Shrimp

* Dairy

Cheddar Cheese, Feta Cheese, Greek Yogurt, (plain), Milk, Mozzarella Cheese, Provolone Cheese

* Pantry Items

BBQ Sauce, Soup, Chipotle Peppers, (canned in adobo sauce), Dried Cranberries, Maple Syrup, Marinara Sauce, Olive Oil, (Extra Virgin), Orange Marmalade, Pancake Mix, Cashews, Peanut Butter, Red Wine Vinegar, Salsa

*The 4-Week Meal Plan and the 2-Week Grocery Shopping Ideas are a starting point for you to choose from when deciding what to eat for breakfast, lunch, and dinner (skip breakfast if you are fasting). The snack options are there, for if and when you need them. Based on whether, or not you will be cooking, ordering food from the meal delivery kit services, eating out or using the food from structured diet programs, your menu will change. Pick the types of food you will enjoy and that will allow you to spend your daily body budget wisely. You can always refer to Chapter 12-13 again for the four key steps to making the *weight loss food shift* more convenient for you and for additional food ideas and recipes.

SMOOTHIES

In the next section is a list of smoothie recipes you can use for your liquid meals. They can come in handy on the days when you decide to incorporate a liquid dinner into your weight loss plan. As, well as, there are a few listed that can be used as a detox for the times when you want to cleanse your body.

Low-Carb Smoothie Ideas: Add Ingredients, Blend and Enjoy!

1. **Blackberry:** ½ Cup of Low-Carb Milk, ¾ Cup Blackberries, 2 Tablespoons Peanut Butter, 1 Scoop Low-Carb Protein Powder, 1 Cup Ice

2. **Raspberry:** ¾ Cup Raspberries, Juice from 1 Lemon, 1 Scoop Vanilla Protein Powder, 1 Cup Low-Carb Milk, ¾ Cup Ice

3. **Chocolate:** 1 Scoop Chocolate Protein Powder, ½ Avocado, 2 Cups Low-Carb Milk, 1 Cup Ice

4. **Green:** ½ Avocado, 1Cup Spinach, 1 Scoop Vanilla Protein Powder, ½ Cup Low-Carb Milk, 5-6 Mint Leaves

5. **Strawberry:** ¾ Cup Strawberries, 1 Cup Greek Yogurt, 1 Cup Low-Carb Milk, 2-3 Mint Leaves, ¾ Cup Ice

Weight Loss Cleanse Smoothie Ideas: Add Ingredients, Blend and Enjoy!

1. **Raspberry:** 1 Cup Frozen Raspberries, ½ Cup Frozen Mango, ½ Cup Frozen Pineapple, 1 Cup Coconut Milk, ¾ Cup Ice

2. **Pina Colada:** 1 Cup Pineapple, 1 Banana, 1 Cup Coconut Milk, 1 tbsp. Shredded Coconut, ¾ Cup Ice

3. **Green Lemon:** 1 Cup Spinach, 1 Cup Frozen Mango, 1 Banana, Juice from 1 Lemon, ¾ Cup Ice

4. **Banana/Peanut Butter:** 1 Cup Frozen Strawberries, 1 Banana, ¼ Cup Peanut Butter, 1 Cup of Milk, ¾ Cup Ice

5. **Mango:** ½ Cup of Frozen Mango, ½ Banana, ½ tbsp Cinnamon, ½ tbsp Turmeric, 1 tbsp Honey, ½ tbsp Ginger, 1 tbsp Chia Seeds, 1 Cup Almond Milk, ¾ Cup Ice

*You can use fresh or frozen fruits and vegetables

LAST WORDS ON GETTING STARTED

My best advice is to start by starting...

I will be totally honest, as I have been throughout the book. Getting started can be challenging, and you will have some tough days. I had several hard days. I lost my motivation and was tempted by family and friends to quit. I fell off my diet a few times. Beat myself up and resorted back to what was comfortable, food, and would give up. Then I remembered those faithful words my grandmother used to say, "Never give up because falling down is not failing."

Please hear me clearly: **IT IS OKAY TO START AGAIN**. Down does not mean out. You can hit the reset button and decide to stand up and fight again. Keep these four key points in mind when you do.

First: Remember to create that weight loss vision board we talked about. The power of visualization is amazing! No one stumbles into success. You must approach this time like a well-executed plan. Start with the end in mind. For your board, cut out and add the things that will make you feel good. Put pictures of yourself at your ideal weight or pictures of you smiling and happy. Make sure you add some positive words and read them to yourself daily, out loud! It is so important to see yourself already at the finish line.

Second: Whatever your weight loss goal is, remember to break it up into five stages. So, the whole number does not look or feel overwhelming. Or you can decide not to set a number at all, but rather a timeframe, to see how much you will lose over a set period of time. Celebrate all wins, big and small.

Third: My all-time favorite and a key step on your journey, be sure to put together your "Weight Loss MRE Kits." These will come in handy. Most of the time we "backslide" is because when we do turn to food, we do not have great choices in our homes or with us when we are out and about. As, we discussed earlier, the grocery store has tons of good snack options for you to choose from. And, of course, you can include fruits and vegetables. You can refer to Chapter 10 for snacks, fruit, and vegetable ideas. Stock your pantry with snacks that are delicious and nutritious for you. I recommend "pre-measuring" out each snack ahead of time and put them in containers or Ziplock bags, so you are not eating the whole package or box (like I used to do).

Fourth: Forgive yourself for the weight gain. It does not matter how or why you got to this size. It does not matter if you fell down seven times, as long as you decide to stand up eight! Decide that this time, will be different because you will silence the internal self-sabotaging thoughts, love your curves just as they are and start walking in the direction of getting healthy. I know, when you are ready, you got this! I have learned so much over the years with weight loss, and one thing I know for sure is, making it up in your mind first can be the hardest part to getting started. Remember to start by starting, Sis! I believe in you. Take it one meal, one day and one pound at a time. And lastly, always take it easy on yourself and be kind to your mind.

WOULD YOU DO ME A FAVOR

Thank you for reading *Slim Down Level Up* and hearing my story. I hope you gained some valuable information and tools you can use on your weight loss journey.

I have a small favor to ask, would you take a moment and write a review on Amazon or Barnes & Noble about this book? I check all my reviews and look forward to hearing honest feedback. Knowing that the information you learned from reading this book will have a positive impact on your weight loss journey, will be the most rewarding thing to hear.

To leave a review, you can:

1. Go to Amazon's or Barnes & Noble's website and search "Slim Down Level Up"

2. Click on the book and scroll down to where it says, "Write a customer review."

Thanks again, and I look forward to reading your feedback!

Visit

www.mylittabutler.com

for additional tips and tools, blog posts, Transformation Success Stories, and more.

I am looking forward to seeing you and hearing how your journey is going in my Facebook weight loss support group: ***Slim Down Level Up.***

9 LITTLE THINGS THAT MAKE A BIG DIFFERENCE

1. **Drink 16-20 ounces of water** every time you eat something. This helps with digestion and can help you feel full.

2. **Do not overeat and slow down when eating**. By slowing down at mealtime, you are less likely to overeat, because the feeling of full (satiety) does not happen until about 20 minutes after the first bite. Try putting your utensil down after each bite and do not pick it back up until you have completely, finished chewing.

3. **Aim for 8,000-10, 000 steps** a day. Try and burn as many, calories during the day through energy expenditure by being more active.

4. **Add 2-3 extra minutes** of exercise bi-weekly to your routine. As your heart, and lungs become more conditioned, you will be able to push yourself longer.

5. **Cut your eating time off 2-3 hours before bedtime**. This will help with reducing late night snacking. (for non-fasters)

6. **Change up your exercise routine monthly**. When you add little changes to your exercise routine, you can increase your weight loss success and fitness goals.

7. **Walk around when talking on the phone, instead of sitting down**. This can help you reach your 10,000 steps a day.

8. **Avoid watching regular TV at night with food commercials**. Doing this and not scrolling through social media, can help you avoid seeing food images, that can cause you to want to eat outside of your normal timeframe.

9. **Reward yourself with things other than food**. It is a common thing to want to celebrate using food. Try and make it a habit to incorporate some form of physical activity in your rewarding process.

THE BONUS MATERIAL DIETS

Yay! Four more eating style options you will have a choice in selecting to use on your journey. They are, Jenny Craig, Nutrisystem, South Beach, and Paleo Diets. Keep in mind, the first three are structured diet options that you do not necessarily have to join to utilize the food and recipes from their programs. You may have used some of them in the past. But, now it is about looking at them differently and seeing how you can use them, as one of your *Remixx Diets.*

A useful benefit from looking at structured diet programs is, you can find a lot of good recipes and food ideas you can use to stay within your daily body budget numbers. Several food ideas can be found on Google, Pinterest or you can order cookbooks that can provide the benefits of the lower-calorie, lower-fat and lower-carb options, they offer. You can enjoy some of the prepackaged food options, without the commitment and cost of joining.

However, I recommend structured programs if you would like a little more guidance and added support while losing weight. They can be a great tool while on your weight loss journey and can also be utilized as a *reset* button. While losing weight, if you are having trouble with meal prepping and measuring your food portions or hit a plateau, you can use the meals from programs like these to get your food intake back on track.

Side Note: The prepackaged food in some of the programs have changed a lot over the past couple of years, aiming at providing better nutritious and delicious options while you are losing weight. As, stated earlier in the book, these are available if, and when you need them and are not required to use any of the *Slim Down Level Up Formulas.*

JENNY CRAIG DIET

WHAT IS THE DIET?

The Jenny Craig Diet is the first on our list of the Bonus Material Diets you can utilize to help you lose weight. They provide prepackaged meals and recipes and put an emphasis on healthy eating and being active. The concept behind wanting to start Jenny Craig came from its founder, Jenny Craig, and started back in the early 1980's. Mrs. Craig, after the birth of her first, child, found herself without the needed support or tools to lose weight. After figuring it out on her own, she was able to take the weight off and started working in a gym. She took her passion for fitness and health and opened her first Jenny Craig Weight Loss Center in 1983. Since then, they have been providing weight loss services, premeasured, prepackaged meals, support, and recipes to their members.

According to their website, they are an evidence-based program designed by Registered Dieticians. Built on the beliefs successful weight loss happens when you develop a healthy relationship with food.

After joining their program, members are personally guided through what their day-to-day weight loss plan will look like. Jenny Craig's main focus is, to provide you with motivation and support needed to lose weight. They also work on teaching members about what a balanced meal looks like and how to use that knowledge to achieve weight maintenance. Your caloric intake budget will typically be anywhere between 1200 to 2300 calories a day. The calculation comes from your current weight, age, gender, and height. As well as your goal weight and fitness habits.

CAN IT HELP YOU LOSE WEIGHT?

By design, the program reduces your overall caloric intake, creating the calorie deficit needed. If you follow their program of eating three of their prepackaged meals and two snacks a day, you can expect to lose up to two pounds a week. They offer four different programs you can use: Rapid Results, Simple Meal Plan, Essential Meal Plan and Jenny Craig for Type 2, for members with diabetes.

The menu options include lower carb choices to help with lowering insulin levels.

IS A JENNY CRAIG DIET EASY TO FOLLOW?

When joining Jenny Craig, you will receive a personalized meal and exercise plan. They will also provide you with weekly one-on-one counseling sessions with a Jenny Craig consultant. You can use the diet for as long as you need to. Some people stick with the program anywhere from three months to two years. When you are at the halfway point of being at your goal weight, your consultant will begin the process of helping you transition to cooking some meals on your own. Specifically using some of the Jenny Craig Diet recipes and other low-fat, low-calorie food strategies, that can be helpful to you in the maintenance stage.

Once you reach your goal weight, your consultant will work with you on prevention strategies of ways to not regain the weight back. Over a four-week period, the goal is for you to transition back to eating a slightly higher number in calories, but with exercise, stress management, and understanding the importance of reading food labels.

Another benefit to being a Jenny Craig member is your consultant will help you plan for social events, holidays and eating out. They offer members the *Jenny Craig Friendly* menus that can help during the holidays. They also provide the *Maintenance Manual* and *Weight Loss Journey Guide* with additional dining-out tips and strategies.

COST AND FOOD OPTIONS?

Jenny Craig has a variety of plan options on their website. They have their Essential Plan for as low as $3.00 a meal, which equates to about $140.00 for the week.

Their seven-day plans include breakfast, lunch, dinner, and snacks for each day. They have other plans that offer more features and more options, at Jennycraig.com. Check for specials before joining.

WHAT ARE EXAMPLES OF JENNY CRAIG FOODS?

Here are a Few Examples of Eating on the Jenny Craig Diet

Chocolate Muffin	Cinnamon Rolls
Egg, Cheese and Turkey Sausage Burrito	S'mores Bar
Ham and Swiss Baguette	Blueberry Pancakes and Sausage
Homestyle Meatloaf and Vegetables	Chicken Cranberry Salad
Vanilla Buttercream Cake	Apple Crisp

Here is an Example of Eating a Jenny Craig Meal

Breakfast: Morning Frittata Sandwich
Lunch: Chicken Carbonara
Dinner: Classic Lasagna with Meat Sauce
Snacks: 1st Lemon Cake 2nd 12 Baby Carrots

SOUTH BEACH DIET
WHAT IS THE DIET?

The South Beach Diet is another option of the structured diet programs you can decide to use while losing weight. The diet consists of food like, non-starchy vegetables, eggs, fish, and full-fat dairy products. It also includes proteins like nuts whole grains, chicken, and turkey. In order, to get the most of out the diet, you will eliminate eating trans fats and omega-3 vegetable oils. However, omega-3 fatty acids from fish are acceptable. As well as olive and avocado oil and plant-based sources like coconut.

The South Beach Diet does not completely, eliminate all carbs, but you will reduce processed, refined, sugary foods from your diet. Like, white bread, candy, soda, and ice cream. The diet offers meals that are higher in protein, which helps with making you feel fuller longer.

They have three levels in their program, Phase 1, 2 and 3. More recently, they have added their *South Beach Keto-Friendly* diet options. With an emphasis on losing weight by reducing your carb intake.

CAN IT HELP YOU LOSE WEIGHT?

Like most other structured programs, the South Beach Diet is designed to help you eliminate a lot of processed refined foods, reduce your carb intake, and lower your daily food intake. The diet can work with helping you lose weight by creating the desired calorie deficit needed each day. According to their website, by following the program's three levels, you can lose between eight to thirteen pounds in the first 14 days because you would reduce your carbs and calories drastically. In Phase 2, you can expect to level off and lose one to two pounds a week. Phase 3 is about maintenance and remembering to not overindulge to keep your body at the desired weight.

IS A SOUTH BEACH DIET EASY TO FOLLOW?

By following the South Beach Diet, you will eat three meals and three snacks daily. However, the program does allow for some flexibility, and you can choose to have three larger meals instead of having the three snacks. Like a Low-Carb Diet, your intake will be at or below 50 net carbs in Phase 1 of their program. Phase 2 allows for a little more carb leg room as you transition up to 75-100 net carbs daily. The goal of the program is to provide premeasured prepackaged meals, support, and recipes to help you with reaching your weight loss goals. They offer meal delivery services with a variety of menu items to choose from. To help you with learning to cook and eat healthier meals twice a week, you are encouraged to plan your own meals at home or eating out. The program offers a user-friendly website to order from and has an app for online members to use for tracking their meals, weight, and diet goals. They offer support via online, email or over the phone as well.

COST AND FOOD OPTIONS?

The South Beach Diet has a variety of plans available to choose from. Their Silver Plan costs about $10.00 a day and includes three meals and three snacks for one-month. The cost is roughly $300.00

for the first month. They have other plan options on their website, at Southbeach.com. Check for specials before ordering. If you are looking for a less expensive way to start using the South Beach Diet program, Walmart sells their seven-day ready-to-go meal kits for about $89.00. Which includes 7 Breakfast meals and 14 Entrées.

WHAT ARE EXAMPLES OF THE SOUTH BEACH DIET?

Here Are Some South Beach Diet Staples

*Lean Beef *Almonds *Pork *Lamb *Black Beans
*Fish *Hummus *Shellfish *Turkey Bacon *Lentils
*Skinless Chicken Breast *Eggs *Low-Fat Hard Cheese *Walnuts
*Greek Yogurt *Soy-Milk *Turkey Breast *Pinto Beans *Avocado

Here is an Example of Eating on a South Beach Diet

Breakfast: Canadian Style Turkey Bacon, Egg & Cheese Muffin
Lunch: Just in Thyme Beef Soup
Dinner: Spicy Chicken & Riced Cauliflower
Snacks: 1st Dark Chocolate Nut Bar 2nd Peanut Butter Cookie Bites 3rd Nacho Puffs

NUTRISYSTEM DIET
WHAT IS THE DIET?

Nutrisystem is the final structured Bonus Material Diet we will go over that you can use to lose weight. They offer their members several different plans to choose from with a variety of breakfast, lunch, dinner, and snack options. Their focus is on providing well balanced nutritional meals in an easy and convenient way and to take the guesswork out of meal prep for you. They have three meal plan options to choose from, all of which include the food and snacks for their 4-Week Meal Plan. Depending on how many meal options, food selections and snacks you would like, you can choose between the Nutrisystem Basic, Uniquely Yours or Uniquely Yours Ultimate.

The first week of the plan you will be provided seven full days of meals and probiotic shakes. Weeks two through four are a combination of Nutrisystem food and snacks and a few recommended grocery store items. Each day consists of three meals and a snack. Depending on your food preferences and eating habits, they offer a new option called Mix and Match Plan. You can customize your order based on how frequently you eat either breakfast, lunch, or dinner. They also offer Nutrisystem D for those living with Type 2 diabetes or who are pre-diabetic.

CAN IT HELP YOU LOSE WEIGHT?

Yes, the Nutrisystem Diet can help you lose weight because the reduction in calories and fat grams will create the desired calorie deficit needed. They put an emphasis on how their meals are well balanced and help to put your body into fat-burning mode. Sticking with their program, you can expect to lose up to one to two pounds a week. According to their website, their new *Nutrisystem Personal Plans* can help customers lose up to thirteen pounds and seven inches overall in the first month, up to eighteen pounds and ten inches overall in the first two months and up to twenty-two pounds and twelve inches in the first three months. They have a *Healthy Living Team* which crafts healthier versions of a variety of foods for you to choose from. Nutrisystem's new initiative is aimed at providing additional weight loss meals without artificial flavors or sweeteners, no colors from artificial sources, no high-fructose corn syrup, and no trans-fat (no partially hydrogenated oils). Following their plan and using their food and snacks can provide you the resources needed to lose weight. They do not require a long-term commitment. You can place a one-time order or set up monthly reoccurring payments.

IS A NUTRISYSTEM DIET EASY TO FOLLOW?

All the plans on the Nutrisystem Diet include 3 meals and 3 snacks a day, and recommendations on how to enhance your weight loss with added grocery store items. They offer support and counseling options from their trained weight loss coaches and registered dietitians. Nutrisystem also has certified diabetes educators. They offer support seven days a week. And provide a user-friendly app that can assist with personalized meal plans and grocery guides. The app provides customers with weekly challenges, where they can potentially win prizes, for keeping track of their progress. Nutrisystem also provides a blog called the *Leaf* where they provide recipes and tips on healthy living.

For those looking to transition to maintenance mode, they have their *Nutrisystem Success Plan* option. They also provide additional options for customers who would like to order their favorite meals at discounted rates through the *Nutrisystem Advantage Plan.*

COST AND FOOD OPTIONS?

The Nutrisystem Diet has a variety of plan options on their website. Their Basic Plan is roughly $9.00 a day and about $260.00 for one month of food. Which includes breakfast, lunch, dinner, and snacks for the four-week program. They have other plan options on their website, at Nutrisystem.com. Check for specials and coupons before ordering. If you are looking for a less expensive option to using the Nutrisystem Program, Walmart has a variety of their products for sale. For instance, they have a five-day Belly Buster Weight Loss Kit for about $45.00. Which includes breakfast, lunch, and dinner for the five days. They also carry a variety of their weight loss snacks. Amazon also sells a few of their products on their website.

WHAT ARE EXAMPLES OF NUTRISYSTEM MEALS?

Breakfast: Turkey Sausage & Egg Muffin

Lunch: Grilled Chicken Sandwich

Dinner: Four Cheese Manicotti

Breakfast: Apple Walnut Oatmeal

Lunch: Steak & Cheese Melt

Dinner: Roasted Turkey & Mash Potatoes

Recap: Joining structured diet programs can be a good option if you need a little more guidance and support while losing weight. They can provide coaching, meal planning and help you transition out of the program and cooking healthier meals on your own. Or, if you do not need the extra support, you can always order the different portion-controlled meals from them, to incorporate into your weight loss plan.

PALEO DIET

WHAT IS THE DIET?

The last of the eleven eating style options in the book, brings us to the Paleo Diet. This diet is based on a premise of eating more unprocessed meat, low-carb, plant-based, meals. Similar, to what our ancestors ate back in the caveman era. Before processed carbs, added sugars, dairy products, legumes, and grains. The diet mainly consists of lean meats, seafood, vegetables, eggs, fruits, seeds, and nuts. It puts an emphasis on eating high quality meats and organic produce. The thought process behind the diet is to reset the body back to what humans ate prior to farming changing the types of food we consumed.

Like the Keto and Low-Carb Diets, carb lovers may find the Paleo Diet a little hard to follow at first. Removing things like bread, sweets, grains, and potatoes are a big part of the diet. However, if you are looking for a diet to improve your overall health and help you lose weight, Paleo can be the way to go. That is because **a Paleo Diet can improve your glucose tolerance, which is tied to your insulin levels. It can also improve your blood pressure, and lower your triglycerides.**

Unlike a Vegan Diet, beans, lentils, peanuts, and peas are not included in the foods to eat. The diet, however, does consist of more nutrient dense whole foods like carrots, celery, tomatoes, broccoli, and avocados. It is a high protein and high fiber diet, which can help decrease your appetite. By following this diet, it will mean saying good-bye to prepackaged processed foods because these would have not been items that were around during the hunter-gatherer stage of mankind.

The goal of a Paleo Diet is to include more foods that can *heal* your body and reduce the intake of overprocessed and empty calorie foods, that can be harmful. By adopting this type of diet, you can improve your health by eating more balanced and complete nutrition meals.

CAN IT HELP YOU LOSE WEIGHT?

Yes, a Paleo Diet can be used to help you lose weight because high-protein diets have a positive effect on weight loss and weight management. Eating a more nutrient dense plant-based diet will allow you to eat more food but, only use a small amount, of your daily calories. That is because most whole-plant foods are calorically diluted. Helping you feel fuller longer and creating the desired calorie deficit to lose weight.

Whether you are looking to lose weight or reduce heart disease related problems, using a Paleo Diet with a healthy micronutrient breakdown of protein, fiber and complex carbs, can be a good decision to make. Consuming smaller amounts of carbs, processed food, and sugar can be beneficial in helping you reach your goal.

However, you do not have to completely dive into the deep end and fully adapt a Paleo Diet. You can still enjoy the benefits of following their principles of removing processed, harmful foods from your diet. By eliminating those types of foods, even over a period, of time, while losing or maintaining weight, you would be making an investment in your long-term health.

IS A PALEO DIET EASY TO FOLLOW?

A Paleo Diet, being plant-based, will make your meal plate breakdown look a little different than it probably has in the past. Which can be a good thing when losing weight, because two-thirds or more of each of your meals will consist of plant foods. The other third of your plate will come from animal products.

Meat consumption is encouraged when following a Paleo Diet. However, the emphasis is put on choosing pasture-raised and grass-fed meat. Also, you are encouraged to shop local organic fruits and vegetables whenever possible and eat wild-caught seafood. Like salmon, octopus, halibut, and scallops.

Following a Paleo Diet has gotten more convenient over the years. There are cookbooks, recipes, Pinterest ideas and easy to follow YouTube videos. Providing meal prep tips and how-to videos on shopping and cooking efficiently. To simplify the Paleo Diet, remember to eat lean meats or seafood with veggies and fresh fruit. A good rule of thumb is to avoid processed, sugary foods and all items our caveman ancestors would have had no access to.

WHAT ARE SOME EXAMPLES OF A PALEO DIET?

Here Arc a Few Paleo Diet Staples

*Beef *Bison *Chicken *Lamb *Pork *Turkey *Wild Game *Catfish
*Cod *Halibut *Salmon *Tilapia *Tuna *Oysters *Lobster *Octopus
*Collard Greens *Kale *Arugula *Lettuce *Spinach *Watercress *Broccoli
*Brussel Sprouts *Napa Cabbage *Radishes *Turnips *Cauliflower *Endive
*Blackberries *Apple *Grapes *Strawberries *Cranberries *Grapefruit
*Lemon *Limes *Oranges *Peaches *Pears *Honeydew *Watermelon

An Example of Eating on the Paleo Diet

Breakfast: Italian Breakfast Casserole with Sausage, Sun Dried Tomatoes, Peppers, Onions, Garlic and Spices
Lunch: Shrimp Fried Cauliflower Rice with Spinach
Dinner: Grilled Chicken Cobb Salad with Honey Dijon; (Seasoned grilled chicken, crispy bacon, sliced eggs and avocado)
Dessert: Sliced Peaches and Pears

CAN YOU EXERCISE WHILE USING ANY OF THE 4 DIETS?

To get the most from using either a Paleo, Jenny Craig, South Beach, or Nutrisystem Diet, it can be beneficial to incorporate some form of physical activities into your routine. Pick the types of activities you will enjoy and aim to workout 3-5 days a week. However, just as with using any of the diets mentioned in the book, in the first week of the *6-Week Program*, you will not add exercising to your weight loss routine. This is done for a very, specific reason. The goal is to reduce your stress and make the transition as simple as possible.

The first week of the program, as stated earlier, will be about getting you ready and accustomed to the new way of losing weight. As you are preparing for the new shift, this will allow you time to shop, meal prep and make necessary arrangements for cooking, as well as if you want to look in to ordering food from any of the meal plans.

To jumpstart your metabolism and to help with reducing your caloric intake, you can work on increasing your daily activities, like walking around on commercial breaks while watching tv, taking a nice walk after dinner and increasing your water intake by drinking 16-20 ounces every time you eat something. This will help you to feel full and cause you to eat less calories.

During the first week or prior to getting started look up and gather all necessary workout items, you will need. You can start searching for fun exercise videos on YouTube, order DVD's and look for local fitness programs you can join as well.

Remember when you do start incorporating exercise into your routine, refer to Chapter 19 for ideas and tips on getting started and on how to increase the duration and intensity as you are losing weight. And of course, if possible, try and incorporate a few morning exercises into your routine, each week to maximize your results.

Provided in the next section, is a quick reference sheet of multiple ways you can incorporate various eating styles. It has all the diets we have reviewed in the book, including the four in this section. As, well as a few other extra ones to provide you even more options, in deciding which food choices you would like to include in your Diet Buffet. Using either option will be about accessing the different food and recipes, from the various eating styles, to give yourself endless choices. They will be another example of how you can take losing and maintaining weight to the next level. There are 15 options using the 2-Step process of combining different diets together and 21 options using the power of either the 3-Step or the 4-Step combination.

SLIM DOWN LEVEL UP COMBINATION IDEAS:

2 Step Combinations

1. Intermittent Fasting with Keto
2. Intermittent Fasting with Low Calorie
3. Intermittent Fasting with Vegan
4. Intermittent Fasting with Weight Watchers
5. Intermittent Fasting with Paleo
6. Intermittent Fasting with Jenny Craig
7. Intermittent Fasting with Akins
8. Intermittent Fasting with No Sugar Challenge
9. Intermittent Fasting with Nutrisystem
10. Intermittent Fasting with South Beach
11. Intermittent Fasting with Slim Fast
12. Intermittent Fasting with Whole30
13. Intermittent Fasting with Mediterranean Diet
14. Intermittent Fasting with Mayo Clinic
15. Intermittent Fasting with The Biggest Loser Diet

3 Step Combinations

1. Intermittent Fasting with Keto and Low Calorie
2. Intermittent Fasting with Vegan and Low Calorie
3. Intermittent Fasting with Weight Watchers and Low Calorie
4. Intermittent Fasting with Paleo and Low Calorie

5. Intermittent Fasting with Jenny Craig and Low Calorie

6. Intermittent Fasting with Akins and Low Calorie

7. Intermittent Fasting with Nutrisystem and Low Calorie

8. Intermittent Fasting with South Beach and Low Calorie

9. Intermittent Fasting with Slim Fast and Low Calorie

10. Intermittent Fasting with Whole30 and Low Calorie

4 Step Combinations

11. Intermittent Fasting with Keto and Low Calorie- No Sugar Challenge

12. Intermittent Fasting with Vegan Low Calorie/3 Liquid Dinners a Week

13. Intermittent Fasting with Weight Watchers/Low Calorie/3 Meatless Dinners a week

14. Intermittent Fasting with Paleo/Low Calorie and 3 Meatless Dinners a Week

15. Intermittent Fasting with Jenny Craig/Low Calorie/3 Liquid Dinners a Week

16. Intermittent Fasting with Akins/Low Calorie/3 Meatless Dinners a Week

17. Intermittent Fasting with Nutrisystem/Low Calorie/3 Liquid Dinners a week

18. Intermittent Fasting with Low Calorie/Low Carb/3 Meatless Dinners a Week

19. Intermittent Fasting with South Beach/Low Calorie and No Sugar Challenge

20. Intermittent Fasting with Slim Fast/Low Calorie/3 Meatless Dinners a Week

21. Intermittent Fasting with Whole30/Low Calorie and No
Sugar Challenge

READING FOOD LABELS

NUTRITION FACTS		
3 servings per container		
Serving size		3 Pretzels (28g)
CALORIES	**110** per serving	**330** per container
	%DV*	%DV*
TOTAL FAT	0.5g 1%	
Saturated Fat	0g 0%	0g 0%
Trans fat	0g	0g
Cholesterol	0mg 0%	0mg 0%
Sodium	400mg 17%	1200mg 52%
Total carb.	23g 8%	69g 24%
Dietary fiber	2g 7%	6g 21%
Total sugars	<1g	3g
Incl. added sugars	0g 0%	0g 0%
Protein	3g	9g
Vitamin D	0mcg 0%	0mcg 0%
Calcium	10mg 0%	30mg 2%
Iron	1.2mg 6%	3.6mg 18%
Potassium	90mg 0%	270mg 5%

NUTRITION FACTS		
16 servings per container		
Serving size		1 Tbsp. (21g)
CALORIES	per serving	60
		% daily value*
TOTAL FAT	0g	0%
Saturated Fat	0g	0%
Trans fat	0g	0%
Cholesterol	0mg	0%
Sodium	0mg	0%
Total carb.	17g	6%
Dietary fiber	0g	0%
Total sugars	17g	**34%**
Protein	0g	
Vitamin D	0mg	0%
Calcium	0mg	0%
Iron	0mg	0%
Potassium	0mg	0%

Important Tip: When picking out your snacks and planning your meals, it is important to pay attention to the food labels. The key is to check *the serving size* first, because one package can have multiple servings inside. At first glance, it could look like the item's amount is the calorie count first seen. I made this mistake before, eating a whole package of chips and drank a bottle of Coke thinking it was only one serving when it was two. For example, the first label on the previous page, is a package of pretzels. It contains three servings. Therefore, if the entire package is eaten, take note of the total calories, fat grams and carbs for that item. Looking at the labels can also be helpful if you are tracking your sodium and sugar intake as well.

The second label on the previous page, is an example of a bottle of salad dressing, and it has a total of 16 servings. Same premise if you are using multiple servings; add that to your calculation. Special care is needed, for instance, when we are using salad dressings, oils, butter, and creams, as they can add up quickly and take up a larger percentage of our budget.

Remember, you can eat almost anything, as long as you plan for it and spend your daily body budget numbers wisely, to get the most out of each meal and snack option.

APPENDIX

35 WEIGHT LOSS TIPS

1. Cook and eat at home more frequently

2. Eat fewer carbohydrates (between 20-50 net carbs or 50-100 net carbs max)

3. Eat less gluten (look for more gluten free recipes and meals)

4. Aim to drink 1 gallon of water a day

5. Eat out less (check nutritional fact information when eating out)

6. Do not go to the grocery store when you are hungry

7. Keep healthy snacks around (MRE'S)

8. Become aware of how many calories, fat grams and net carbs you eat a day (Calorie/Fitness Tracker Apps)

9. Try to eat more protein

10. Drink a glass of water with lemon when you wake up

11. Have meat-free days (meatless dinners can make you thinner)

12. Eat slowly (the feeling of full takes 20 minutes from the first bite)

13. Limit your sweets and added sugar intake as much as possible

14. Reduce the amount of junk food you eat (find healthier snack ideas in Chapter 12)

15. Avoid white rice (try brown rice or cauliflower rice)

16. Avoid white bread (use whole grain and Low-Carb wraps instead)

17. Hungry? Try drinking a glass of water, you may be thirsty and not hungry

18. Find a healthier alternative to using regular mayonnaise

19. Drink herbal teas (green tea, ginger tea, hibiscus tea, sage tea, lemon balm tea)

20. Drink your tea with honey on an empty stomach in the morning

21. Take a shot of apple cider vinegar or with a glass of water, daily

22. Eat more vegetables and use fruits as your desserts

23. Do push-ups and sit-ups (2-3 days a week)

24. Have a pool at home? Do a few laps a couple of days a week

25. Play your favorite music, to get motivated while exercising

26. Walk as much as possible

27. Do weight training exercises during TV commercials

28. Are you a smoker? Try to smoke less gradually over time

29. Get at least 7-8 hours of sleep nightly

30. Set an alarm clock one-hour early to wake up and workout

31. Write down your goals (weight loss vision board)

32. Watch motivational YouTube clips

33. Weigh yourself only once a week on Wednesdays

34. Find inspirational stories online about people who lost weight (social media)

35. Form a support group (your support team, family, friends, workout programs)

BOOK RECOMMENDATIONS

The Obesity Code by Dr. Jason Fung

The book better explains the scientific role insulin levels and insulin resistance plays in your ability to lose weight and the benefits to fasting as a long-term weight loss solution.

Fast Feast Repeat by Gin Stephens

A weight loss success story about learning a variety of ways to work intermittent fasting into your lifestyle and change your approach to when you are eating.

The Power of Appetite Correction by Dr. Bert Herring

Teaching you to train your body to reach the point where it corrects your, eating patterns and digestion, by using a variety of fasting schedules, until your body is well adjusted and continues to lose weight.

The Every Other Day Diet by Dr. Krista Varady

This gives a better understanding to the alternating day approach to fasting and the science behind the benefits towards your health and fitness.

Chasing Cupcakes by Elizabeth Benton

A weight loss story of triumph after years of struggling with obesity and being in debt. She shares her story of how she broke through, got out of debt, and transformed her life, from the inside out.

The Forks Over the Knives Plan by Alona Pulde M.D.

A four-week meal plan makeover on how to transition to a whole-food plant-based diet and all the benefits to improving your overall health with making changes to the way you eat.

The Body Keeps the Score: Brain, Mind, and Body in the Healing of *Trauma* by Bessel van der Kolk M.D.

A mental approach to healing years of trauma and stress that is carried in the body and has a profound effect on the mental and physical well-being. Stress causes weight gain and learning to control it by dealing with past and current pains can be key for your long-term success.

COOKBOOK RECOMMENDATIONS

The Super Easy Air Fryer Cookbook by Brandi Crawford

One-Pot Keto Cooking by Charlotte Smythe

Cooking That Counts: 1200-1500 Calorie Meal Plans to Lose Weight Deliciously by The Editors of Cooking Light

Vegan For Everybody by America's Test Kitchen

The 30-Minute Low Carb Cookbook by Pamela Ellgen

Mediterranean Diet Cookbook for Beginners by Wilda Buckley

Unbelievable Paleo 60-Wholesome One Dish Recipes by Kelsey Preciado

The SkinnyTaste Cookbook: Light On Calories Big On Flavor by Gina Homolka and Heather K Jones

Keto Meal Prep for Beginners by Kira Peterson has over 600 recipes

Plant-Based on a Budget by Toni Okamoto and MD FACLM Michael Greger

Healthy Quick and Easy Smoothies 100 No Fuss Recipes Under 300 Calories by Dana Angelo White MS RD AT

Weight Watchers Complete Cookbook SmartPoints Addition over 500 Recipes by Weight Watchers

South Beach Cookbook Main Course 60+Breakfast Lunch Dinner and Desserts for Healthy Weight Loss by Noah Jerris

***If you have not already done so, look into downloading the app PINTEREST for access to endless free recipes, weight loss tips and snack ideas.

REFERENCES

1. Klempel M C et al. Intermittent fasting combined with calorie restriction is effective for weight loss and cardio-protection in obese women. Nutr J. 2012; 11:98. Doi"10.1186/1475-2891-11-98. Accessed 2015 Apr 8.

2. Shiffer Emily, (2020) "I did a Low-Carb, 18:6 Intermittent Fasting Diet and Camp Gladiator Workouts to Lose 70 LBS". "I Combined Keto and Intermittent Fasting with HIIT Workouts to Lose 55 Pounds." Published online at Womenshealthmag.com (online resource)

3. S. Linda. (2020) Weight Loss Success Story. Received through INSTAGRAM. (social media resource)

4. Poorman Elisabeth Dr. (2016) Why I Stopped Telling My Patients to Lose Weight. Published online at WBur. org. Retrieved from: https://www.wbur.org/common-health/2016/10/14/why-stopped-telling-patients-lose-weight (online resource)

5. Hannah Ritchie (2018) – "Cause of Death". Published online at OurWorldInData.org. Retrieved from: https://our-worldindata.org/causes-of-death (online resource)

6. Fung Jason M D, The Obesity Code. Chapter 19-page 217.

7. Wing Rena Ph. D National Weight Control Registry Project. Published online at Weightresearch.org. Retrieved from: http://www.weightresearch.org/publishedresearch.aspx (online resource)

8. Shiffer Emily, (2020) "With Keto and Intermittent Fasting, I lost 90 Pounds in 9 Months and Erased My Joint Pain and Discomfort". Published online at Womenshealthmag.com (online resource)

9. Medscape Medical Report. (2019) Intermittent Fasting Combined with Lower-Calorie Diet is the Best Plan for Weight Loss. Published online at Timesnownews.com. Retrieved from: https://www.timesnownews.com/health/article/intermittent-fasting-combined-with-lower-calorie-diet-is-the-best-plan-for-weight-loss-flat-belly-5-tips-for-beginners/352298 (online resource)

10. Editing Staff. (2020) "I Lost 42 Pounds Combining Weight Watchers and Intermittent Fasting". Published online at parade.com. (online resource)

11. Sabate J, Wien M. Nuts, blood lipids and cardiovascular disease. Asia Pac J Clin Nutr. 2010; 19(1):131-6. Dr. Fung-The Obesity Code 2016.

12. Flegal, PhD. Kit, MD Orpana PhD; et al. Association of All-Cause Mortality with Over-Weight and Obesity Using Standard Body Mass Index Categories. Doi.10.1001/jama.2012.113905. 2013;309(1):71-82.

13. Brownell K D, Robin J Medical, metabolic, and psychological effects of weight cycling. Arch Intern Med. 1994 Jun 27;154(12):1325-30. PMID: 8002684.

14. Natural Heart, Lung, and Blood Institute. BMI Calculator. https://www.nhlbi.nih.gov/health/educational/lose_wt/BMI/bmi_tbl.htm

15. Maheshwari Sapna, (2014). "Old Navy Explains Why It Charges More For Women's Plus-Size Clothes." Published online at Buzzfeednews.com. Retrieved from: https://www.buzzfeednews.com/article/sapna/old-navy-explains-why-it-charges-more-for-womens-plus-size-c (online resource)

16. George-Parkin Hilary, (2018) "Size By the Numbers." Published online at Racked.com. Retrieved from: https://www.racked.com/2018/6/5/17380662/size-numbers-average-woman-plus-market (online resource)

17. Jakubowicz, Barnea, Wainstein, Froy, High Caloric Intake at Breakfast vs. Dinner Differently Influences Weight Loss of Overweight and Obese Women. Doi.org/10.1002/oby.20460. March 2013.

18. Klempel, Kroeger, Bhutani, Trepanowski, Varady, Intermittent Fasting Combined with Calorie Restriction is Effective for Weight Loss and Cardio-Protection in Obese Women. Nutrition Journal: Volume 11 Article Number:98 (2012). Published online at Biomedcentral.com. Retrieved from: https://nutritionj.biomedcentral.com/articles/10.1186/1475-2891-11-98/metrics

19. H. Sophia. (2020) Weight Loss Success Story. Received through FACEBOOK. (social media resource)

20. V. Nancy. (2020) Weight Loss Success Story. Received through LINKEDIN (social media resource)

21. Fung Jason M D (2017) Intermittent Fasting vs. Caloric Reduction-What's the Difference? Published online at Dietdoctor.com. (online resource)

22. Nutrition and Healthy Aging Report. (2018) Weight Loss: All You Need to Know About the 16:8 Diet and 6 Tips to Burn Belly Fat Using Intermittent Fasting. Published online at Timesnownews.com. Retrieved from: https://www.timesnownews.com/health/article/follow-16-8-diet-to-boost-weight-loss-6-tips-to-lose-belly-fat-fast-with-intermittent-fasting-plan/244923 (online resource)

23. Shai, R.D., Ph.D., Schwarzfuchs, M.D., Henkin, M.D., Shahar, R.D., Ph.D., et.al. Weight Loss with a Low-Carbohydrate, Mediterranean, or Low-Fat Diet. N Engl j Med DOI:10.1056/NEjMoa0708681. 2008 July 17; 359:229-241.

24. Mayo Clinic Staff (2020). Low-Carb Diet: Can It Help You Lose Weight? Published online at Mayoclinic.org. Retrieved from: https://mayoclinic.org/healthy-lifestyle/weight-loss/in-depth/low-carb-diet/art-20045831 (online resource)

25. Gunnars Kris BSc (2016) 10 Evidence Based Health Benefits of Intermittent Fasting. Published online at Healthline.com. Retrieved from: https://www.healthline.com/nutrition/10-health-benefits-of-intermittent-fasting (online resource)

26. Young Lisa Dr. (2012). Charts/Benefits of Fruits and Vegetables. Published online at Huffpost.com. Retrieved from: https://huffpost.com/entry/healthy-food_b_1665279 Pages, 165-168. (online resource)

27. Mayo Clinic Staff (2019) Dietary Fiber: Essential For a Healthy Diet. Published online at Mayoclinic.org. Retrieved from: https://www.mayoclinic.org/healthy-lifestyle/nutri-

tion-and-healthy-eating/in-depth/fiber/art-20043983 (online resource)

28. Fast Food (2020) Nutrition & Cost of Fast Food Items. Published online at Fastfoodmenuprices.com. Retrieved from: https://www.fastfoodmenuprices.com/ (online resource)

29. Fast Food Fun Facts (2020). Fast Food Industry Analysis 2020-Cost and Trends. Published online at Franchisehelp. com. Retrieved from: https://www.franchisehelp.com/ industry-reports/fast-food-industry-analysis-2020-cost-trends/ Page 185. (online resource)

30. Ready Store (2020) Meals Ready to Eat. Published online at TheReadyStore.com. Retrieved from: https://www.thereadystore.com/mre

31. Park Madison (2010) Twinkie Diet Helps Nutrition Professor Lose 27 Pounds. Published online at CNN.com. Retrieved from: https://www.nurtitionunplugged.com/2010/11/ whats-the-point-of-the-twinkie-diet/ (online resource)

32. Varady K A. Intermittent Versus Daily Calorie Restriction: Which Diet Regimen is More Effective for Weight Loss? Obes Rev. 2011 Jul;12(7):e593-601. Retrieved from: https://pubmed.ncbi.nlm.nih.gov/21410865/

33. T Janet (2020) Weight Loss Success Story. Received through FACEBOOK (social media resource)

34. Shiffer Emily (2020). "I Did Intermittent Fasting and Used a Calorie Counter App to Lose 122 Pounds." Published online at Womenshealthmag.com (online resource)

35. McGrice Melanie, Porter Judi. The Effects of Low-Carbohydrate Diets on Fertility Hormones and Outcomes in Overweight and Obese Women: Systematic Review. 2017 Mar; 9(3): 204. Doi: 10.3390/nu9030204. Retrieved from: https://www.ncbi.nlm.nih.gov/pmc/articles/ PMC5372867/

36. Po-Ju Lin Katarina T. Borer. (2016) Third Exposure to a Reduced Carbohydrate Meal Lowers Evening Postprandial Insulin and GIP Responses. Retrieved from: https://

journals.plos.org/plosone/article?id=10.1371/journal.pone.0165378

37. Mawer Rudy, MSc, CISSN. The Ketogenic Diet: A Detailed Beginner's Guide to Keto. Published online at Healthline. com. Retrieved from: https://www.healthline.com/nutrition/ketogenic-diet-101

38. Masood, Annamaraju P, Uppaluri KR. https://www.ncbi. nlm.nih.gov/books/NBK499830/. Ketosis, (2020) Published online at Webmd.com. Retrieved from: https://www. webmd.com/diabetes/type-1-diabetes-guide/what-is-ketosis

39. Shiffer Emily (2020). "Combining Intermittent Fasting and Paleo Diet Transformed My Body". Published online at Womenshealthmag.com. (online resource)

40. J Wendy. (2019) WW and Intermittent Fasting How and Why I'm Doing it! Published online at Wendysweightjourney.com. Retrieved from: https://wendysweightjourney. com/ww-weight-watchers-and-intermittent-fasting-how-and-why-im-doing-it/.

41. Missy Jen (2020) WW Point System Explained. Published online at Wonkypie.com. Retrieved from: https://wonkypie.com/ww-point-system/ (online resource)

42. Missy Jen (2020) WW Point System Explained. Published online at Wonkypie.com. Retrieved from: https://wonkypie.com/ww-point-system/ (online resource)

43. Craig Jenny (2018). Body Clock Circadian Rhythm for Obese and Overweight Individuals in a Four Week Case Controlled Weight Loss Study for Commercially Weight Loss Program. Published online at JennyCraig.com. Retrieved from: https://statics.jennycraig.com/pdfs/ Jenny-Craig Rapid-Results-Study-2018-updated-compressed.pdf?ga=2.56007595.181097709.1606761483-1099968266.1606761483 (online resource)

44. CDC Staff (2019). Centers for Disease Control and Prevention Benefits of Physical Activity. Published online at CDC.

gov. Retrieved from: https://www.cdc.gov/physicalactivity/basics/pa-health/index.htm (online resource)

45. Yeager Selene, Crevling Mallory (2020) How to Run When You're Just Getting Started. Published online at Runnersworld.com. Retrieved from: https://www.runnersworld.com/training/a20845020/how-to-get-started-as-a-runner/ (online resource)

46. Honerkamp John (2020). Running and Weight Loss Goals. Published online at Verywellfit.com. Retrieved from: https://www.verywellfit.com/running-weight-loss-overview-4581848 (online resource)

47. Marcin Ashley (2018). Benefits of Jumping Jacks and How to Do Them. Published online at Healthline.com. Retrieved from: https://www.healthline.com/health/fitness-exercise/jumping-jacks

ABOUT THE AUTHOR

Mylitta Butler is a former 300-pound New Yorker who is the CEO/Founder of MyLegkini® Swimwear Inc. Her patented swimwear designs slims a woman's stomach, hips, waist, legs, and thighs. The brand story behind her designing swimwear came from years of dealing with being obese and having body insecurities, which drove her to want to change how women felt wearing swimwear.

Mylitta is a mother and a wife who has struggled with her weight since she was nineteen years old. At her heaviest, she tipped the scale at 304 pounds. Was suffering from high blood pressure and high cholesterol, as well as being borderline type 2 diabetic. After a visit to her doctor and hearing her blood work results were getting worse, she faced the reality of the unhealthy relationship she had developed with food. It was a hard pill to swallow, but Mylitta came to realize, she was not only eating when she was hungry but rather when she was hurting.

After some much-needed soul searching, Mylitta was able to go from 304 pounds down to 143 pounds in less than 15 months. By using the power of combining different diets together like Keto, Vegan, Low-Calorie, Weight Watchers and Intermittent Fasting, she successfully conquered the mountain many feel they cannot climb. Since the beginning of 2020, Mylitta has set out to motivate and inspire thousands of women with her words of encouragement through a series of YouTube videos, social media and on her blog.

Her goal is to continue inspiring women who are struggling with losing weight. She is adamant about empowering them with the right information and tools. So, they too, can stand in the ring and fight for their health and win.

Mylitta lives in Tampa, Florida and between writing, and designing, empowering swimwear, that encourages women to feel beautiful, Mylitta spends time with her husband, son, and their two Doberman Pinchers.

SLIM DOWN LEVEL UP INDEX

Made in the USA
Columbia, SC
22 April 2021